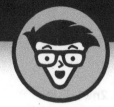

Parkinson's Disease

2nd Edition

by Michele Tagliati, MD
and Jo Horne, MA

FOREWORD BY Deborah W. Brooks

CEO and Co-Founder of The Michael J. Fox Foundation
for Parkinson's Research

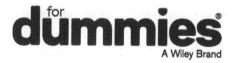

for dummies®
A Wiley Brand

Parkinson's Disease For Dummies®, 2nd Edition

Published by: **John Wiley & Sons, Inc.,** 111 River Street, Hoboken, NJ 07030-5774, www.wiley.com

Copyright © 2022 by John Wiley & Sons, Inc., Hoboken, New Jersey

Published simultaneously in Canada

For general information on our other products and services, please contact our Customer Care Department within the U.S. at 877-762-2974, outside the U.S. at 317-572-3993, or fax 317-572-4002. For technical support, please visit https://hub.wiley.com/community/support/dummies.

Wiley publishes in a variety of print and electronic formats and by print-on-demand. Some material included with standard print versions of this book may not be included in e-books or in print-on-demand. If this book refers to media such as a CD or DVD that is not included in the version you purchased, you may download this material at http://booksupport.wiley.com. For more information about Wiley products, visit www.wiley.com.

Library of Congress Control Number: 2022940644

ISBN 978-1-119-89358-5 (pbk); ISBN 978-1-119-89359-2 (ePDF); ISBN 978-1-119-89360-8 (epub)

SKY10069044_030624

Contents at a Glance

Table of Contents

Foreword

A diagnosis of Parkinson's disease (PD) is a life-altering event. There is no one way to deal with it. Everyone has a unique set of circumstances, and every person and family experiences Parkinson's differently. One book on PD could never be all things to all people. That remains as true today as when *Parkinson's Disease For Dummies* was first published.

Fortunately, little else in Parkinson's research and care has stayed the same. In fact, over the past decade our field has seen astonishing momentum. Parkinson's drug development today is overflowing with promise and possibility. Scientists are making real progress in understanding the disease. Tidal waves of data and insights are flowing directly into the R&D pipeline to accelerate better treatments on their path to pharmacy shelves.

Over the same period, the national and international community of people and families living with Parkinson's has become more energetic and engaged than ever before. It's a growing community, unfortunately, with some estimates suggesting that the number of people living with Parkinson's could double by 2040. But here's the good news: While no one joins this community by choice, once they are here, many find it to be a source of tremendous richness, comfort, and support.

The Michael J. Fox Foundation is privileged to work closely with people and families living with Parkinson's, and we partner with them on new ways to help you, too, live well with this disease. You may be surprised by the voracity of your appetite for up-to-date, trustworthy, and just plain *more* information about PD. And since Parkinson's — for now, at least — stays with you for life, your information needs will change over time. That's why we offer informational and support resources including events, guides, webinars, videos and podcasts, our Parkinson's Buddy Network to foster social connections, and much more.

But we know PD can still feel overwhelming on your best day. That's why *Parkinson's Disease For Dummies, 2nd Edition* continues to represent something incredibly important: a place to start. We commend its emphasis on tenets that Our Foundation also strives to embody: an action orientation, a problem-solving mentality, and the distillation of complicated information into clear, logical next steps. And most importantly, a commitment to keep those living with Parkinson's front and center in everything we do.

I am continually inspired by the people I meet who are endeavoring to live their lives beyond the potentially limiting effects of this disease, defining themselves by their achievements, not their struggle with PD. But no one who knows Parkinson's would suggest that a positive outlook is achievable all the time. So do everything you can to put the odds on your side. Build relationships with care providers you trust; participate in research studies that urgently need you; eat well and exercise as much as you can; invest in your family and friendships; practice stress reduction techniques that work for you.

And know that work is continuing aggressively to make this disease, finally, a thing of the past.

Debi Brooks

CEO and Co-Founder, The Michael J. Fox Foundation for Parkinson's Research

Introduction

I f the very idea of a Parkinson's disease (PD) diagnosis scares the bejeebers out of you, take a deep breath and pay attention. Although Parkinson's is a chronic and progressive condition that has no cure (yet), the strides made in just the last decade to control and manage symptoms are impressive and hopeful. Also, the number of national organizations (not to mention big-name celebrities) that are placing the spotlight squarely on the need for a cure is unparalleled in the history of PD.

And we're here to help: An experienced movement disorders specialist, researcher, and lecturer on the treatment of Parkinson's disease (PD), and a writer of books on aging and caregiving who has years of experience as a care partner for members of her own family. Together, we give you the facts you need, resources you can rely on, and tips on how best to structure your life so that even though you may need to face living with PD, PD does not define you.

This book is your guide to understanding and living with PD. Although we assume that you — the person with Parkinson's (PWP) — are the primary audience, feel free to share *Parkinson's Disease For Dummies, 2nd Edition* with family, friends, and especially that person who will most likely make this journey with you — your care partner.

Neither of us — the writer who's followed dozens of people living with PD, and the doctor dedicated to those living with movement disorders such as PD — are in the business of giving up. We wish you the strength to persevere, the will to keep fighting for a cure, and the physical and emotional stamina to enjoy a long, productive life.

About This Book

At first glance, the idea of a *For Dummies* guide to Parkinson's disease may seem ludicrous or even downright insulting. But those of you who have used these guides understand that the Dummies reference indicates a guide that presents its topic in simple, straightforward terms. Although PD doesn't have a cure, you and your healthcare team can manage it well for years before you face its more challenging aspects. And that's what this guide is about — practical ways that you can control and manage the symptoms of your Parkinson's so that you can get on with your life.

Now, we won't insult you by offering some sugar-coated Pollyanna guide to living with PD. You deserve a realistic look at what you're facing. This guide provides solid information and resources to help you and your family come to terms with PD as a factor in all your lives. It offers proven techniques and tips to help you prepare for the future without projecting the worst. And most of all, it reminds you that you can possibly — even probably — live a full and satisfying life, in spite of PD.

We designed each chapter of *Parkinson's Disease For Dummies, 2nd Edition* to be self-contained so that you don't have to read the book sequentially; don't worry about reading the first parts first if you want to understand any later chapters. You can dip in and out wherever you please and concentrate only on what you need. The Table of Contents and the Index can help guide your search.

Foolish Assumptions

In putting together this guide to living with PD, we assumed the following about you:

>> You have (or suspect you have) PD yourself or are close to someone who does.

>> You want reliable information about PD, and you're looking for proven ways (techniques and resources) to treat and manage its symptoms.

>> You intend to take a proactive role in facing this challenge and not simply (blindly!) do everything the first healthcare provider you see tells you to do.

>> You're open to lifestyle adjustments, and complementary or alternative techniques, proven to manage symptoms and prolong functions.

>> You realize PD isn't just a physical condition that affects only you; it has elements that impact you — and everyone who cares about you — physically, mentally, and emotionally. You all need to be proactive in preparing for and meeting the challenges head-on.

Icons Used in This Book

REMEMBER

This icon signals essential information that's important enough to pull out of the general discussion and highlight.

This icon identifies information that may save you time, offer a resource, or show you an easier way of doing some task or activity.

This icon flags essential information that cautions and protects you against potential pitfalls and problems. Don't skip over these paragraphs.

This icon marks the paragraphs that take a deeper look into the medical info surrounding Parkinson's disease. This icon doesn't appear often in this book, but where it does, you can feel free to skip that text if you don't want to take a deeper dive into the technical side of the disease.

Beyond the Book

In this book, we talk often about your journey of living with PD, and just like with any journey, you need more than a roadmap (or GPS). When you take an actual road trip, you likely pick up brochures or check out additional resources online to enrich your trip. To guide you on your PD journey, we offer a Cheat Sheet (go to www.dummies.com and search for "Parkinson's Disease For Dummies Cheat Sheet") — a kind of digest version of key tools for you to have on hand. We've also compiled a list of resources (see Appendix B) for you to explore — not all at the same time, but certainly little by little while your journey continues.

And one more thing: When you travel, connecting with others — locals or fellow travelers who have similar interests — always makes for a better trip. Your journey with PD is no different. Connecting with others through support groups (in-person or online), staying informed by signing up for newsletters and updates from groups such as the Michael J. Fox Foundation (www.michaeljfox.org), and perhaps becoming an active advocate for finding a cure can give your journey deeper meaning and purpose.

Where to Go from Here

Where you open this book — Chapter 1, Chapter 24, or somewhere in between — depends on where you are in your Parkinson's journey. If you suspect PD is the cause behind some troubling symptoms, you may want to start with Chapter 4 for tips on the best way to get an accurate diagnosis. If you've already been diagnosed, then Part 3, where we discuss treatment options, may be your first stop.

Use this book as a guide, a roadmap to help you on the path to living with PD. We offer information and resources that you can trust — tools that help you adapt to life with PD without making PD your whole life. In the long run, however, your resolve to face each day with renewed strength and energy will see you through. And your example will set the stage for those people who intend to partner with you in the fight.

1

Getting to Know PD

Chapter **1**

Parkinson's Disease: The Big Picture

he National Center for Health Statistics (a division of the Centers for Disease Control and Prevention) reports that approximately 1 percent of all Americans over the age of 65 receive a diagnosis of Parkinson's disease (PD). Doctors diagnose 60,000 new cases every year. But you didn't pick up this book because you're interested in mass numbers. You opened it because you're only interested in one number — for you or someone you love. You opened it because maybe you noticed some symptoms that made you think, "Parkinson's," or you just got a confirmed diagnosis and you're wondering what's next.

What's next is for you to go into action mode: Understand the facts (rather than listen to the myths) about PD — what causes it, how it's treated, and of huge importance to anyone diagnosed with PD, how to live with it. (Notice we said *live*, not just *exist*.) In this chapter, you can find the big picture of the rest of the book and (more to the point) where to find the information that you need right now.

Defining Parkinson's — A Movement Disorder

Parkinson's disease falls into a group of conditions called *movement disorders* (disorders that result from a loss of the brain's control on voluntary movements). The normal action of several neurotransmitters in the brain may be affected by PD. The best-known neurotransmitter is *dopamine*, which relays signals from the substantia nigra to certain brain regions that control movement, balance, and coordination. In the brain of people who have Parkinson's (PWP), cells that produce this essential substance (dopamine) die earlier than normal.

TECHNICAL STUFF

The brain regions that receive signals from the substantia nigra are the putamen, caudate, and globus pallidus — collectively named the *basal ganglia* — in the *striatum*; see Figure 1-1.

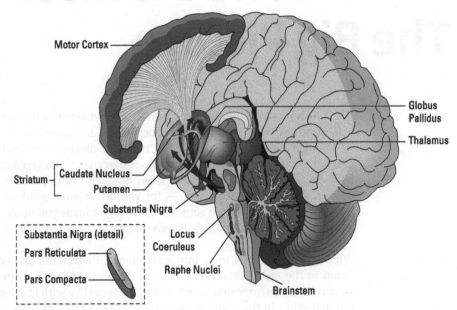

FIGURE 1-1: The dopamine pathway.

Motor Cortex

Globus Pallidus

Thalamus

Striatum — Caudate Nucleus / Putamen

Substantia Nigra

Substantia Nigra (detail)
Pars Reticulata
Pars Compacta

Locus Coeruleus

Raphe Nuclei

Brainstem

REMEMBER

Although a whole group of conditions can cause parkinsonism (as defined by rest tremor, bradykinesia or slowness of movement, rigidity or stiffness, and postural instability or propensity for falling), the exact cause of parkinsonism is unknown and therefore you will see the disease defined as idiopathic PD. *Idiopathic* is a Greek word that means *arising spontaneously from an unknown cause*. As the term suggests, the jury is still out as to the underlying cause (although theories do exist).

Navigating the unpredictable path

Go into a room filled with 50 people with Parkinson's (PWP), and they all vary when it comes to

>> How they first suspected they had PD

>> Signs of PD progression — from almost no progression to rapid onset of symptoms

>> Attitudes and outlooks from the individuals dealing with their PD

REMEMBER

When you're diagnosed with PD, you set out on a unique journey — one where your outlook, lifestyle changes, and medical treatment can be key directional maneuvers along the way. In truth, this disease is one that you can live with, surrender to, or fight with everything you've got. The road veers and curves differently for each person. Some people may choose one path for managing symptoms, and some people choose another. Sometimes, the disease itself sets the course. The bottom line? No one can give you a clear roadmap. But you can count on one thing: Understanding the chronic and progressive nature of PD can take you a long way toward effectively managing your symptoms and living a full life.

Accepting the chronic progressive factors

Chronic and *progressive* can be scary words when you're talking about your health. But keep the words in perspective. Any number of chronic conditions occur with age — arthritis, high blood pressure, and high cholesterol, to name three. So, take a realistic look at the terms, accept them for what they are (and aren't), and move on.

Chronic: It's part of you now

In medical terms, illnesses are either *acute* (develop quickly and usually go away with treatment or time) or *chronic* (develop over time, may be managed with treatment, but have no cure at this time). In short, a chronic illness such as PD (or arthritis or high blood pressure) is now part of you — a fact that can help or hinder you as you work to build and maintain quality of life.

REMEMBER

If you refuse to accept that PD is a fact of life for you, then you're wasting precious time and energy in denial. Remember that most people face many challenges in life; if you can accept that PD is yours, then you're ahead of the game. Facing PD is no different than facing any situation that changes the way you think your life will turn out.

Progressive: It will get more challenging

Progressive, advancing, worsening — scary stuff. But to give you some good news: For millions of PWP, the progression takes years, even decades. Many PWP live relatively normal life spans following their diagnosis. However, two factors are essential for successfully containing PD's progressive effects: your attitude and your willingness to attend to lifestyle and medical therapy.

Throughout this book, we address both factors in multiple ways, but for now, remember

>> **Your attitude:** Refusing to allow this diagnosis to color every part of your routine and life gives you a huge assist in coping with the management of new symptoms through the years.

>> **Your willingness to take lifestyle changes seriously:** Also, get involved in the fight to find a cure (see Chapter 24 for how). Being proactive can make all the difference between you managing the disease or the disease managing you.

Recognizing symptoms that raise questions

First things first: Do you have PD? Although researchers may not yet have a clear idea of the cause(s) for PD (see Chapter 3), they have established that the neurological symptoms of idiopathic PD usually start only on one side of the body and include at least two of these four key symptoms:

>> **Tremor at rest:** Trembling in the hands, arms, feet, legs, or chin when you aren't engaging that body part in activity

>> **Rigidity:** Stiffness in the limbs and trunk, usually detected by the doctor and different from the joint stiffness typical of arthritis

>> **Abnormal movements:** reduced dexterity and slowness of fine movements (*bradykinesia*)

>> **Postural instability:** Impaired balance with tendency to fall or near fall

The first letters of the symptoms spell out the handy acronym *TRAP* to help you remember (like you need to be reminded!). The symptoms of PD can sometimes make you feel trapped inside your body. In this book, we work hard to show you a number of ways to fight back and maintain control of your life in spite of the TRAP.

TIP

Chapter 3 discusses symptoms (what you report to the doctor) and signs (what the doctor observes) in more detail.

Distinguishing between Parkinson's Disease and Related Conditions

Several neurological conditions may at first appear to be *idiopathic* PD (without known cause), but doctors can sometimes eventually trace the symptoms back to some other neurological condition (essential tremor, for example). Such variants progress differently and respond differently to therapy. (Chapter 4 has more on the distinctions.)

REMEMBER

The subtleties of diagnosing idiopathic PD may lead your family doctor to send you to a *neurologist*, a specialist in the treatment of neurological conditions or a *movement disorders specialist*, who is specifically trained to treat patients experiencing loss of motor function. If that happens, don't panic, because it is actually a good thing. Getting the correct diagnosis, discussed in Chapter 4, is the first step toward figuring out what comes next for you and how to effectively deal with it.

A real condition or syndrome, but not PD

Non–PD conditions that can have similar symptoms include the following:

>> **Essential tremor (ET):** Perhaps the most common type of tremor, affecting as many as five million Americans. ET differs from the tremor in idiopathic PD in several ways: ET occurs when the hand is active (as in eating, grasping, writing, and such). It may also occur in the head, voice, and legs.

   The renowned actress, Katherine Hepburn, had ET, not PD. You need to figure out whether you have ET or PD because each condition responds to completely different sets of medications.

>> **Atypical parkinsonian syndromes:** May initially have the same symptoms as PD. But these syndromes will also cause early (within three years) and severe problems with balance, blood pressure, vision, and cognition. In addition, they do not respond to medications as well as PD and have a much faster progression than does PD.

>> **Secondary parkinsonism:** Can result from traumatic brain injury or from damage to the brain due to multiple small strokes (*atherosclerotic* or *vascular parkinsonism*). Doctors can rule out both forms through scans (CTs or MRIs) that produce images of the brain (see Chapter 4).

>> **Drug- or toxin-induced parkinsonism:** Taking antipsychotic medications (drug-induced) or being over-exposed to toxins, such as carbon monoxide and manganese dust (toxin-induced), can cause parkinsonism. Drug-induced symptoms are usually (but not always) reversible; toxin-induced symptoms usually aren't.

>> **Pseudoparkinsonism:** A person displaying PD symptoms when in fact they have another condition (possibly caused by severe depression, a reaction to medications, or the onset of dementia, such as Alzheimer's disease) that can mimic PD symptoms (such as the inexpressive face of PWP).

Debunking some commonly held myths about PD

REMEMBER

Getting a grasp on some of the more commonly held myths about PD — understanding what's true and what's fiction — can help you develop a plan for how you will confront your diagnosis and build a quality of life in spite of having PD.

This list tells you what PD *is*:

>> **Chronic:** When you have it, you have it — like arthritis or diabetes.

>> **Slowly progressive:** Over time — often years, even decades with proper treatment.

>> **Manageable:** For many years, if you receive proper treatment and make key lifestyle changes.

>> **Life-changing:** For you, your family, and your friends (either good or bad, all depending on how you decide to face it).

You also have to understand what PD is *not*:

>> **Contagious:** It's human nature, when learning about an unfamiliar medical condition, to worry about giving it to others. Rest assured you can neither infect someone else with PD nor *catch it* like a cold.

>> **Curable:** At the time of this writing, we don't have a cure for PD, but research is definitely getting closer!

>> **Normal:** PD is not a normal condition for people of any age.

>> **For old folks only:** While it is more common in older people, younger people might also develop PD.

>> **Immediately life-changing:** Don't make life-changing decisions (such as assuming you can't work or that you need to move) as soon as you're diagnosed.

>> **Inevitable:** No, PD isn't necessarily going to get you if you live long enough.

If you take any key messages away from this book, we hope you take these debunkers. If you have PD, you have an enormous challenge before you, but tens of thousands of people successfully face it every day. You can live a full and satisfying life in spite of having PD — and we're here to show you how.

Seeking the Care You Need

Perhaps more than any other chronic condition, managing PD is a team effort. You're going to be working with an entire front line of healthcare professionals (doctors, therapists, and the like), as well as non-professionals like your family and friends, and other PWP that you'll meet along the way.

From medical professionals

You probably have at least two doctors intricately involved in your care: Your primary care physician and a PD doctor, usually a neurologist or a *movement disorders specialist* (a neurologist with additional fellowship training in movement disorders). Over time, you may connect with several other healthcare professionals: your pharmacist; physical, occupational, and speech therapists; counselors, and advisors to help you manage any depression, anxiety, diet changes, and exercise regimens; advisors to help manage financial, legal, housing, and other major decisions that will affect you and your family over the long term. Chapter 6 offers more information about this group.

From loved ones

You also have a personal care team: your spouse or significant other; your children (and possibly grandchildren); your close friends and (if you're diagnosed with young-onset Parkinson's — YOPD) your parents and siblings. Benchwarmers who may surprise you with their willingness to help out include neighbors, coworkers, members of groups you belong to, and others. In Chapters 7 and 16, we talk more about how to break the news and get these folks involved. Chapter 8 covers questions and situations specific to YOPD.

While your PD progresses

One of the toughest truths you have to face while your PD progresses is that you have to rely on other people's help to some degree. Years may pass before you need significant help, but you and your loved ones need to plan for it. In Chapter 18, we discuss the symptoms that can crop up while your PD progresses. Every case of PD is different, though; symptoms that occur in another person may never be a problem for you. Knowledge is good, but don't assume that you'll have to endure every symptom in this book — that's just wrong on so many levels.

The more positive approach is to *prepare* without *projecting*. For example, will you have swallowing difficulties? Maybe, but you can have a speech therapist as a part your care team, as we talk about in Chapter 6. The therapist is sitting there on the bench, ready to get in the game if you need help. Will your spouse, significant other, or other caregiver have to dress you, feed you, bathe you? At some point, in the advanced stages of your PD, a care partner may need to assist you in these basic daily activities, but not necessarily. We cover that step in Chapter 19. Bottom line? You need to give some thought to "what if," of course, BUT at the same time, don't lose sight of living your best possible life in the here and now.

REMEMBER

Reaching decisions about advanced PD questions before they occur (such as identifying a caregiver and having a family meeting to plan an extended network of support) is just smart planning. (That's in Chapter 19, too.)

Treating Parkinson's — Previewing Your Options

After you educate yourself with facts (not myths or hearsay) and draft your care team, you need to get down to the serious business of treating your PD and managing symptoms when they appear. In this book, we cover the options — in fact, a growing number of options — for treating and managing your PD symptoms. In addition to medications (Chapter 10) and — in some advanced cases — surgery (Chapter 11), you can find relief in complementary treatments (such as physical and occupation therapies) and alternative treatments (such as yoga or acupuncture). See Chapter 12 for more about these complementary and alternative options.

In the beginning, if your symptoms are mild and do not impact your daily life in significant ways, your doctor may want to prioritize some lifestyle changes — for example, sleep hygiene (habits that help you get a good night's sleep), diet and exercise (see Chapter 9), and counseling for your PD-related anxiety and depression (Chapter 13). With today's bright spotlight on research for a cure, you may even want to participate in one of the many clinical trials for new disease modifying treatments (Chapter 14).

TIP

When new symptoms appear (often years after your initial diagnosis), check out Chapter 18 to understand the difference between PD-related symptoms and symptoms related to the aging process or another condition entirely (such as high blood pressure).

Starting the Course, Staying the Course

Not surprisingly, for many people and their families, the diagnosis of PD comes as a shock. *Progressive* and *incurable* are likely to be the words that register in these early hours. But while the news begins to sink in, you have choices to make. The following sections provide advice.

Dealing with the here and now

As Debi Brooks, CEO and Co-Founder of the Michael J. Fox Foundation (an organization funding PD research and offering PWP the latest information on dealing with their condition), notes in the foreword to this book, if you're going to truly have a life with PD, you need to do three things: develop an attitude of action, form a problem-solving mentality, and possess the ability to take a great deal of information coming at you from all directions and distill it into clear, logical next steps.

TIP

Here are some tips to get you on the road:

>> **Stay in the here and now** — not the distant future. You can successfully manage PD, perhaps for many years, before you must rely on other people.

>> **Work with your healthcare team** to focus on your PD, specifically, and how you can most effectively manage those symptoms.

>> **Don't compare your situation, symptoms, or ability to manage** to other PWP. The progression of PD varies from person to person, and their situation may not compare to yours.

>> **Get organized.** What are your questions? Write them down. Who are the best medical professionals to treat your PD? If finding that doctor means traveling to another community, at least consider it. This is your life, after all.

>> **Maintain some sense of control over your destiny** by educating yourself. Use only reputable sources, such as those we list throughout this guide and in Appendix B.

>> **Use the lingo.** Everyone else will — your doctors, the people in your support group, the authors of the articles you read. We define terms while we go, but Appendix A is a glossary for your convenience.

>> **Live your life well.** Learn as much as you can, lean on the support of other PWP who have been there (done that), exercise, eat well, and sleep well. Laugh with other people and at yourself, love those people who offer you love in their support and care, and live with the single determination that you won't be reduced to a PD-only identification.

Exceling as a team player

After you put your medical and personal PD care team in place (which we get specific about in Chapter 6), you yourself have to be a team player. Join the team by

>> Taking the time to prepare for doctor appointments by making a list of questions and information about your current symptoms.

>> Taking charge of your own health by making changes to your sleep, diet, and exercise routines, as needed — and sticking with it.

>> Understanding that, although you have every right to maintain independence and autonomy over your decisions, you also have a responsibility to care for the people who will care for and eventually speak for you.

>> Encouraging a shift in thinking in your health team, your family and friends, and yourself. (For example, if you used to love playing jazz saxophone but your tremor makes that impossible, does that mean you have to give up loving jazz?)

>> Celebrating even the smallest victory and allowing yourself a decent interval to mourn the greater losses.

>> Remembering that your PD affects more than just you; some people in your life will also experience major life changes themselves because of your diagnosis.

>> Advocating for new and more effective treatments and a cure. (See Chapter 24.) You can't be more effective than when you're speaking out for those 60,000 PWP diagnosed each year.

Working, playing, and having a life

Okay, you have the medical experts in place (flip to Chapter 6 for the details on creating your Dream Team), and they have you on a regimen customized to manage your symptoms (check out Part 3). What's next? How about getting a life — at least, getting back to some semblance of the life you had before the diagnosis?

Part 4 of this book talks all about living with PD: keeping up with the relationships that are so vital to you as an individual (Chapter 15), maintaining a job (even continuing to build a career, if that's important for you; see Chapter 16), and getting out and about — you know, *living* (Chapter 17).

Making plans for your future

Any diagnosis of a chronic and progressive condition — no matter how slowly it progresses — is a wake-up call for attending to those financial and legal matters everyone needs to address. For you, that time is now. You and your family need to get together with an experienced team of financial and legal consultants; take steps to protect you and your loved ones in the event that you become incapacitated.

TIP

If at some point you can no longer speak for yourself or make the complex decisions in managing finances, your care partner, trusted friend or family member, or a professional advocate (such as an attorney) must know your choices and have the power to act on your behalf. This advice is just common sense whether a person has PD or not. Chapter 20 offers guidelines and tips that can save you and your family a lot of stress and worry in the future on these matters.

If your current housing becomes an issue later on (for example, the bedrooms and the only bathroom are on the second floor), Chapter 21 takes a look at the growing range of options, including adapting your current residence so you can stay there.

REMEMBER

In the course of our individual careers and our collaboration on this book, we have seen case after case of people living full and satisfying lives in spite of PD. We understand that you can't always do it easily, but we have seen the incredible results when PWP succeed in living beyond their disease.

Although no single resource can provide all the answers, we believe that in these pages, you can find the information you need to make the best decisions for living your life with PD.

Chapter **2**

Considering Possible Causes and Risk Factors

A lthough James Parkinson described the disease nearly two centuries ago, and research has been ongoing ever since, doctors continue to describe the underlying cause — the factor that sets Parkinson's disease (PD) in motion — as *idiopathic*, meaning of unknown cause. But scientists continue to discuss and research a number of theories, any one of which may lead to the breakthrough in managing symptoms or even curing the disease.

The medical community has also made progress in recognizing symptoms that may precede the neurological manifestations of PD and how these symptoms may correlate with the risk of developing PD in the future. In this chapter, we cover these potential causes and risk factors so that you can better understand them while the hunt for a cure continues.

Considering Causes: What Is Known and What Is a Mystery

The underlying event behind the onset of PD is a loss of *neurons* (nerve cells) in various parts of the brain, including the substantia nigra region of the brain (see Chapter 1 for an image of the brain). Neurons in the substantia nigra produce *dopamine*, a neurotransmitter that helps the brain coordinate the performance of common movements (such as walking, handling objects, and maintaining balance) almost automatically. What we don't know is why such loss occurs in PWP and not others. Other parts of the brain can also be affected by PD, impairing the production of other neurotransmitters that explain the appearance of non-motor symptoms (see Chapter 3).

PD is a little like diabetes because in both diseases

>> You lose a vital chemical (insulin in diabetes; dopamine in PD).

>> Your body needs that chemical to function properly.

>> You can replace the chemical with medication (insulin injections for diabetes; dopamine promoters for PD).

Of course, the diseases are more complex than the preceding list suggests, but you get the idea. While we age, all of us partially lose dopamine-producing neurons, and that loss results in slower, more measured movements. But the decline of dopamine in people with Parkinson's (PWP) is not a normal part of aging because it happens more rapidly.

Why PD targets the substantia nigra at the stem of the brain remains a mystery. But the damage results in abnormal protein deposits that can disrupt the normal function of the cells in that area. These protein clumps are called *Lewy bodies*, named for Friedrich H. Lewy, the German physician who discovered and documented them in 1908. (For more about Lewy bodies, see Chapter 4.)

REMEMBER

Theories on causes abound — family history, environment, occupation, and so on. Today's researchers generally agree, however, that the onset of PD is a *multi-factorial* process; meaning that several conditions may be at play in the onset of PD depending on the individual, rather than one specific and single cause explaining all cases. But we still don't know the true causes behind the onset of PD in one person and not another — in one family member and not another. Much of the research today focuses on environmental and genetic factors that may contribute to the onset of PD.

Digging into environmental factors

According to the National Institute of Environmental Health Sciences, PD is the second most prevalent neurodegenerative disorder behind Alzheimer's disease. Of the three primary risk factors for PD (age, genetics, and environmental exposures), a line of research that began in the 1980s shows an increasing association between environmental factors and PD. The following sections explore the variety of environmental exposures that may play a role in triggering PD.

Although environmental factors and cellular interactions (of the living cell type, not the cellphone type) appear to significantly contribute to the onset of PD, the Parkinson's Foundation notes that we currently have "no conclusive evidence that any single environmental factor, alone, can be considered a cause of the disease." Indeed, environmental toxins may contribute to the pathological process but are insufficient for PD to develop. Other factors must be present to ignite the initial environmental trigger. Go to the foundation website's discussion of causes of PD (www.parkinson.org/understanding-parkinsons/causes) for more information on this topic.

Location, location, location

For the overwhelming number of PD patients who get Parkinson's, certain environmental factors seem to put a person at higher risk for getting the disease. Consider that family members share not only a genetic history (you can read about the role of genes in the section "Examining possible genetic factors," later in this chapter), but also an environmental history — at least, for a portion of their lives. They live in the same house, drink the same water, eat the same food from the same sources, have exposure to the same chemical compounds, and so on.

Therefore, researchers are studying geographic environmental factors as a possible link to the onset of PD. These factors include living in a rural area and using well water for drinking, cooking, and such.

Exposure to toxins

Toxins that people inhale or ingest can damage the body in many ways, including cell function interference. Research shows that excessive exposure to specific environmental or industrial toxic chemicals, such as pesticides and herbicides, can increase the risk of developing PD. For example, the damage by the pesticide rotenone is directed at the *mitochondria* (the power plant of our body's cells, including brain cells) and can critically reduce the energy produced by the cell until the cell dies.

Farming and agriculture workers are those most at risk of excessive exposure to pesticides and herbicides, which may explain the unusually high incidence of PD in some rural areas. However, everyday exposure to chemical toxins can range from the chemicals that you use to control weeds on your lawn to the unseen sprays that coat and polish fresh produce from overseas.

Because prolonged or consistent exposure to such toxins can possibly contribute to developing PD, take the following precautions:

>> Wash all fresh produce thoroughly — even those items such as melons or citrus, where you normally discard the skin.

>> Limit your exposure to toxins such as pesticides and insecticides.

>> Use all chemical materials in open areas and wear a protective mask.

TIP

If your job requires you to work with chemical compounds, such as those in industrial pesticides and herbicides, talk to your employer about precautions to protect you and other employees from exposure and contamination.

TECHNICAL STUFF

It is possible that environmental toxicity and genetic factors (see "Examining possible genetic factors," later in this chapter) may operate in tandem. For example, scientists have discovered that the gene CYP2D6, when functioning normally, produces an enzyme that breaks down the toxicity of pesticides. But in some people, the gene is less effective, leaving those people more sensitive to the toxicity of pesticides. Researchers need to conduct more studies to verify whether a correlation between genetic predisposition to pesticide toxicity and PD means that the predisposition — and exposure to pesticides — contributes to the development of PD.

Professions possibly linked to PD

Another class of work associated with onset of PD is the welding profession. While an absolute connection between prolonged exposure to metallic fumes or dust and the onset of PD-like symptoms has not been incontrovertibly proven, the link between welding and PD appears to be the chemical element manganese (Mn). Also, miners who are exposed to manganese commonly show signs of parkinsonism. Manganese is an essential element for neuronal function, but excessive exposure may lead to accumulation in the basal ganglia and cause symptoms and signs of PD.

Oddly enough, in more than one occupational study, teachers and healthcare workers showed a higher incidence of PD — as much as two to three times higher than other professions. Researchers are puzzled because the major factor that the two professions seem to share is exposure to infection, even though PD is clearly not a contagious disease.

Head trauma

Many people theorize that Muhammad Ali's PD was brought on by his years in the boxing ring. "Too many times getting hit in the head," they assert. Indeed, some studies suggest an association between head trauma and the development of PD. But possibly, Ali's years in the ring brought the underlying presence of his PD to light.

Studies over the last decade show evidence related to a person suffering one or more concussions or traumatic brain injuries (TBI) in their life and the later development of PD. Definitely make your doctor aware of any such past injuries, especially if you lost consciousness during the event. But in all likelihood, that information doesn't affect your options for treatment. Check out the online article "Traumatic Brain Injury and Parkinson's" (`https://apdaparkinson.org/article/traumatic-brain-injury-pd`), from the American Parkinson Disease Association (APDA).

Aging

Perhaps the greatest risk factor for Parkinson's disease is simply growing older. Recent predictions by researchers in the field suggest that because the global population is aging, the number of PWP will likely double by 2040. Living a healthy lifestyle that focuses on regular sleeping patterns, exercise, and nutrition can help keep your brain in the best shape it can be.

Examining possible genetic factors

Every human being plays host to a gazillion genes in their DNA molecules. Genes determine everything from the color of your eyes to the possibility of developing a certain disease or condition. Note the use of the word *possibility*. You carry genes in double copies, so if one of your genes has the propensity for a condition, the other copy may offset that vulnerability.

REMEMBER

Keep in mind that only about 15-20 percent of PWP appear to have inherited it. However, the study of genes enhances our ability to understand the mechanisms of the disease and the molecules a scientist may target for treatment. If you have a family history of PD or are interested in more information on genetic research, check out the article "The Genetic Link to Parkinson's Disease," on the Johns Hopkins Medicine website (go to `https://hopkinsmedicine.org/health` and search for "genetic link to parkinsons disease").

Just a slight genetic link

According to the National Human Genome Research Institute (NHGRI), evidence now shows a genetic factor in the development of PD. People who have a close relative (parent or sibling) who has PD are slightly more likely to contract Parkinson's than someone who has no family history of the disease. But, according to the Mayo Clinic, the link is relatively small and more common when the onset of PD occurs before age 50, which is also less common. (For more information about early onset PD, check out Chapter 8.)

So why waste time and money studying genes? Oddly enough, the very fact that PD is one of the most typical nongenetic diseases makes the genetic study of PD patients interesting. In other words, if PD is typically *not* inherited, then what else is going on?

Gene mutation may contribute

Over time, scientists have identified specific gene mutations that have definite links to the onset of PD in families where PD is present in multiple generations. An abnormality in one such gene, which scientists have named *Parkin*, may predict the onset of Parkinson's at a young age (before age 50). Because Parkinson's is present and progressing for several years before any symptoms become obvious, a gene predictor can mean earlier diagnosis and earlier intervention.

Another discovery shows that a *mutation* (change) in the gene producing the protein alpha-synuclein (SNCA) may increase the amount of protein produced and thereby contribute to the development of *clumps* (multiple proteins bonding together) in dopamine neurons, eventually damaging or destroying them. Interestingly, alpha-synuclein is part of Lewy bodies, the hallmark protein deposit in dopamine cells affected by Parkinson's disease. If researchers can find a way to break up those clumps and get rid of the excess proteins, then they may have found a way to slow or even stop the progression of PD. (See the section "Occupational causes," later in this chapter, for more about clumping.)

TECHNICAL
STUFF

Other genes with established correlation to PD include LRRK2 and GBA, which may lead to the disease in opposite ways. The first gene variant (LRRK2) is believed to cause increased levels of an enzyme that will result in toxic gain of function. The second (GBA) will result in a decrease of the enzyme glucocerebrosidase, with resulting accumulation of abnormal proteins in the neuron. Potential treatments (which are under investigation) will therefore try to slow down LRRK2 activity and enhance GBA activity. Sounds confusing? Welcome to the world of neuroscience research.

TIP

You can use 23andMe (a genetics-based health and ancestry service at www.23andme.com) to perform a test for these genes.

YOUNG-ONSET PARKINSON'S DISEASE: A UNIQUE PD SUB-GROUP

People diagnosed with young-onset Parkinson's disease (YOPD) experience many of the same motor symptoms (stiffness, impaired balance) and non-motor symptoms (sleep disturbances, depression) as people whose PD manifests later in life. Those diagnosed before age 50 have some differences from those diagnosed later in life. People with YOPD

> Often have a family history of PD, meaning that the genetic mechanisms reviewed in the chapter may play a larger role

Potentially have more difficulty just getting a diagnosis, and doctors more commonly misdiagnose them (for example, a doctor may attribute a stiff shoulder to a sports injury or arthritis)

Experience more troublesome side effects from medications

But the major difference for the PWP is that a person with YOPD is in the prime of their life when PD strikes. The impact of receiving a chronic debilitating diagnosis such as YOPD affects every facet of that life — socially and professionally. Maybe the PWP is on track for a major job promotion or has just found out about a significant life-changing event (such as pregnancy). The PWP may be raising a family and looking forward to life as an empty-nester and retiree. The list goes on, and the questions are endless. But you get the idea: This is not going to be a walk in the park — or a 5K run.

However, if you or someone you care about is diagnosed with YOPD, you have time to prepare for what may come because the progression of YOPD is usually slower than PD progression in older people. In Chapter 8, we do a deeper dive into this unique topic, offering ideas for how best to cope with your diagnosis.

Checking out other possible causes

If your PD wasn't caused by family history, the environment, or head trauma (see the preceding sections for discussions of all these possible causes), what did cause it? Unfortunately, researchers can't really answer that question at this stage. And any time a chronic illness has no definitive cause, theories fly. At the moment, PD has its fair share of such theories. The following sections describe instances where the jury is still out regarding whether a link exists between certain factors and the onset of PD.

Latent effects of war

PD researchers continue to explore links between PD and both Agent Orange (an herbicide used during the Vietnam War) and chemical weapons during the Gulf War, but the evidence is still far from conclusive. Age is a consideration in the onset of PD, and Vietnam vets are reaching the age that onset of PD is more common simply because of their generation. We still don't have definitive proof whether exposure to Agent Orange during the Vietnam War or chemical weapons in the Gulf War may also be a contributing factor.

The Veterans Administration (VA) is conducting ongoing research. If you're a veteran of either war, you can find out more information at the U.S. Department of Veterans Affairs website (www.va.gov) by entering "Parkinson's" in the search text box and clicking the Search button.

Over-medication and drug use

If you take certain drugs to excess or over a long period of time, you may display the symptoms of PD. Some of the conditions and their drugs include

Condition	Drugs
Schizophrenia, major depression, or agitation in older people	haloperidol (Haldol), chlorpromazine (Thorazine)
Nausea	metoclopramide (Reglan), prochlorperazine (Compazine)

These medications can cause Parkinson-like symptoms and should not be prescribed for someone already diagnosed with PD (they could be potentially very dangerous). Fortunately, side effects of such medicines usually subside after the medicine leaves the body's system. We still don't know whether a drug reaction of this nature can predict later development of PD, but some postulate that the exposure to dopamine-blocking agents may unmask latent PD. *Note:* Symptoms brought on by drug use may occur on both sides of your body at the same time, unlike primary PD. Your PD doctor (neurologist or movement disorders specialist) may consider obtaining a special imaging test called a DaTScan to aid in the diagnosis of PD versus drug-induced PD.

WARNING

Illicit drug use may also be a factor in whether a person develops PD. In the early 1980s, a group of young people injected a heroin-like drug that contained the toxin 1-methyl-4-phenyl-1,2,3,6-tetrahydropyridine (MPTP). It headed straight for the substantia nigra, destroying dopamine cells in its path and leaving the youngsters with signs of advanced PD. As a silver lining, this tragedy opened up a new line of research to model possible causes of PD.

SOUNDS LIKE SCI-FI, BUT A WORD ABOUT NEUROPROTECTORS

The brain has two types of cells: *neurons* (nerve cells) and *glia* (cells that respond to injury and regulate the chemical composition surrounding them, among other tasks). Although glia cells are far more prevalent, the neuron cells do the heavy lifting when it comes to brain work. According to the National Institute of Neurological Disorders and Stroke (NINDS), the three classes of neurons are

Sensory neurons: Carry information from the senses (eyes, ears, and such) to the brain

Motor neurons: Carry messages from the *central nervous system* (comprised of the brain, spinal cord, and network of nerves running through the body) to the body's muscles and glands

Interneurons: Communicate only within their immediate location

Within each category, hundreds of neuron types operate with the very specific messaging abilities that make each person unique. But the neurons affected by PD control the body's ability to move. When those neurons die in large enough numbers, the brain's ability to signal the body to move is compromised.

Researchers are working hard to understand the death of these neurons and to develop treatments and therapies that can protect them. One potential value of stem cell research is that neural stem cells may reproduce the variety of neurons in the brain. Scientists could then figure out how to maneuver these new neurons to become

A protector of healthy neurons (preventing or at least slowing further damage or loss)

A replacement for damaged or dead neurons

In addition, ongoing research considers whether certain therapies — such as certain drugs, vitamin supplements, and rigorous exercise therapy — may act as a protector and slow the loss of these vital neurons. For more information on the role of neuroprotection in the battle against PD, check out Chapters 11 and 12.

Weighing Your Risk Factors

Your suspicion that you have PD (or an actual diagnosis from your doctor) can raise all sorts of questions, starting with, "How did this happen to me?" It's perfectly normal to look back and consider the risk factors in your past (although you didn't know they were risk factors at the time) while you also look forward to help protect your children and others around you from those same risks.

Start with what's known for sure:

>> PD isn't contagious — you can't get it from or give it to another person.

>> Most cases (at least three-fourths) show up after age 60, and incidence increases every decade after that.

>> Head trauma (a serious fall or accident involving injury to the head) can be a risk factor for PD.

>> Most cases are random, meaning that most cases show up in the absence of a family history of the disease and are likely due to a combination of factors rather than a single cause.

>> Men are more likely to get PD than women.

Your particular *risk factors* (or family members' risks if you suspect you have PD) are the life and lifestyle details that can increase the chances of developing PD. The risks may be *multi-factorial* (meaning it's believed that people get PD due to a number of factors and not just a single cause).

Considering your age and gender

Currently, the one concrete (and greatest) risk factor for developing PD is age. Most people develop symptoms in middle age, but the risk for developing PD increases simply because dopamine production declines with age. The average age for onset is 60, and risk increases until around age 75. Some research has shown a significant decrease in the number of people who develop PD after age 75.

At least three studies have confirmed that men are more likely to develop PD than women — in some studies, twice as likely. One theory suggests that the production of estrogen may protect women. In recent observational studies, estrogen seems to have a mild to moderate neuroprotective effect against dopaminergic neurons in the substantia nigra. As always, researchers have more work to do, but estrogen (in combination with other medications) might play a part in the prevention and treatment of PD.

Taking a look at ethnicity

Studies have shown that non-white populations, such as African Americans and Asian Americans, have a lower risk of developing primary Parkinson's disease but may be more vulnerable to other forms of parkinsonism, such as essential tremor (see Chapter 1) and multiple system atrophy (see Chapter 4). However, these studies haven't fully considered whether this difference is tied to an economic and class-based imbalance in the delivery of medical care — especially specialized medical care, such as seeing a neurologist or movement disorders specialist.

Regarding other risk possibilities

Although scientists don't yet know of any definitive causes, some factors we discuss in this chapter may contribute to your risk for developing PD. In an eat-on-the-run fast-food society, people may be denying their bodies' needs for key vitamins and nutrients, or disregard proper exercise and sleep routines. And what about the dangers of such evils as smoking and caffeine? Can these factors put people at greater risk for getting PD?

Looking at diet and exercise

Face it: Being overweight sets you up for all kinds of health risks. However, a 2020 study published in *Neurology* by the American Academy of Neurology found no significant link between inactivity and obesity, and the risk for developing PD. That said, the benefits of a diet rich in antioxidants and a regular program of exercise can't hurt. In some cases, these benefits prolonged the time before PWP needed to treat their PD symptoms with medication (see Chapter 9).

Checking out other signs

A *prodromal* sign, or symptom, is an early symptom signaling the onset of an illness or disease. When a person presents all three of the *prodromal* signs listed here, the risk of developing PD increases over 150 times. These three signs are

>> **REM sleep behavior disorder (RBD):** When people dream their bodies are naturally paralyzed, with the exception of respiratory (fortunately!) and ocular muscles. A loss of this necessary motor inhibition results in sleep behaviors like *acting out* dreams, which can range from simple vocalizations to complex and organized movements such as sleepwalking. RBD is a strong predictor of PD: most people with RBD will develop PD within 10 years of the diagnosis.

>> **Loss of smell:** Almost every PWP experiences some degree of reduced sense of smell, which is however often discounted as a recurrent cold or sinusitis. Most importantly, loss of smell can occur years before the onset of motor difficulties typical of PD. When loss of smell occurs in association with RBD, the chance of developing PD increases to 65 percent within five years.

>> **Constipation:** Irregular or difficult bowel movements are not uncommon with advancing age, and they are often experienced by PWP, particularly after taking levodopa. Similar to RBD and loss of smell, constipation can occur years before neurological symptoms of PD.

Smoking and caffeine

Get this: As many as 50 published studies over two decades have shown that smoking cigarettes reduces the risk of Parkinson's in people who have smoked steadily most of their adult lives. *But* the negative effects of smoking (such as lung cancer) can greatly shorten your stay on this planet; a two-pack-a-day habit doesn't make sense to lower your risk of developing PD.

As for caffeine? Many studies have firmly established a neuroprotective effect of caffeine intake, which can reduce the risk of developing PD by several folds. Caffeine action appears to be facilitated by adenosine receptors in the brain (a new target for PD treatment, see Chapter 10) and is shown to have other benefits as well.

Knowing What We Don't Know

The more researchers tackle the problems of PD, the more complex the challenges become. The following sections take a quick look at the unknowns of PD and offer ways that PWP and the general public can help PD research move forward.

The need-to-know info

Questions for PD researchers abound, but one of the greatest challenges is simply getting a good handle on the accurate numbers and extent of PD. For example, scientists don't yet know

» How common Parkinson's is because there is no universal database for recording new cases

» Whether the numbers of PWP are increasing over time or whether those larger numbers simply reflect longevity and an aging population

» Whether geographic cluster patterns exist (places around the globe where PD is unusually prevalent or absent)

TIP

In 2010, the Michael J. Fox Foundation launched the Parkinson's Progressive Markers Initiative (PPMI) to better understand how PD develops and affects PWP. The initiative relies on participation on all fronts: PWP, doctors, researchers, caregivers, and even people who don't have a direct connection to PD. You can play a role. Go to www.michaeljfox.org for more information and become a partner in the fight to find a cure.

As of this writing, PD has no national registry where doctors can report the diagnosis of PD in the United States, and only a few states require doctors to report cases of PD. Research could take an enormous step forward with a mandatory national registry for the diagnosis of PD (a global registry would be even better!), helping researchers gather the knowledge and data that they need.

A mandatory registry of PD diagnoses may seem an invasion of your privacy, but information that allows researchers to track patterns is the best way to gain vital knowledge that can lead to new treatments — and even a cure.

The attitude that busts research barriers

At the 2006 World Parkinson's Congress in Washington, D.C., Joan Samuelson (founder of the Parkinson's Action Network, now an integral part of the Michael J. Fox Foundation) said that when first diagnosed, she believed her job was to be a *patient* patient. That attitude quickly changed when Joan understood more about the knowns and unknowns of PD. Today, her motto is that patients need to be *in the room* — the PD patient community needs to take a vocal and proactive role in helping research move forward.

You may not be ready to take on this larger fight but keep it in the back of your mind while you find out more about PD. *Note:* In many ways, you've taken a key first step — you're educating yourself about Parkinson's and what a diagnosis may mean for you and your loved ones. But getting involved with the greater Parkinson's community at a local, state, and national level is one of the most empowering steps you can take to live a full and productive life in spite of PD. (And when you're ready to get more involved, see Chapter 14 for more information on clinical trials and Chapter 24 for ideas on advocacy roles.)

IN THIS CHAPTER

» Getting the PD terms straight

» Taking stock of your symptoms

» Working with your doctor to identify signs

» Categorizing the progression of PD in stages

» Keeping your care partner in the loop

Chapter **3**

Sizing Up Symptoms, Signs, and Stages

Whenever you have a concern about your health, you usually first take note of certain troubling (and unexplained) symptoms. Perhaps you seem clumsier than usual, or your posture seems unusually stiff and rigid. If these symptoms trouble you enough, you probably make an appointment with your primary care physician (PCP) to have them checked out. After you describe your symptoms, your doctor conducts a clinical exam, looking for signs that may explain your symptoms.

In this chapter, we describe the *symptoms* you observe that can signal Parkinson's disease (PD), as well as the *signs* that your doctor looks for to reach a diagnosis.

REMEMBER

Many chronic, progressive conditions move through defined stages, but progression in PD and associated symptoms are unique for each patient.

Familiarizing Yourself with the Lingo

In the medical world, a *symptom* is

>> What you feel or perceive before you see the doctor

>> The reason you ultimately decide to make an appointment

>> The details (vague or specific) that you give when the doctor or nurse asks why you've come in

For example, you may say that you're more tired than usual or moving more slowly because you lack energy. Or perhaps you're depressed or experiencing dizziness or shaking.

In contrast, medical *signs* are what your doctor observes during the examination. The best doctors use their senses, in addition to the data from the usual medical imaging techniques and screening tools (see Chapter 4 for more about these instruments). For example, a doctor's touch may sense tightened muscles, their eyes may observe a fine tremor when your hand is at rest, they may note that you have a slight shuffle or don't swing one arm when you walk, or their ears may detect softer speech, a searching for words, or unusual sounds in your lungs or intestines.

REMEMBER

Simply put, symptoms make up the subjective report of your experiences, and signs contribute to your doctor's objective basis for a diagnosis.

Disease *staging* divides a chronic and progressive illness into levels that usually correspond to the advancement of symptoms and disease. Generally, stages have the following labels:

>> **Early stage:** The disease is manageable with little outside assistance.

>> **Moderate stage:** The patient needs more assistance and lifestyle changes.

>> **Advanced stage:** The disease has advanced to the point that the patient can find it difficult to manage without significant assistance; the patient may face the need for major lifestyle changes, extra care, and planning for the end of life.

Symptoms — What You Look For

Let's cut to the chase. You suspect that you or someone you love may have PD; otherwise (unless you're writing a school report about Parkinson's), you wouldn't be flipping through this book, and you definitely wouldn't have turned to this chapter. Ask yourself what's behind those suspicions:

>> **A slight shakiness in the hands:** Does it occur in only one hand? If the shaking occurs while the hand is at rest, does it stop when that hand picks up a cup of coffee, a pen, or a tennis racket? If you notice the shakiness in both hands and it mostly occurs when you grasp something, then PD probably isn't the cause (but get it checked out to figure out what is causing it).

>> **A general slowing down of movement:** Does it take longer to walk from one place to another or to get in and out of the car? Have you noticed an increase in stumbling, clumsiness, or loss of balance? Do you (or does the person) feel tired, stiff, or just not yourself (or themselves)?

>> **A significant change in energy level or outlook:** Everyone experiences days when they're more tired or weaker than usual. And everyone has the blues from time to time. But if you've been feeling unusually weak, fatigued, depressed, or anxious for longer than two weeks, those symptoms need attention — even when you have a plausible cause (such as an unusually busy week at work or the death of a loved one).

>> **Sleep disturbances:** Research has shown that *REM behavior disorder* (or acting out your dreams vocally or physically) is an important early indicator of PD or related neurological conditions. This can happen before the typical neurological symptoms of PD develop. In general, most PWP report poor sleep years before the emergence of classical symptoms of the disease.

>> **Gastrointestinal (GI) problems or psychological problems:** In some cases, patients show none of the usual symptoms, so don't stop with the more traditional PD symptoms. You can also see GI symptoms such as constipation or abdominal pain and issues such as increased nervousness or anxiety.

These symptoms — the feelings, aches, and pains — might make you think something's not right. PD may be causing your symptoms, or it may not. Either way, you owe it to yourself to get your doctor's assessment.

Signs — What Your Doctor Looks For

When you see a doctor, they listen while you describe your symptoms, and then they conduct an examination to determine what those symptoms indicate. While you talk about your symptoms, your doctor begins a *differential diagnosis*, listing the diagnostic possibilities while they try to determine what disorder your symptoms indicate. For example, if your symptoms could be caused by PD, your doctor also looks for signs that indicate PD. But any doctor worth their salt doesn't offer a firm diagnosis before seeing the results of several tests and getting confirmation from a specialist.

In addition to four primary signs of PD (discussed in the following section), which may or may not be evident when you first go to the doctor, your doctor considers several other possible indicators (see the section "Secondary signs and symptoms," later in this chapter). And because PD is a *syndrome* (not just one symptom, but a number of problems that tend to occur together), it doesn't affect only your physical movements; it can also trigger other issues, such as cognitive or sleep problems, or even pain. (Find out about such symptoms in the section "Non-motor signs and symptoms," later in this chapter).

Four primary signs

Although the actual causes and risk factors for getting PD are still mysterious (see Chapter 2 for more on these factors), the primary signs that signal the neurological presence of PD are clear. You may have noticed one or more of these signs but then dismissed them as something slight, easily explained, or due to an entirely different condition.

TIP

Several resources use the acronym *TRAP* (tremor, rigidity, akinesia, postural instability) to illustrate the four primary signs of PD. And because PD seems to trap your body with your brain's compromised ability to communicate, the acronym makes the top four symptoms easier to remember.

T = Tremor at rest (uncontrolled shaking)

PD was originally called *shaking palsy* because the *resting tremor* (it goes away as soon as the hand is engaged in an activity) rarely occurs in other illnesses. Characteristically, the resting tremor begins in one hand and moves to the other hand later in the disease. The tremor may extend to the leg or foot on the same side and sometimes to the lips and jaw. Tremor in the head and neck, however, virtually never occur in primary Parkinson's disease and it points to a diagnosis of other movement disorders such as dystonic or essential tremor (ET).

Other types of tremor — which may or may not be part of PD — include

>> **Postural tremor:** Obvious when arms are extended to hold a position or posture

>> **Action tremor:** Present when certain tasks, such as writing or bringing a spoon to the mouth, are performed

>> **Internal tremor:** The patient feels the tremor but can't show it, almost as if it's coming from inside

Although tremor is the most obvious symptom of PD, you don't need to have a tremor to be diagnosed with PD.

R = Rigidity (stiff muscles)

Rigidity is probably the most ignored and easy-to-explain-as-something-else sign. In plain English, *rigidity* means stiffness. (Who doesn't experience stiffness in joints and limbs that makes movement more difficult while they age?) If your doctor observes rigidity (without other signs of PD), they may first suspect arthritis and prescribe an anti-inflammatory medication. But if anti-inflammatory medicine doesn't relieve the stiffness, or if other symptoms emerge, let your doctor know.

A = Akinesia or bradykinesia (absence or slowness of movement)

Especially early on, people with PD (PWP) may experience unusually slow and clumsy movements, technically known as *bradykinesia*. Much later in the progression, that slowed movement may become virtual inability to move, known as *akinesia*. *Bradykinesia*, like tremor and rigidity, is typically present only or predominantly on one side of the body.

Get to know these terms because, if indeed you or a loved one has PD, you'll hear these words again and again. *Kinesia* means movement, in the sense of knowing what you want your body to do. So *akinesia* and *bradykinesia* indicate problems initiating or continuing an action. For example, to walk across the room, you stand up, and your brain tells your foot to step out — but with bradykinesia, your body doesn't move right away.

The problem can extend well beyond simply walking from here to there. Bradykinesia can also affect

>> **Facial expression:** It slows the blinking eye movement and the ability to smile.

>> **Fine motor movements:** The fingers progressively lose the necessary speed and coordination to perform detailed actions, such as managing buttons or cutting food. In addition, fingers may curl or stiffen because of rigidity (discussed in the preceding section).

>> **Sequential movements:** Lack of coordination between the various parts of the body that need to move in sequence can, for example, make it difficult to turn over in bed. Again, muscle stiffness and rigidity may further complicate this normally routine task.

See a discussion of how bradykinesia and akinesia can lead to other issues in the section "Secondary signs and symptoms," later in this chapter.

P = Postural instability (impaired balance)

In a healthy person, the natural walking movement involves alternately swinging the arms and stepping forward with assurance. For PWP, however, the swing slowly decreases, particularly on one side; in time, the person moves by using small, uncertain, shuffling steps. (PWP may compensate the resulting balance shift forward by propelling themselves forward with several quick, short steps.) Other PWP experience episodes of *freezing* (their feet feel glued to the floor).

Problems with balance (resulting in falls that can cause major injuries, hospitalization, and escalation of symptoms) usually don't become a factor until later in the progression of symptoms (see Chapter 18 for info about PD progression). In time, PWP may lose the ability to gauge the necessary action to regain balance and prevent a fall. They may grasp at doorways or other stationary objects in an effort to prevent the loss of balance. Unfortunately, someone watching these maneuvers might think that the PWP is under the influence of alcohol or other substances.

Secondary signs and symptoms

Although you don't need to display the indicators in Table 3-1 for your doctor to diagnose PD, you may observe many of them early on, and they can contribute to the diagnosis of PD. During your appointment, tell your physician anything that you find troublesome regarding these secondary symptoms. They're part of your symptomatic history, which helps your doctors see the total picture of your condition.

TABLE 3-1

Secondary PD Indicators

Sign/Symptom	Presentation	Additional Info
Facial mask	A lack of facial expression or change in facial expression; decreased animation or emotion; appearance of staring due to less frequent eye blinks.	Can lead people to assume that you're not listening or not understanding. Maybe someone has said, "You don't smile as often," and you're thinking, "I'm smiling just as often as before!"
Slowed or slurred speech	A voice that is softer or fades away after a strong start; lack of normal variations of tone and emotion; hoarseness; slurred speech.	Issues with speech (such as stuttering or speaking very rapidly) or swallowing difficulties can appear while PD symptoms advance. See Chapter 18 for more info about advanced symptoms of PD.
Small, cramped handwriting	Once smooth handwriting appears increasingly cramped and jerky.	Called *micrographia,* this symptom typically appears as handwriting that becomes progressively smaller (for example: Parkinson) and closer together.
Changes to skin	Increased sweating; excessively oily or dry skin. Increased danger of skin cancer.	PD could be a culprit here; even if it turns out not to be PD-associated, changes in skin condition need your attention. Again, consult your doctor.

Non-motor signs and symptoms

Although seeing the *TRAP* signs (check out the section "Four primary signs," earlier in this chapter) often gives you enough evidence to raise the possibility of PD, you may see non-motor factors before those primary signs appear. Your doctor may ask questions to discover underlying symptoms that you've been ignoring or simply discounting.

REMEMBER

Keep an open mind and answer your doctor's questions as honestly and fully as possible. Any one of the symptoms in Table 3-2 or a combination of them may indicate a condition other than PD. Don't jump to conclusions or try to self-diagnose. Trust your doctor on this!

TABLE 3-2

Non-Motor PD Indicators

Sign/Symptom	Presentation	Additional Info
Anxiety or depression	Anxiety episodes, ranging from a mild feeling of uneasiness to a full-blown panic attack; depression may show up as a lack of interest in normal activities or a severe condition that calls for counseling or medication.	Anxiety and depression are such an integral part of PD that they get their own chapter (Chapter 13). These feelings may be some of the earliest symptoms of PD.
Constipation and urinary incontinence	Unusual changes in bowel or urinary habits, including slowing bowels, and *urinary frequency* (having to urinate often) and *urinary urgency* (NOW!).	Many people (even doctors) associate these symptoms with aging or other conditions, but they can be signs of advancing PD. Bring these symptoms to your doctor's attention. Constipation can occur *before* typical motor signs of the disease.
Sleep disturbances	Mostly difficulty staying asleep, with multiple unprovoked awakenings during the night, resulting in excessive daytime sleepiness and tendency to nap throughout the day.	In some cases, the PWP has vivid dreams or REM sleep behavior disorder (RBD), manifesting as acting out their dreams. RBD can occur *before* typical motor signs of the disease. Sleep apnea is also a frequent problem.
Loss of smell	Perhaps tricky to recognize, reduced sense of smell can often be chalked off as chronic sinusitis or simply not perceived as an issue.	In many cases, reduced sense of smell precedes the onset of the typical motor symptoms of PD by several years.
Executive dysfunction, inattention, spatial disorientation, and other cognitive abnormalities	Difficulties with keeping track of your monthly bills, following directions, or making decisions; needing reminders (called *cue-dependent function*); problems with memory, thought processing, and word finding.	Use task reminders (for example, an alarm that tells you to take your medicine) or labels on cabinets and drawers to remind you of their contents. Mention any escalation in the need for reminders or other cognitive problems to your doctor. These symptoms are usually more pronounced as PD progresses (see Chapter 18).
Dizziness or lightheadedness	Standing up may cause dizziness or lightheadedness due to a drop in blood pressure caused by abnormal fluctuations of blood pressure due to dysfunction within nervous system signals.	Although dizziness can indicate a number of conditions (especially in warm weather or over-heated rooms), mention it to your doctor if it's one of your symptoms.

Sign/Symptom	Presentation	Additional Info
Pain	Shoulder pain, hip or back pain can occur very early in PD, usually on the same side of tremor and/or bradykinesia.	Pain is usually described as muscle spasms or intense stiffness and is likely associated with muscle rigidity. Unfortunately, a misdiagnosis of rotator cuff tear or pinched nerve may lead to unnecessary surgery.
Sexual dysfunction	Decreased sexual desire and performance can often occur, usually later in the progression of the disease.	If you experience this dysfunction as part of your PD, proper medication and treatment can help.
Visual hallucinations	Some medications for PD may have the side effect of making you see people or objects that really aren't present. These hallucinations are usually benign such as believing something (like a cat) just scurried past or the feeling someone is there but is not.	If you experience hallucinations before the PD diagnosis and before taking PD meds, the doctor can look for other medications or causes.

Stages — Understanding the Unique Path PD Can Take

To live with any chronic, progressive illness, you need to take responsibility to maintain your life beyond that condition. We discuss the specifics of this responsibility in much greater depth throughout the book. But here's a significant question: If you do have PD and it does progress, then how fast and to what extent?

Some *chronic* (long-lasting) and *progressive* (advancing or worsening) diseases have clear-cut divisions between *stages* (obvious, and even predictable, changes in the patient's condition). However, PD isn't one of those diseases — it affects each patient differently. For most PWP, the progression of neurological symptoms takes years. With proper treatment and management of new symptoms, PWP can live independently for quite some time before they need close care. A rapid progression of PD — in which the PWP quickly becomes dependent on others for assistance in performing basic daily activities — is less common. PD may progress more rapidly if other *comorbidities* (diseases or medical conditions that are simultaneously present with others) such as diabetes, hypertension, or obesity are present.

Don't let yourself or others try to project the future. Do *prepare* — plan for what may happen. But don't *project* or assume that it will happen and on a certain timetable. Projecting only adds to your anxiety and may actually prevent you from taking some measures that prolong the time between stages.

In spite of PD's lack of clearly defined and timed steps, your doctor may describe your condition in terms of stages. This breakdown is a common practice in the medical profession because it permits doctors to use a medically accepted language when making notes about your condition. If you need to change doctors midstream, the new physician's ability to understand the previous doctor's notes can save you valuable time and enhance the new doctor's ability to address your needs.

The length of each stage is unique to each PWP. With lifestyle and medical therapies, and even with certain interventions (a change to more practical housing; the use of aides such as walking sticks) along the way, PWP can maintain the early-stage status quo for several years. Even so, the disease does have some broad outlines of progression. (For a fuller discussion of PD rating scales that determine its various stages, turn to Chapter 4.)

Early-stage PD: When life can be fairly normal

You may have experienced (and ignored) certain warning signals from PD for several years before you went to your doctor. Maybe you were constantly tired or had a vague, don't-feel-good sensation. While your general movement slowed, maybe you dismissed it as getting older or just lack of energy today.

Then you began to notice some troubling (not to mention, annoying!) symptoms: stiffness that was different from the not-as-young-as-I-used-to-be version, shakiness, dizziness, or mood changes. (If you don't know the list, flip back to the section "Signs — What Your Doctor Looks For," earlier in this chapter.)

If you have tremor, you may have barely noticed it at first, or maybe you dismissed it as a spasm. It may have appeared in one finger, so you noticed it only when you were performing a certain task, like tying your shoe or buttoning a jacket.

In early-stage PD, here's what you can probably expect:

>> Symptoms are mild, and you can often easily explain them to yourself and others.

>> You find symptoms annoying when they occur, but they don't significantly interfere with normal activity.

- » Symptoms typically occur on only one side of the body.

- » If you have tremor, it is likely present in one limb — usually the hand — and it occurs most often when the hand is at rest.

- » You may notice trouble with fine motor tasks, like tying your shoe or writing.

- » Your loved ones may notice you are walking at a slower pace or that there is a reduction in your arm swing with walking.

- » Other people may comment on changes related to appearance, posture, energy, and facial expression.

REMEMBER

In the early stages of PD, you can probably manage for some time with no pharmacological intervention. In other words, you may not need pills to control the symptoms. However, do not be afraid to take medications if your doctor believes that you may benefit from them.

Moderate-stage PD: When you need to accept help

The defining signal of progression in PD occurs when you begin to see symptoms on both sides of the body. However, even at this stage, some primary care physicians have missed the diagnosis of PD in some cases simply because your PCP took the symptoms (rigidity, gait change, tremor) as normal signs of aging.

Other factors that may signal the moderate stage of PD include the following:

- » **Your posture becomes stooped.** Your head more often bends forward with your chin toward the chest.

- » **You move all of your body parts significantly slower.** When you walk, you may experience *freezing* (your feet feel glued to the floor); your hand tremor may now affect your entire arm, making activities such as shaving or brushing your teeth more difficult.

- » **You experience slower cognitive and executive function.** You have issues with your short-term memory, and you have difficulty putting thoughts into words, keeping track of monthly bills, and making decisions. (See the section "Non-motor signs and symptoms," earlier in this chapter.) This slowdown may also include trouble with attention and spatial orientation.

- » **You have an increased reliance on medicines and need for assistance.** PWP must rely on medicines, and occasionally assistance from other people, to pursue many of the activities they took for granted before PD. Examples of these activities include driving, getting in and out of a chair or bed, and going to the bathroom.

As your symptoms become more troublesome, you and your doctor can discuss strategies and pharmacological options to address your symptoms so that you can continue to live your best life now.

TIP

Balancing the dosages and timing of medications early on can mitigate the more serious side effects as your PD progresses. After you begin taking them, antiparkinsonian medicines can be amazingly effective. (For more about PD meds and their side effects, check out the discussion in Chapter 10.) Also, new medicines become available every year, medicines that — ideally — can be more effective with fewer troubling side effects.

Late-stage PD: When planning keeps you in control

When a PWP reaches the point of serious disability (meaning that you can no longer lead a normal, independent life without major assistance), the medical community describes the stage as *late* or *advanced*. At this stage, even the medications that worked so well in the earlier stages start creating problems and complications, and the PWP may face unprecedented challenges.

For most patients, the late stage begins many years after the initial diagnosis; when all your planning and preparing (which we preach about throughout this book) pays off for you and your family. In spite of the potential for advancing frailty, you're still in control. You made the decisions necessary to see you through this time during earlier stages of PD, and your family understands and accepts your wishes. You can probably guess the signs of late PD:

>> The PWP has significantly reduced mobility and compromised balance.

>> The PWP can walk only by using a walker and for short distances, if at all.

>> The PWP can no longer manage the basic activities of daily living (such as grooming, dressing, and bathing) without considerable assistance.

>> Cognitive impairments worsen; physical limitations increase.

>> Other non-motor symptoms (such as interrupted sleep, difficulty swallowing, or poor bladder control) may become prevalent.

>> The benefits of medication wear off earlier between each dose.

>> In the most advanced stage, the PWP is usually confined to bed and requires round-the-clock care.

A Few Words for You and Your Care Partner

If you're living with someone whom you suspect has PD, encourage that person to seek a definitive diagnosis. The symptoms may or may not be PD. Many symptoms associated with PD are also factors in illnesses and conditions that are treatable and curable. Neither you nor the other person should jump to conclusions, but you shouldn't ignore the warning signs, either.

REMEMBER

If the diagnosis is PD, don't panic. You and the PWP are now members of a unique, extraordinarily proactive, well-organized community. If you open yourself to that community, you become richer for the friends you make, the information you exchange, and the comfort you share.

Understand the impact first

If the diagnosis is PD, then first and foremost you need to understand that this person you love can continue to live an independent and self-reliant life for some time, even many years.

If you're the PWP's care partner, here are some tips:

>> **Don't be a superhero.** Don't put on your cape and assume you need to be Super-Caregiver. Resist the urge to go into full-on nurturing mode; encourage independence and self-reliance.

>> **Incorporate care into your life.** Understand that adding PD to your already busy life can lead to problems if you aren't proactive and don't take the necessary steps to care for yourself and integrate your new role into the rest of your life.

>> **Watch out for depression.** Be aware that a decline in the PWP's self-reliance and confidence may be a sign of depression — a common symptom of PD. While you are at it, don't fail to address your mental health. You are taking on a role that carries extra stress. Be open to support and help from others.

If you're the PWP

>> **Maintain your independence** and refuse to permit PD to rob you of the normal roles you've always played in all your relationships.

>> **Understand that depression is perfectly normal** when you first hear that you have PD; however, don't let depression continue for so long untreated that it actually escalates the progression of your PD and your need for hands-on care. Seek out a support group and be open to the support and care you can receive from others.

Embrace coping strategies second

For each of you — the PWP and their care partner — the second task involves realizing (and accepting) that all the medicines and physician advice in the world can't help unless the PWP follows treatment recommendations, including changes in lifestyle. Self-management (the ability to take responsibility through changes in attitude and behavior) is the key to living with chronic illness of any type — and vital for living with PD. If you're the partner, consider what changes you can make in your own routines and habits that support and encourage the PWP to fight this disease.

The following tips may help both of you cope in these early stages:

>> **Find out everything you can** — from reliable and respected sources — about PD. (See Appendix B for many of the best resources.)

>> **Ask questions.** Chapters 4 and 5 deal specifically with the diagnosis and the steps immediately following it.

>> **Take an active role** in partnering with the PWP and medical professionals to consider treatment options and manage symptoms (See Chapter 6 for teaming up with the pros and Chapters 9, 10, and 11 for more about treatment options.)

>> **Maintain emotional balance** while you each cope with your fears and anxieties about the meaning of this diagnosis for you and other people close to the PWP. (Chapter 7 offers ideas on dealing with other people. Chapters 15 and 19 address relationship questions you may be asking.)

>> **Remind each other** of times when the PWP faced a difficult situation and didn't just cope but triumphed in handling it.

>> **Don't wait to get help for obvious anxiety and depression,** whether you're the PWP or the care partner. (Chapter 13 covers this piece of PD in more detail.)

2

Making PD Part — But Not All — of Your Life

Find the best professionals to give you an accurate diagnosis.

Educate yourself about living with PD.

Assemble a great healthcare team for the PD long haul.

Decide the best way and time to tell others about your diagnosis.

Deal with a diagnosis of young onset PD or even Lewy body disease.

Chapter **4**

Getting an Accurate Diagnosis

O kay, perhaps you've checked out Chapters 2 and 3 to see the causes and risk factors of Parkinson's disease (PD), as well as its signs and symptoms. And maybe the more you read, the more you worry that you (or someone you care for) may actually have it. Before you freak out, get to a doctor and find out for sure. Your imagination about PD and its consequences is far worse than living with it. In reality, many people who have PD live relatively normal and fully active lives for many years after diagnosis. It's your call, but you can set this book aside right now and go bury your head in the sand, or you can take a measured, proactive approach to checking out those symptoms.

Ah, you're still here — great! (Okay, so the book's a little sandy. No problem.) First, get an accurate idea of your symptoms, starting with a comprehensive list of your current symptoms and a thorough medical history. Take that information with you on a visit to your primary care physician (PCP), who may recommend that you see a specialist. No doubt, the doctors will prod and test you, but you can finally have a diagnosis. Last step? You want to get that diagnosis confirmed by a neurologist or a doctor who specializes in diagnosing and treating movement disorders (of which PD is one).

Bringing Up the Subject with Your Doctor

This isn't going to be the usual appointment with your doctor. You're not going for an annual check-up or some routine test. You're making this appointment because you have symptoms that you can't explain and that don't seem to be going away. And you made this appointment because you're concerned something is seriously wrong. When you need an appointment for these reasons, carefully plan it all along the way, from scheduling the appointment, to gathering information, to preparing questions you want to ask. Do all of this preparation before the appointment.

Scheduling an appointment

When you call your doctor's office to schedule the appointment, ask to speak to the doctor's nurse or assistant. Then follow these steps:

1. **Tell the nurse or assistant why you're scheduling the appointment.**

   Yes, go ahead and say it: "I'm concerned that I may have Parkinson's disease."

2. **Add that you want an appointment when the doctor will have sufficient time to discuss your symptoms and concerns.**

   You especially want plenty of time to talk with your doctor if your suspicions are correct.

3. **Ask the nurse or assistant what information you should bring with you.**

   They may ask you to bring your most recent medical records and imaging data, so ask any other doctors you have to send them to the PCP.

4. **Make the appointment, usually through the office manager or receptionist.**

   When you do, only you can weigh accepting the possible wait (perhaps several weeks until the doctor has the extra time you need) against taking the earliest available appointment.

TIP

You may opt for the earliest available appointment with your PCP, instead of waiting for an extended appointment. If so, consider also booking a later appointment in case you want to follow up in more detail with the doctor. In either case, ask to be on the cancellation call list; in the event of a cancellation, you can then get to see the doctor sooner than your scheduled appointment.

Preparing for your initial exam

Before seeing your PCP, plan to take the steps discussed in the following sections to make that first meeting as productive as possible.

Gathering your medical records

Be sure that your PCP has copies of all your medical records. For example, if you see a cardiologist, your PCP needs copies of any lab work or stress test results, as well as that doctor's notes on observations and treatment. Today, many medical systems use an online charting system that makes it easy for you to collect all of your data in one place. If the PCP whom you're seeing doesn't have access to the system that holds your records, then go ahead and print out, save as a PDF, or take a screenshot of key information — lab results, test results, or current prescription medications. Then send them electronically or via fax.

TIP

If you're not part of an online system, then as soon as you schedule the appointment with your PCP, ask the office staff of any specialist you're seeing to send copies of recent lab results to your PCP's office. Preparing and transferring such information can take time. So, if time is short, call the clinic where you had the tests done or the doctor who ordered the tests, and ask them for a copy of the results. You can pick up these reports and take them with you to your appointment.

Prioritizing your symptoms

Next, make a list of your symptoms and prioritize them. For example, maybe the following is your list of symptoms:

>> Anxious and not my usual upbeat self

>> Shaky — especially in my right hand

>> Unusually fatigued — no get-up-and-go

>> Not sleeping well

If you suspect PD because you've noticed a slight tremor, you may want to move the second bullet (shaky) to the top of your list.

REMEMBER

Keep in mind that the doctor's staff may interview you first. When the nurse asks you why you came in, the first words out of your mouth get their attention. So, if you say, "I haven't been sleeping that well," rather than "Over the last few weeks, I've noticed a slight shakiness in my right hand," the nurse writes that your primary issue is *sleep disturbance*. And that statement can take matters in a whole different direction, wasting precious time.

Your doctor refers to the first symptom as your *chief complaint*. When they follow up on your answer with some form of "What makes you suspect Parkinson's?" then you can offer the rest of the symptoms on your list.

TIP

For heaven's sake, if you suspect PD, don't be afraid to introduce it into the conversation right away. Life — and doctor's appointments — are too short to beat around the bush!

Compiling your medical history

Writing down your personal medical history helps you prepare for the many questions along the way to your diagnosis. Preparing your history in advance also gives you time to think carefully about the specifics, instead of trying to remember details on the spot.

If you've seen a doctor recently, you know that the questions are usually the same — no matter how many times you give the information. First, one or two members of the staff gather your information, and then the nurse or physician assistant (PA) may ask the same questions. But, with a trusty printout of your history, you can provide a clean copy for their file and still have a copy in-hand (you made two copies, right?) to prompt you on dates and details. This step saves everyone precious time during the appointment and spares you the frustration of recalling every detail for every question.

TIP

Don't let multiple quizzing sessions frustrate you. Medical professionals have a method to the madness of having three different people asking you the same question — usually some form of "Why have you come to see the doctor?" They know that the second (or third) time patients answer that question, they may provide additional information without even realizing it.

Many doctors send a questionnaire to help patients gather essential information about themselves and their medical histories. Even if you don't receive such a document, be prepared for your doctor's questions by writing down the following information and taking it with you to your initial exam:

» Patient's legal (full) name (including maiden name, if applicable)

» Date and place of birth

» Parents' names, as well as parents' dates and causes of death

» Family history of PD or other movement disorder such as essential tremor (ET), as well as family history of dementia (Alzheimer's, for example)

» Medications, dosing routine, and purpose (listed separately), including

- *Current prescribed (Rx) medications:* For example, dyazide, 10 mg 1 x day for hypertension

- *Current over-the-counter (OTC) medications:* Those you take regularly, including vitamins, supplements, and such (for example, calcium + Vitamin D, 600 mg 2 x day)

- *Any historical medications (Rx or OTC):* Anything you've taken over the past year but don't currently take

» Known allergies or adverse reactions to medications or common medical equipment (for example, latex gloves)

» Other physicians whom you see regularly (for example, an allergist or a cardiologist) — name, address, and telephone number

» Current health problems and approximate dates of onset

» Dates and circumstances of past illnesses or medical events (for example, when you fractured a rib, had a heart attack, or were in an accident)

» Dates and reasons for hospitalizations and surgeries

» Recent changes in physical, mental, or emotional health

» Current situations that may contribute to health changes (consider family, work, and other factors)

Stepping through your initial exam

TIP

Okay, you have everything in order (if not, flip back to the section "Preparing for your initial exam," earlier in this chapter), and today's the appointment. Take someone with you. If you think you have PD (and it turns out that your doctor agrees), you need that extra set of ears to hear what you're bound to miss after you hear that you may have a chronic and progressive condition. Most likely, a friend or care partner can provide you support if the diagnosis turns out to be PD. This person should take notes and listen during the appointment, and then help you digest and decipher that discussion after the appointment. Alternatively, in this day of technological advances, you may want to take out your trusty cellphone and ask whether the doctor minds if you record the appointment and discussion.

You already know much of what happens at the doctor's office: the wait in the waiting room (complete with dog-eared selections of last year's magazines); the weigh-in, blood pressure reading, and updating of your medical history, conducted by the nurse or PA; the wait for your doctor (this time, in the exam room). Use your wait time to go over the information and questions you've prepared. The doctor will ask why you think you have PD, and you need to be prepared to offer specifics (your symptoms, when and how often they occur, when they began, what seems to relieve them, and so on). If you've made a list, you're ready and can just review it.

REMEMBER

The doctor may be giving you extra time for your appointment, but that's not the same as endless time. You need to use the time you have wisely by coming to the appointment as well prepared as possible. Your goal is to leave with either a clear diagnosis of something that is not PD, or barring that, a referral for further testing and discussion with a specialist. For more tips on knowing what to expect from a diagnostic appointment and getting the most from that appointment, see the section "Working with Your PD Doctor to Determine Whether This Is PD," later in this chapter.

Leaving with the answers you need

You probably arrive at your initial appointment with a gazillion questions, and you probably can't think of a single one while you're actually in the exam room. So, be prepared. Create a list of questions in advance and use that list. You may even want to hand a copy to your doctor.

TIP

If you bring another person with you to listen and take notes, they may want to speak up and ask questions also. You can use the questions in the following sections as a guide during the appointment. But feel free to add your own.

A pretty clear diagnosis

Although your PCP may feel confident in the diagnosis, they most likely deliver this news as *possibly* or *likely* Parkinson's. The PCP may then recommend that you see a *neurologist* (a specialist in disorders of the central nervous system) or a movement disorders specialist.

Your PCP may talk in lingo that you don't know (*parkinsonism, bradykinesia, postural instability,* and such). Don't be afraid to get a clear, layperson's explanation by asking the following questions:

» What's the diagnosis — in plain English?

» What's the prognosis (how quickly will the condition progress)?

» How do you plan to confirm the diagnosis?

» Does this diagnosis require me to see a specialist?

>> Can you recommend a specialist and help set an appointment for me?

>> In the meantime, what should I do?

Tests

Even if your doctor feels confident in the diagnosis, they may want to rule out other possibilities. For example, maybe some of the medications you've been taking can produce a slight shaking (tremor) in your hand. Or maybe your PCP and you feel that your primary symptom seems to be depression and apathy; the doctor may want to refer you to a psychologist for evaluation. If you receive a referral or recommendations for other tests, ask the following questions:

>> What are the tests and why are you ordering them?

>> What's the procedure for each test?

>> How quickly will you have the results?

>> What are the next steps after you have the test results?

Treatment

Especially if you live in a small community or rural area, your PCP may be the only name in town for treating a wide variety of complex conditions. Even if you live in a larger community that has several specialists, including neurologists, your doctor may know that your economic situation and/or lack of adequate insurance could keep you from seeking these services. In any case, if your PCP doesn't recommend seeking a specialist as a next step but does recommend a plan of treatment, or if they recommend a specialist but offer you the alternative of a plan of treatment with them, ask the following questions:

>> What treatment do you propose, and why are you choosing this option?

>> What are the risks or possible down sides of taking the prescribed medicines or following the recommended therapies?

>> What's the cost, and will my insurance cover the therapies or medication?

>> What are the potential benefits of the treatment?

>> How quickly will the treatment work?

>> How will you monitor and follow up on the treatment plan?

>> What are the alternatives to this treatment plan?

Connecting with a Neurologist or Movement Disorders Specialist

The initial suspicions of you and your PCP likely lead you to an appointment with a neurologist or movement disorders specialist who can administer further tests to confirm the diagnosis. This is the doctor who will guide you through the process of potentially confirming a diagnosis and establishing a plan for treating and living with PD; we'll call this your PD doctor. (If your PCP has already diagnosed PD, then this specialist can validate that and help manage your care.) The following sections suggest how to find a specialist in your area and how to know whether you'll make a good team.

Locating an experienced and qualified specialist

TIP

If possible, look for a PD doctor who specializes in movement disorders (such as Parkinson's). A neurologist with this specialty is called a *movement disorders specialist* and has done additional fellowship training in movement disorders. If you're very fortunate, you live in or near a community that has a Parkinson's Foundation Center of Excellence. To find out, visit the website at www.parkinson. org, hover over the Expert Care link, click the Global Care Network link from the drop-down that appears, and then click the Centers of Excellence Listing link on the resulting page. These centers' programs — often in a medical university or institution — take part in clinical research specifically for the benefit of PD patients.

The following sections suggest resources that you can use to find a doctor specially qualified to help you deal with your PD — now and down the road.

Surfing the web

The Internet can offer you a huge help in locating a doctor. Several sites locate physicians by specialty, as well as by location, and the sites provide important information about a doctor's training, expertise, possible ethical or treatment violations, and so on. Try an online search with the phrase "neurologists finding" or "movement disorders specialist finding."

You can also get information by checking with the local or regional chapter of a national PD organization. (See the following section, as well as Appendix B, for the national organizations' info.) Ask whether your area has a local PD support group. If it does, ask for the name and contact information of the group's facilitator.

When you call the facilitator, ask whether the group has compiled a list of specialists that members have recommended through personal experience.

Checking with the local chapter of PD groups

The following organizations have chapters and support groups in communities across the country. You can call them to get names of doctors who specialize in treating PD in your area:

>> **Parkinson's Foundation:** www.parkinson.org; 800-473-4636

>> **American Parkinson's Disease Association (APDA):** www.apdaparkinson. org; 800-223-2732

If you live in a small community, you may have to connect with the group in a larger community nearby (or even at the state level), but you can get invaluable information from these experienced groups while you look for a PD doctor who's right for you.

Asking your family doctor

Your PCP may be an internist or, if you live in a small community or rural area that has limited access to medical care, a general practitioner. For some women, an Obstetrician/Gynecologist (OB/GYN) is their PCP. Whatever your doctor's focus, they're probably aware of local leading doctors in various specialties.

Here's a key question to ask your PCP: Which specialist do you recommend for working in tandem with you (the PCP) and me to manage my overall health and PD? The answer to this question is important for many reasons, but mainly because you absolutely must consult with your PD doctor before any other doctor prescribes medications or treatment that may adversely affect your PD medication routine or worsen your symptoms.

When your town has no neurologists

Speaking of small communities, what are your options if the closest PD specialist is some distance away? First, consider that after you confirm the diagnosis and begin routine treatment, you don't have to see the specialist every week, or even every month. Second, assuming the PD doctor and your PCP can work together, you have the emergency back-up of your PCP if you need immediate attention. Third, consider the possibility of virtual medical appointments (telemedicine) when travel is not convenient.

WARNING

Don't let your PCP manage your PD just for the sake of convenience. At the very least, have your PD doctor reevaluate your treatment and status two to four times a year, depending on how much change you experience between visits. If you have questions between appointments, try calling or e-mailing your PD doctor's office. If you take a day every two to three months to see the specialist treating your PD in person or virtually, it's time well spent. You're worth every minute of it!

Evaluating your specialist

First things first. You can't expect a neurologist or movement disorders specialist to cure you: A cure for PD doesn't exist — yet. But you can and should expect a professional partnership. You and your PD doctor (as well as other team members that we introduce in Chapter 6) work together to manage your PD symptoms and maintain your physical, mental, and emotional health to the highest possible levels during the years ahead.

REMEMBER

You're looking for a specialist who seems curious about your Parkinson's, in particular:

>> How it's affecting you now

>> How you can manage those symptoms best

>> How to postpone the onset of new or worsening symptoms for as long as possible

Along with expertise, you're looking for a certain quality of empathy — a chemistry between the two of you. (See more discussion on this relationship in the following section.) You don't want a godlike figure who makes decisions for you rather than with you. After all, who has to live with your PD? Not the doctor.

Preparing for that first visit

Use the following checklist while you prepare for meeting the neurologist or movement disorders specialist:

>> **Ask for the first or last appointment of the day.** Having no one before or no one after your appointment should assure additional time with the specialist for you to ask questions.

>> **Make sure your PCP sends copies of your records to the PD specialist's office.** Assuming that your PCP who referred you to the specialist, you may think that the records are transferred automatically. Guess again. You need to stay on top of this transfer and follow up with both offices to make sure the transfer actually takes place.

>> **Take a copy of your personal medical history and the results of any recent lab work with you.** Bring them along, even if you believe that the offices have already successfully exchanged records. (Refer to the section "Preparing for your initial exam," earlier in this chapter, for more advice about your medical history.)

>> **Be sure to update your medical history to include your medications.** Include the strength and dosage routine for your meds (or pack up and take along the actual meds in a plastic bag — seriously!). Also, list any vitamins, supplements, or other OTC meds you take on a regular basis.

>> **Call the office to confirm the appointment and the receipt of your records.** Make this call a few days prior to the appointment. If the office hasn't received your records, follow up with your PCP. You may need to pick up copies of the records and take them with you to the appointment.

>> **Arrive half an hour before your scheduled appointment.** With a little extra time beforehand, you can complete their paperwork without cutting into your time with the doctor. Better yet, if possible, complete the paperwork online, but still arrive early to give yourself time to review your questions for the doctor.

Interviewing the good doctor

Everyone wants the best PD doctor out there. But, because of PD's chronic and progressive nature, you also need a specialist who's a good fit for you and your care partner. Start with the basic nuts and bolts. The following list contains the most essential factors you need to consider:

TIP

>> **How special a specialist:** Of course, the PD specialist has a medical degree, but are they *board-certified* (have they completed and passed nationally recognized exams to test expertise)? If they also have special training in movement disorders (a list that includes PD), count yourself ahead of the game.

>> **Professional groups:** What professional organizations and societies does the doctor belong to? You can often find this kind of information online if you do a search for the doctor by name.

>> **The doctor's PWP roster:** How many people with Parkinson's (PWP) are currently under their care?

>> **Familiarity with treating PD:** How long has the doctor been treating PWP? (If the good doctor is a good older doctor, how long do they plan to continue their practice?) If the doctor is relatively young, check their background and experience. Has this person worked with more experienced PD specialists?

>> **Professional partners:** Who are the partners in this specialist's practice, and what are the partners' backgrounds? If the specialist doesn't have partners, does another practice see patients when the doctor is unavailable?

>> **Office hours:** What days and hours does the practice see patients? (If the doctor is well known and sought after, but has really limited office hours, that situation may send up a red flag about your ability to get appointments when you need them.)

>> **Relative convenience:** Are the office hours and location convenient for you? If not, is that a deal breaker for you? Keep in mind that in the early stages of your PD (see Chapter 3) you probably see your PD doctor infrequently, perhaps every six to eight weeks or more.

WARNING

If the distance and schedule still seem inconvenient, you can look elsewhere, but please try not to sacrifice experience and skill for convenience.

>> **Running labs:** If the doctor orders lab work, does the office provide the service? If not, is the office part of a hospital-physician complex where they can easily get labs done? If the answer is "No" to both questions, you probably need to go to your area hospital or walk-in clinic for the lab work.

>> **Price:** What's the cost of an office visit?

>> **Insurance compatibility:** Does the practice accept your insurance? If you're on Medicare, does the practice *accept assignment* (charge only what Medicare assigns as the cost)? See Chapter 20 for more help on those sticky insurance questions.

>> **Telemedicine:** If you need to consult with the doctor by phone, email, or online, does the practice charge you for it?

You can gather much of this information either online or by asking the person you speak to when scheduling the appointment.

Reviewing your first impressions

After getting the details on the doc (see the preceding section), the PD specialist passes your basic tests. Now for the tough part: How well will the two of you work together? First impressions can say a great deal, so pay attention to details like the following:

>> **Does the doctor seem rushed or distracted** when meeting you?

>> **Does the specialist listen and ask questions** that draw out additional information, or do they cut you off and make pronouncements rather than recommendations?

>> **How does the practice approach treatment of PD?** Medication right away? Medication only after symptoms start to interfere with life routines? Do they have a multidisciplinary approach? Do they offer the opportunity to participate in clinical trials? What about the use of new or proven surgical procedures?

The right answer, of course, includes a reminder that all patients progress differently and under varying circumstances, so the treatment regimen varies person to person.

>> **How does the doctor feel about partnering** with the patient and care partner? (Eventually, your care partner becomes your advocate and spokesperson.)

>> **Do you have chemistry?** (We're not talking magic here, just good vibes.) Do you feel an intangible connection — where you can rely on this doctor's partnership to explore ways to manage symptoms and maintain functionality as long as possible?

Moving forward if it's a good fit

Finally, if this doctor seems a good fit (see the preceding sections), you have just a few more questions to ask:

>> **Appointment prep:** How does the practice prefer that you prepare for an appointment? For example, does the doctor want you to e-mail questions or concerns in advance, or can you bring written questions to the appointment? Can you record the conversation you have with the specialist at your appointment so that you can listen to it again later?

>> **Communication:** How does the doctor prefer communicating with you between appointments: by phone or e-mail; through their nurse or physician assistant; or through a patient portal online? (If you have to contact the nurse or physician assistant, be sure you meet this person and get direct contact information.)

>> **Hospital affiliation:** What hospital does the doctor use for treating patients?

And what if, after all of this, the doctor just doesn't offer a good fit? Of course, you can move on and start the whole process with another doctor. On the other hand, if all your research tells you that this doctor is the best in your area, perhaps you should give the relationship a chance. After all, the two of you are relative strangers. How well did you click with other professionals in your life on first meeting?

REMEMBER

Keep in mind that the relationship you have with your specialist is first and foremost professional; you rely on this expert to plot the course you navigate through the challenges of PD. This doctor may not necessarily want to see pictures of your first grandchild, but if the treatment plan that they put together clearly focuses on your individual journey through PD and helps you enjoy that grandchild for years to come, do you really need anything more?

Working with Your PD Doctor to Determine Whether You Have PD

PD specialists use a variety of methods to make a definitive diagnosis of PD:

» The physical examination

» An assessment of your function through mental and performance testing

» Sophisticated imaging equipment that permits a look inside your brain

Despite all these methods, your doctor may still need to rule out other explanations for your symptoms before they're prepared to state, without question, that you have PD.

The following sections take you through the usual steps of that first visit, tools for confirming PD or scoring the stage and severity, and ways to evaluate signs and symptoms to exclude other conditions.

Navigating the clinical exam

No single diagnostic test (such as the ones that doctors have for measuring blood pressure or cholesterol levels) can establish a diagnosis of Parkinson's disease. Such diagnosis relies to a large degree on your PD doctor's skilled observation and experience in diagnosing and treating PWP. Your initial appointment probably includes the three levels of examination discussed in the following sections.

History taking

The first level of examination involves a discussion about your complete medical history. You can provide a printed copy (see the section "Compiling your medical history," earlier in this chapter, for help with this step), but expect to hear some questions two or three times in this first appointment. Be a *patient* patient (pun intended). A good PD doctor asks these questions not only to review your symptoms, but also to rule out less-typical types of parkinsonism or other neurological conditions, which sometimes entail radically different management. (See the section "Parkinsonism, But Not PD," later in this chapter.)

Physical exam

After recording your medical history, the doctor performs a physical examination that may include such standards as

>> Measuring your blood pressure (while you're lying down and then again standing up)

>> Checking your pulses, heartbeat, lungs, and abdomen

The doctor makes such routine observations to confirm that problems in other parts of your body aren't causing your symptoms.

Neurological exam

The final level is the neurological examination, which is largely a process of observation. The doctor tests your strength, coordination, and balance while observing you walk, stand, sit, turn, extend your arms and hands, and so on.

This exam may also include any of the following tasks:

>> Opening and closing your fists or tapping your fingers several times

>> Touching the doctor's finger and then your nose with your index finger (It looks silly but can give the doctor valuable information related to hand/eye coordination)

>> Recovering your balance after the doctor pulls you gently from behind your shoulders as you stand with your eyes open or closed

>> Answering several simple questions from the doctor to test your attention and memory

>> Drawing a figure on a piece of paper and then duplicating it

Don't be surprised by the apparent simplicity of these questions and tests; they're all part of a standardized exam designed to rule out other possibilities (like some form of dementia or possibly the aftereffects of a small undiagnosed stroke)!

Establishing the severity and staging the progression of your PD

After the PD doctor has completed the initial interview, the physical exam, and neurological observations, they (or an assistant) may use a variety of tools for establishing your PD's progression through the various stages or levels. (See Chapter 3 for more about these stages.) The rating scales in the following section help the doctor set a benchmark for staging your PD at this time. Neuroimaging tools can also help track progression and rule out other possibilities for symptoms you may experience.

REMEMBER

You doctor can use rating scales and neuroimaging tests to assist in establishing the progression of your PD. These tools can't confirm the diagnosis. (See the section "Working with Your PD Doctor to Determine Whether You Have PD," earlier in this chapter, for how a doctor reaches a diagnosis.)

Rating scales

In any major disorder like PD, doctors may use standardized rating scales to measure symptoms and stage the disease. (For a refresher on *staging*, flip over to Chapter 3.) These instruments can help your doctor determine how advanced your symptoms are and how best to address them. The scales also form the basis for a more extensive medical history if you need to change doctors in the future. In addition, clinical researchers frequently use these scales to monitor the effects of new and experimental therapies on patients. (See Chapter 14, where we discuss clinical trials more completely.) Here are the scales that doctors commonly use to evaluate PWP:

>> **Hoehn and Yahr rating scale:** This diagnostic tool stages the level of a person's PD by using broad measures of disability. This scale was originally devised by Drs. Margaret Hoehn and Melvin Yahr following a detailed study of the natural progression of untreated PD in the late 1960s. They observed five general stages in PD, ranging from Stage 1 (unilateral disease, limited to one side of the body) to Stage 5 (wheelchair bound or bedridden unless aided). However, as we mention often in this book, PD doesn't progress in neat little predictable stages and proper treatment, either pharmacological or surgical (later on), can greatly reduce for many years the disability associated with PD.

>> **Movement Disorder Society Unified Parkinson Disease Rating Scale (MDS-UPDRS):** This more complex, more informative scale usually accompanies and complements the Hoehn and Yahr scale. It consists of a painless interview and a focused neurological exam, with a score for each of the 50 items from 0 (normal) to 4 (severe). Therefore, the higher the MDS-UPDRS score, the greater the disability from PD.

The MDS-UPDRS is a revision of the original Unified Parkinson Disease Rating Scale (UPDRS), created in the 1980s. The scale can be used in the clinic and for research. According to the National Institutes of Health, the updated MDS-UPDRS specifically

- *Covers a greater number of PD manifestations,* including nonmotor symptoms (NMS)

- *Better discriminates slight/mild manifestations of PD* when compared with the original UPDRS

- *Resolves ambiguities and gives clear instructions* for both raters and patients

- *Assesses all items in a uniform way*

>> **Schwab and England Activities of Daily Living:** This tool uses a percentage rating to quantify a person's ability to perform the normal routine activities of daily living. Patients usually rate themselves with the help of set definitions presented by their doctors.

For example, people who consider themselves to be completely independent and functional qualify for a 100-percent rating. They can perform all activities without difficulty. In contrast, a person who takes three to four times longer than the normal time to perform a task (such as dressing) has a 70-percent independence rating. And a person who can manage only a few chores from time to time (and always with great effort) has a 30-percent rating.

>> **Parkinson's Disease Questionnaire (PDQ-39):** This tool is a 39-item questionnaire that evaluates the impact of PD on quality of life. Similar to the Schwab and England tool and some portions of the MDS-UPDRS, patients usually rate themselves with the help of set definitions presented by their examiners.

Neuroimaging

A doctor can usually diagnose a new case of PD through a neurological exam and the proper administration of the MDS-UPDRS (see the preceding section). However, neuroimaging techniques now permit PD specialists to determine whether there is radiographic evidence of dopamine deficiency. Such tests can be very helpful to distinguish between Parkinson's disease and essential tremor (ET), or between drug-induced parkinsonism and a neurodegenerative parkinsonian disorder.

Two advanced imaging techniques — positron-emission tomography (PET) and single photon emission computed tomography (SPECT), can confirm the diagnosis of PD and distinguish PD from other Parkinson-like disorders (See the section "Parkinsonism, But Not PD," later in this chapter, for more discussion of other disorders.) Both scans use low levels of radioactive materials and pose very little, if any, risk for the patient.

TIP

The DaTscan (SPECT) is most frequently used and (most importantly) is FDA approved, which makes it always covered by insurance when properly indicated. Most hospitals nowadays have the equipment and the expert staff needed to perform and interpret a DaTscan.

Ruling out the red herrings: What else can it be?

What else looks like PD? That answer may depend on your *presenting symptoms* (the information you tell the doctor) or on other signs that the doctor gathers through interviewing and examining you.

Here are a couple of examples of your doctor and you sleuthing the cause of symptoms:

REMEMBER

>> Even if you first saw a PD specialist because of a hand tremor, that symptom — by itself — is not enough to make the diagnosis of PD. Determining whether the tremor happens in one hand or both, as well as whether the tremor stops after you engage the hand in activity (or continues regardless of whether you're using it) is important. But most importantly, a diagnosis of PD also needs the simultaneous presence of bradykinesia and/or rigidity (symptoms described in Chapter 3).

Not every tremor means Parkinson's disease.

>> If you don't present with any of the *TRAP* symptoms (check out Chapter 3 for a quick review of these) but you talk about a loss of energy, the doctor may want to explore that symptom more. After further questioning, your doctor may see that depression plays a role in your loss of energy. Now, the doctor and you need to determine whether the depression is associated with PD or is related to some other life-changing event, such as the death of a loved one or the loss of a job.

Alternatively, the doctor may test your vitamin B12, folate, or testosterone levels (if you're male), all factors that may lead to fatigue if deficient in your body.

WARNING

Don't try to second-guess your symptoms. Is it PD? Maybe. Is it something else — something easier to treat and cure? Possibly. Either way, you need to know. Why postpone treating a curable condition simply because you think it may be more serious? And if it does turn out to be PD, then you want to get a jump on managing symptoms as early as possible — when you have the greatest opportunity to maintain independence and flexibility.

Parkinsonism, But Not PD

If it walks like a duck and quacks like a duck, it's a duck, right? So if it looks like PD and acts likes PD, then it's PD, right? Not always.

The same symptoms that indicate PD can also indicate other conditions. The generic term *parkinsonism* refers to slowness and mobility problems that look like PD. Parkinsonism is a feature in several conditions that have different (and perhaps known) causes, but those conditions don't progress in the same way that PD does. As a result, years may go by before you can clearly see the differences between PD and the other disorder; at that point, your doctor may reverse the PD diagnosis to atypical parkinsonism and revise your treatment plan to address what they believe is the real problem.

REMEMBER

You may get your first indicator that parkinsonism isn't actually PD when you start taking antiparkinsonian medications (such as levodopa). As a rule, PD is expected to promptly respond to levodopa, which improves many of your PD symptoms in a consistent way, at least for a while. But, in atypical parkinsonism, you often see erratic improvement or no improvement at all from the beginning. In fact, your PD doctor always closely monitors your response to treatment in order to rule out the possibility that your condition is a disorder other than PD.

Two categories of non-PD disorders manifesting with parkinsonism are

>> **Atypical parkinsonism:** This group of neurodegenerative disorders has parkinsonian features, such as *bradykinesia* (slowness), *rigidity* (stiffness), *gait disturbances* (balance), and less frequently, *tremor* (shaking). See Chapter 3 for more about these PD symptoms. However, these features are also associated with other complex neurological symptoms that reflect problems in brain areas other than the *dopaminergic system* (the network of neurons able to make and release the neurotransmitter dopamine). These conditions progress more rapidly than PD and don't respond as well (or at all) to antiparkinsonian medications.

The most common atypical parkinsonism disorders are *multiple system atrophy* (MSA), characterized by early onset of blood pressure problems; *progressive supranuclear palsy* (PSP), characterized by early onset of balance problems and falls; and *cortico-basal degeneration* (CBD), characterized by severe muscle stiffness and cognitive abnormalities. Last but not least, what looks like PD could in fact be Lewy body dementia (LBD), characterized by early onset of cognitive decline.

>> **Secondary parkinsonism:** The symptoms of these disorders relate to well-defined lesions in the brain from strokes, tumors, infections, traumas, or certain drugs. Like atypical parkinsonism, these syndromes usually respond

less to levodopa. However, if you can control the primary cause of parkinsonism, these symptoms tend to be less progressive and, in fact, if caused by reaction to a medication (such as an antipsychotic), may even resolve once the medication is stopped.

In addition to atypical parkinsonism and secondary parkinsonism, *essential tremor* (ET) is another frequent source of possible confusion. ET, the most common movement disorder (as much as 10 times more common than PD), has as its only symptom a tremor that affects the hands (usually both of them and only while they're moving or holding a posture) but may also affect the head or voice. ET can run in families and is usually annoying but less commonly disabling. The much-admired actress, Katherine Hepburn, may have suffered from ET — not PD.

Getting a Second (or Even Third) Opinion

Whatever the diagnosis, if you have concerns, questions, or doubts, then you have every reason to get a second or even a third opinion. After all, you know your body and its symptoms better than anyone else. So if you live within a reasonable distance of a medical center that has a reputation for excellent care for and research into movement disorders and PD, see whether you can get an appointment and check out what those folks say. Even if you have to travel some distance, the information will be worth the trip.

You might also want to seek a second or third opinion so that you can find a PD doctor with whom you click. The doctor who delivered the initial diagnosis may be a fine doctor who has great credentials and experience; but maybe the two of you had no connection, and you don't anticipate a valuable partnership. If you're living with PD, you don't want to be switching from one doctor to another. So, find a doctor that you can build a real partnership with now — one who has a proactive and optimistic philosophy about meeting the challenges of living with PD.

WARNING

The danger lies in seeking one opinion after another just because you didn't like the first (or second or third) answer — even though, in your heart-of-hearts, you know it's true. That's called denial (not to be confused with *The Nile*, a beautiful river in Egypt). Because you may not want to face the future, you keep running after more opinions, hoping that someday, some doctor will say you don't have PD.

After a doctor has confirmed the diagnosis (and perhaps another doctor has reconfirmed it), you need to accept it and prepare yourself and your family for the journey. Your first step is to find a PD doctor that you and your PCP can partner with to maintain and manage your health for the long term. Chapters 5 and 6 help you out with your next steps.

IN THIS CHAPTER

» **Facing your fears about Parkinson's disease**

» **Establishing your long-term vision and short-term goals**

» **Gathering information about PD from trusted sources**

» **Caring for the future: Advice for your partner**

Chapter **5**

You've Been Diagnosed — Now What?

kay, it's official — you have Parkinson's disease (PD). In these first days following that blow, no doubt your emotions are rocketing. And like a pinball, they're bouncing moment to moment and hour to hour around those five stages of grief that Elisabeth Kubler–Ross introduced:

» Can't be (denial)

» Shouldn't be (anger)

» Don't let it be (bargaining)

» Why me? (depression)

» IS! (acceptance — or at least, realization)

A sixth stage to consider in facing a diagnosis of PD is hope. You can find some measure of control while you continue toward the future you had already planned — one that didn't include living with a chronic and progressive illness.

And that's the purpose of this chapter — to help you move beyond those first jumbled emotions of diagnosis toward a clearly focused, take-charge attitude of this disease. In this chapter, we first talk you through the emotional steps and then guide you toward healthy goals and plans for coming to grips with PD. We also address your care partner or partners, those people (even if they are mostly your medical team) who will walk that walk with you and offer support for these early months after the diagnosis.

TIP

The Parkinson's Foundation has developed a series of webinars for the PWP who is living alone. The series is available on YouTube at www.youtube.com/watch?v=F0N66n9Q73U, and includes a link to more information on the Parkinson.org website.

Sorting Out Your Emotions

Depending on your past awareness or experiences with PD, either you have some idea of how your life is going to change or you have no idea at all. In either case, your imagination can get carried away with all the what-ifs.

Stop! This is a new challenge, but it's not so different from other challenges that have taken your life in unexpected directions. Every day, people face unplanned events that change the path they thought they were on — job losses, break-ups in relationships, unplanned moves to different locations, the death of a loved one, hurricanes, and frogs falling from the sky. Life happens.

Take a breath. Any challenges that you faced (and survived) in the past (such as raising children, building your career, caring for aging parents, and so on) gave you key building blocks and tools to face this new challenge.

Now, give yourself time to

>> **Understand** that a PD diagnosis is not a death sentence. You have a life to live and choices to make about how you want to face each day, probably for years and even decades to come.

>> **Believe** that past experiences have given you the tools you need to cope with PD.

>> **Accept** the difference between what you can and can't control. Focus on what you can.

>> **Connect** with people who are positive and upbeat.

>> **Banish** negative self-talk ("I can't" or "I won't") and turn the negative to a positive ("I can" and "I will").

>> **Embrace** the joys in your life — your partner, children, and friends; your work or avocation; your love of music, art, and sports; and so on. Check out Part 4 for ideas.

>> **Help** yourself by helping other people — volunteer, get involved, make a difference.

>> **Recognize** the opportunities you have to educate others, advocate for change (and a cure, see Chapter 14), make new friends, and know your deeper self.

REMEMBER

You have two choices: Let PD define you or live life to the fullest in spite of PD.

Dodging denial and meeting your diagnosis head on

When you get the confirmed diagnosis, you and those most likely to be part of your care and support network need time to digest the news and react. And the first reaction may be denial. Your friends may become overprotective and treat you like you're gravely ill. Financial concerns may pop up; you may wonder about facing the costs and sacrifices. At times, your partner may feel cheated out of the life the two of you had planned and then angry at such a selfish thought when you're facing a debilitating illness. (For more help in dealing with such difficult feelings, see Chapter 22.)

WARNING

Neither you nor your partner may admit any of these feelings (such as anger) or reactions (such as denial) initially. Big mistake. Your fastest route to coping is to work through such feelings and reactions together by openly communicating your fears and concerns, and then working through possible solutions to each.

Denial can take two forms:

>> **Dismissal of symptoms:** First, many people who receive the diagnosis of PD — or any other serious illness — soon realize that they've been experiencing the early symptoms for some time. Perhaps you dismissed those early warning signs for weeks or even months because you were afraid or didn't want other people to know you had some troublesome symptoms.

>> **Refusal to believe:** The second form of denial comes after you receive the diagnosis. Now, you have the facts. You're human, and no doubt the actual news that you have PD has come as a real blow. Initially refusing to believe the diagnosis is your mind's way of giving you time to gather the necessary strength to go forward.

REMEMBER

Sustaining denial takes an enormous amount of energy — energy that you can better spend facing the actual challenge. Refusing to acknowledge the truth means you're forcing yourself to keep a secret from other people and yourself.

In spite of your denial, deep inside, you know this diagnosis is real. You may even be surprised to realize you have a slight feeling of relief because the enemy has a name, and now you can begin to fight it. You can't go back and not have PD. But you can decide how best to move forward.

Allowing yourself to get angry

Anger is an understandable reaction to news like this. The question is: Who's on the receiving end of that anger? The world, in general? Your friends and family, who've never taken care of themselves in the careful manner you've always cared for yourself and still seem to get a pass when it comes to any kind of serious health issue? Your significant other (who you fear — in your current, warped state of mind — may leave you)? God? How about yourself?

Go ahead — rant, rave, and howl at the moon. A little healthy anger is good for you, and certainly you deserve to indulge that anger — within reason. Try these tips for giving anger your best shot:

>> **Keep the focus on the true object of your anger — having PD.** You may not realize how easily your focus can broaden until suddenly everything and everyone makes you mad. You do not want to go down that road.

>> **Figure out ways to confront this enemy that's attacked your perfectly good life.** Think of it like taking that great new job offer after previously being passed over a promotion.

Frame your anger as a way to show PD who's boss. For example, you can say to your Parkinson's, "I'll show you that I can still lead my life in spite of the challenges you throw my way!"

>> **Set limits.** When you're overwhelmed by your fury at the unfairness of this diagnosis, set a timer for 10 minutes. When the bell dings, you're done fuming — at least, for today.

>> **Find the humor** — black though it may be — in this unexpected and unwanted situation, and defuse your anger with that humor.

TIP

Permit yourself some time to work your way through this news. (Some people can work through this diagnosis in a matter of days; others need a couple of weeks.) If the feelings continue longer than a couple of weeks, you need to get some help to resolve the anger. Anger (like denial and a bunch of other normal reactions to news of a chronic, progressive illness) is non-productive — unless it leads you to fight back. Throughout the course of your PD, the disease is going to make you upset and angry from time to time. We have all learned at some point that life is not fair. Instead of dwelling on anger or other non-productive feelings, transform that energy into determination to regain control and move forward.

Admitting you're scared

Chances are good that you still don't have a handle on the full impact of this diagnosis. Getting your head around the concept of a lifelong, progressive illness is a pretty tall order, especially in the beginning. It's enough to scare the bejee-bers out of anyone! You have so many questions and fears. How do you deal with them?

REMEMBER

There's no shame in admitting you're scared. The title song from the musical *Cabaret* says, "Start by admitting from cradle to grave, it isn't that long a stay." In other words, you get what you get in life — no promises and no guarantees. You can find the unknown intriguing, exhilarating, or frightening. And certainly, when that unknown is PD, you may find yourself even feeding any fear through your responses to the diagnosis.

Instead of further terrifying yourself by reading every case study or article that you can Google (or book that you can buy) about PD, place limits on how much information you need and can handle — especially at the beginning. Instead of smiling politely while some well-meaning clerk or neighbor relates a horror story about a fifth-cousin-twice-removed who had PD back in the Dark Ages, give thanks for the concern but walk away. Instead of allowing other people to educate you based on hearsay, observations from afar, and an article they read about actor Alan Alda or musician Neil Diamond, educate yourself.

By using the reputable and frequently updated resources listed in Appendix B, you can gather the information you need to become the true expert on what is and isn't possible with PD. Then, when people start telling you about your condition and how to manage your life, quietly but firmly correct them. Trust us; nothing silences a know-it-all like someone who really does know. And nothing helps you get a handle on that gut-wrenching fear like educating yourself on the realities, possibilities, and opportunities for expanding your life — of living with PD.

Getting to acceptance

No one is denying that you need to work through a whole range of emotions, but you can't stay locked in those emotional prisons. When you move through them, you free yourself to fully live your days.

You have a chronic and progressive illness, but you likely

>> Have years ahead of you

>> Are still productive

>> Have time to pursue dreams and goals

>> Can live life on your terms if you accommodate PD as part of that life, not all of it

Taking charge of your life with PD

How do you go about living your best life going forward? Start with these key steps:

>> **Get the best treatment that you can after you have the PD diagnosis.** Part 3 of this book talks all about treatment options, some of which you may find surprisingly easy to incorporate into your life.

>> **Deal with the emotional roller coaster of living with a chronic progressive illness.** Chapters 13 and 22 offer tips on facing the depression, anxiety, and other difficult feelings that come as part and parcel of living with any chronic progressive condition.

>> **Manage your inevitable lifestyle changes and social adjustments with family and friends.** Check out Chapter 7 for tips on who, how, and when to tell about your PD; then look at Chapter 15 for more in-depth advice on maintaining key relationships.

>> **Protect your unique sense of self-worth and identity.** Well, we could just remind you to read this whole book because our key message in every chapter is that you can live with this condition. In fact, you can have a full and satisfying life — it just won't be the life you thought you were going to have. (But couldn't that be true for most people?)

Sometimes, acceptance comes most easily when you turn your attention to the people who love you and have heard your diagnosis. They're wrestling with high anxiety, too. Of course, their first concern is for you, but a part of that concern is PD's effect on their relationship with you. How will their lives change with yours? When you acknowledge their fears (as well as your own) and explore those fears with them, you create an environment of "we're in this thing together," which goes a long way toward sustaining everyone when times get tough. (Look for tips on ways you can best communicate with other people in Chapters 7 and 15.)

Mentoring via your PD

By taking the lead in figuring out how to live with PD, in many ways, you become a mentor. You're the person others look to and trust to show the best way to face this life-changing situation. For many of us, actor Christopher Reeve and his wife, Dana, were the poster couple for finding grace in the face of unspeakable adversity. Think about it: If you built your career playing Superman and ended up unable to move (much less leap over tall buildings), wouldn't you be tempted to feel sorry for yourself? Instead, Christopher Reeve found the will and the courage to use his adversity to inspire and motivate people and to make a real difference in the world.

No one expects you to become a national icon now that you have PD. But you can become that mentor for people closest to you. Through your attitude and approach, you can set the tone for the way others interact with you and incorporate PD into the relationship.

Taking charge and moving forward

Prepare but don't project needs to be your mantra. You may be overwhelmed by the temptation to look ahead and worry about the future. Our advice: Fight that instinct! Given a diagnosis of a chronic and progressive disease that has no cure, a person's natural tendency is to try to foretell the future. Major mistake!

With PD, every patient's journey is unique, so projecting what may happen can only increase your anxiety. You and your care partner can go crazy, racing around and trying to cover all the possible challenges even before they develop.

Just realize that you have a disease that will require — like most health conditions — changes to your lifestyle. For example

>> **Emphasis on exercise, nutrition, and sleep:** Paying attention to and making good choices in these three lifestyle areas can help you keep your PD at bay; check out Chapter 9 for specifics about each area.

- *If exercise is not currently part of your routine, start dedicating at least 30 minutes a day to purposeful movement.* Doctors recognize exercise as the only known and accepted way to modify the natural progression of the disease; exercise slows down progression.

- *If your approach to diet and nutrition is haphazard, get organized.* Doctors and researchers continue to learn about the type of foods that may help your body fight PD better.

- *Last but not least, make sure to nurture good sleep habits.* Yes, we know that it's easier said than done, but those eight hours of night sleep become a dream (pun intended) after a certain age. Sleep can be your best friend, and PWP commonly experience fewer symptoms after a night of good sleep than after a night of tossing and turning until dawn.

>> **Adaptations to your environment:** What can you do if you can no longer manage the stairs in your current home, but the bedrooms (and the main bathroom) are all upstairs?

In Chapter 21, we explore many options for staying in your current residence in spite of obstacles such as the dreaded stairways. For example, you may have a room on the first floor that you can adapt as a bedroom; maybe you can convert a half-bath into a full bathroom (with the addition of a shower); or your stairway may be wide enough to accommodate an electric chair lift.

>> **Outlining emergency procedures:** While your ability to move decreases, how can you handle an emergency such as getting out of the house in the event of a fire?

Even if you didn't have PD, common sense should move every family to have an emergency plan in place. So sit down with the family and figure this one out — for you and everyone else in the household. You can even talk to people at your local fire and police department to get their suggestions for effective emergency procedures.

We guess that throughout your life (and certainly as an adult), you've planned for the possibility of unexpected changes or events. And even though those changes may come in a year or not at all, you still consider the options and prepare to act, just in case.

Taking Action

Think of PD as a 400-pound lineman constantly in your face — there when you wake up and when you go to sleep, getting in your way, blocking you when you try to work or play and when your friends come around. Sometimes, he's well-behaved, maybe even sitting on the sidelines for a while. But mostly, he's charging, blocking, and even tackling to keep you from doing what you want.

How do you get around this lineman? Well, sometimes you won't. But other times — most of the time — you can find new and innovative ways to live life on your terms. Managing a chronic illness means you need to give up control over some parts of your life and take control in new ways. Some of those new controls are

>> Educating yourself and your family about your PD

>> Developing a long-range strategy for managing the unpredictability of your PD

>> Turning negatives into positives through creative problem-solving to improve fine motor skills, try coloring in one of the many adult coloring books available these days. Not only will you strengthen your fine motor skills, but you'll also be making art (even if it is only coloring). This creates a sense of accomplishment and satisfaction—a win-win!

>> Being a real team player — with your healthcare team (see Chapter 6), your care partners, and other PWP

Arming yourself with good information

When you start gathering information, make sure you get that information from trustworthy and evidence-based sources. The Agency for Healthcare and Research (an agency within the Department of Health and Human Services) recommends the resources listed in Table 5-1.

TABLE 5-1

Recommended Informational Resources

Name	Online Address	Focus
Parkinson's Foundation	www.parkinson.org	Improving care, providing information, advancing research
The Michael J. Fox Foundation	www.michaeljfox.org	Advancing PD research and offering the latest information on dealing with PD
U.S. Department of Health and Human Services	http://hhs.gov	Offering links to programs for managing day-to-day health
Office of the National Coordinator for Health Information Technology	www.healthit.gov	Supporting the secure exchange of health information at the local, state, and national levels
MedlinePlus (sponsored by the NIH's National Library of Medicine)	http://medlineplus.gov/healthtopics.html	Amassing extensive information and other trusted resources for more than 650 diseases and conditions

For a complete list and contact information for PD-related nonprofit organizations like the Parkinson's Foundation and the Michael J. Fox Foundation, see Appendix B.

TECHNICAL STUFF

In addition, try checking with medical libraries in your area (but keep in mind that this information is for physicians, medical students, and researchers — the reading can get fairly technical).

WARNING

Ignore information from

>> Product advertisements that

- Make extraordinary claims, such as *scientific breakthrough* or *secret formula*.

- Claim to work just as well for a number of different conditions that don't have much in common (for example Parkinson's, multiple sclerosis, and epilepsy).

- Claim the product is available from only one source or for a limited time.

>> Well-meaning friends who have

- Heard of some therapy but can't recall the source.

- Had a relative who tried *x-treatment*. It worked for that person, so it's bound to work for you!

>> Well-meaning strangers who, in their zeal to show sympathy for your condition, rattle off several ideas about treatment.

Jotting down the questions you have

You were probably pretty numb when you sat in the doctor's office and received the news. (See Chapter 4, where we cover the initial doctor visits.) But now you realize you have all sorts of questions. Or perhaps you asked questions at the time and your doctor offered information, but you really didn't take it in.

Schedule a second appointment (if you haven't already) and let your doctor (or the nurse) know that you want to be able to ask questions and discuss issues that have come to mind since the diagnosis. At that appointment, bring your list of questions (as well as your care partner or a good friend, for that second set of ears), and be ready to record the discussion or take notes. The following questions give you a sampling of some concerns you may want to cover:

>> What's the technical name of my condition, and what does that mean in plain English?

>> What's the *prognosis* (my outlook for the future)?

>> How soon do I need to make a decision about treatment?

>> Will I need additional tests? If so, what kind and when?

>> What are my treatment options, and what are the pros and cons of those treatment options?

>> What changes will I need to make in my daily life?

>> What resources and organizations do you recommend for support and information?

>> What resources can your office provide (books, pamphlets, website addresses, and such) that I can review right away?

>> And the question that's probably uppermost in your mind: Am I going to die from this?

Establishing realistic and attainable goals

If PD is to be part of your life but not your entire life, then you need a game plan.

REMEMBER

Fact: If you don't have a plan for dealing with PD, then it will dominate every facet of your life. This section takes you through specific steps toward making and living that plan.

In the world of business, executive teams meet regularly. Their purpose? To plan for the future success of their business. Their process, which you can apply to building a successful life with PD, usually follows a three-step course:

1. **Establish a long-term vision.**

   Your vision is already established: to live a productive and satisfying life for as long as possible, in spite of PD.

2. **Set short-term goals toward achieving that vision.**

   Set aside sentimentality. As much as people wish otherwise, PD has no cure (as of this writing). So don't set the unrealistic and unattainable goal of being cured. But you can modify the progression — making it slower — so that you are in charge. While you consider your goals, remember that you want to keep your goals simple, practical, and specific.

3. **Identify and prioritize tasks necessary to attain those goals.**

   Executives call this step the *plan of action* (POA). Did you ever see a milk stool, the three-legged variety farmers sat on to milk cows? That three-legged approach is the way you need to think about your POA over the long term because living with PD is not only a physical challenge; it's also a mental and emotional one. And, just like the milk stool, if one leg is missing, the plan topples.

The following sections provide examples of three goals and their POAs that support a long-term vision for PD.

Goal 1: Maintain maximum physical function

PD has no magic pill. So, after confirming your diagnosis, your PD doctor will probably have a number of recommendations that may include management of symptoms with proven medications, physical and occupational therapy, and perhaps a program for diet and exercise.

Although medications and traditional medical interventions may help minimize your symptoms, you enhance your opportunity to achieve your long-term vision when you maintain your best physical condition. Developing (and sustaining) a regular exercise routine is what doctors refer to as *disease-modifying*, meaning that doing so can actually slow the progression of your PD. On the other hand, if you ignore the doctor's prescription for changes in your lifestyle (such as maintaining regular sleeping patterns, adjusting your diet and activity routines, or enacting a specific timetable for taking your medications), you compromise your overall vision. (See Chapter 9 for a full discussion of exercise and nutrition, and refer to Chapter 10 for more about the importance of sticking to your medication schedule.)

REMEMBER

No one has all possible PD symptoms. Although PD is a chronic, progressive condition, its path varies tremendously from one person to the next. You are unique — as a person and as a person with Parkinson's (PWP). You and your medical team need to keep that in mind while together you select those options (medications, therapies, and lifestyle changes) that have the greatest effect on maintaining your physical functioning for as long as possible.

Goal 2: Keep your mind sharp

You're certainly going to have a lot on your mind in the days and weeks to come while you and your medical team put together a viable plan for managing your PD symptoms. And you're going to hear a lot of new words — words that PD specialists, PWPs, and their care partners throw around as easily as *apple* or *orange*.

You can refuse to follow that technical PD jargon (and everything else about this intruder), or you can become an authority, someone who actively seeks out background information about PD, understands and uses the technical lingo, and keeps up with the research and new treatment options. Although you can become an authority on PD, that doesn't mean PD has to become your life's work. You have more important (and fun!) ways to spend your time.

Knowledge is power, and seeking out that knowledge exercises your brain. Get started using the resources listed in Appendix B. Getting a grip on PD (what it is and isn't, which we talk about in Chapter 1) is a good place to start — but don't stop there.

What are your interests, and how did you challenge your mind before you had PD? Are you a sports enthusiast who enjoys statistics and box scores? Do you like brainteasers, such as crossword puzzles, jigsaw puzzles, or word games? Do you love music, art, and theater? Then continue these pursuits, even if you need to adjust when and how!

TIP

Continuing to engage your mind in enjoyable ways has as much impact on successfully following your POA as pushing yourself physically. Don't turn your back on the intellectual life you enjoyed before PD.

Goal 3: Embrace the power of emotional and spiritual well-being

You go through a range of emotions post-diagnosis. But anxiety and depression can be symptoms of PD, as well as responses to its diagnosis. Your doctor needs to know if you're experiencing persistent (longer than a couple of weeks) sadness or apathy. (See Chapter 13 for a full discussion of the effects of anxiety, depression, and apathy in PD.)

Although your PD doctor or primary care physician (in consultation with each other) can prescribe medication and professional counseling to help you through these negative emotions, you can also be proactive by

>> Acknowledging that persistent negative feelings are abnormal

>> Finding a support group where you can discuss feelings with other people who

- Perhaps have similar emotions

- Recognize these emotions as part of the adaptive process in dealing with PD

>> Accepting the support of family and friends while you come to terms with PD and its effects on all your lives

In concert with your medical team, you can address physical, mental, and even emotional needs as part of your POA. However, one facet of your care plan that only you can develop is a plan for your spiritual health. This facet goes beyond faith and religious rituals, although those resources certainly help.

Spiritual health means going inside yourself and coming to terms with your illness day by day. For some PWP, coping comes through challenging activities: participating in sports, continuing to pursue a career, traveling, and so on. If these challenges help you find inner peace and comfort, great!

Other PWP may find spiritual healing in quieter pursuits: a walk in the park or along the beach; music; reading; meditation; or just sitting quietly in a secluded, deserted place. These activities also offer excellent opportunity for maintaining spiritual health.

WARNING

Take care that your solitude doesn't become a regular hiding place to wallow over your losses. Be aware that seclusion can sometimes lead to depression.

Living your life to the fullest

You can do a lot of things to fight PD and its effects. But thousands of PWP believe that a huge part of fighting PD is to approach it as only a piece of their lives. The point is this: You're still defined by those facets of your life that defined you before you were diagnosed — at least, for the most part. If you were a parent before, you're still a parent; and your child (or children) needs you as much as before. If you had a career that you enjoyed (even loved), don't allow PD to become your new, full-time occupation. If you enjoyed sports, music, and other leisure activities, get creative about finding new ways to enjoy those pastimes. In short, live!

REMEMBER

You face a challenging road, but as actor and PD advocate Michael J. Fox wrote in his biography, *Lucky Man* (Hyperion), first published in 2002, "If you were to rush into this room right now and announce that you had struck a deal — with God, Allah, Buddha, Christ, Krishna, Bill Gates, whomever — in which the ten years since my diagnosis could be magically taken away, traded in for the person I was before, I would, without a moment's hesitation, tell you to take a hike."

The First Next Steps: Gathering Info

You need to get information that you can trust so that you can form the questions to ask and establish some clear goals for managing this condition — a pretty tall order! Consider these three concrete steps that you can take right now to get started:

1. **Go online and bookmark the sites listed in Appendix B if you have access to the Internet.**

    These national organizations provide your best resource for the latest updates on treatments, as well as tips for managing your PD symptoms. Get into the habit of regularly checking in on the sites that you find most useful. If the site offers an e-list or newsletter, sign up.

2. **Call the toll-free numbers for the PD organizations if you don't have access to the Internet.**

   Ask them to send you their printed materials and add you to the mailing list for new materials in the future.

3. **Keep reading this book.**

TIP

If you're fortunate enough to have family and friends supporting your journey, take a moment to read through the following section with those closest to you — especially the person who's most likely to act as your primary care partner. Even though sections (scattered throughout this book) include *for the care partner* in their headings, try to read them together. The information applies to both of you because you have a responsibility to acknowledge that your care partner has a life beyond helping you manage your PD. (You may also want to check out Chapter 24 for more tips about how to give and receive care and support.)

A Word for the PD Care Partner

In many chronic, progressive illnesses (for example, Alzheimer's disease), family members must increasingly take charge. With PD, however, the person with Parkinson's (PWP) can remain in charge most of the way. As the care partner, you may be tempted to take over, especially when tasks become more difficult, and decisions take longer for your partner to process. But resist that urge. Partnering-in-care is not doing *for* — it's doing *with*.

So, where does that leave you, the care partner, while you face your own fears and anxieties about living with someone who has a chronic, progressive condition that won't go away but will color your lives for years to come? Go back and read this chapter. Everything we suggest for the PWP applies to you, as well:

>> **Sort through your emotions.** Deal with the anger, the fear, and the realities of how life is going to change (see Chapter 22).

>> **Adopt a take charge/move forward/don't look back outlook.** Start preparing for eventualities that may occur down the road. (You may especially want to read Chapters 20 and 21 about housing options and financial and legal matters.)

>> **Be proactive.** Educate yourself; go to doctor and therapy appointments with the PWP and take notes; become a combination of cheerleader and coach while your loved one faces new challenges.

>> **Set specific goals** that allow you to maintain a life and identity beyond your role as care partner.

To provide the best support you can over the long term, be a fierce advocate for your loved one's autonomy and independence. The next best way to show support involves taking care of yourself and making sure that you also meet your own needs. By working together — in partnership — the two of you can take something that could have destroyed you and turn it into a life experience that enriches you in ways you can't yet imagine.

Chapter **6**

Drafting Your Healthcare Team and Making a Game Plan

Knowledge may be power, but with today's constant bombardment of information, you need a team of experts that can answer questions and address unexpected situations by knowing the latest research and the most-advanced procedures.

People with Parkinson's (PWP), like people with other chronic-care needs, must rely on the expertise of several different professionals throughout the course of their illness. In this chapter, you can find out about these professionals and their roles in managing your Parkinson's symptoms. You can also take a look at how best to handle hospitalizations, emergency room visits, and other unexpected medical predicaments and complications that are possible for PWP. Last, but not least, your care partner can get ideas for building their own team.

Recruiting Your Teammates

Each member of your professional Parkinson's disease (PD) team has special talents and expertise that can help you manage symptoms and maintain normal function and quality of life, often for years following the initial diagnosis. The following sections offer a list of professionals and their roles in your care, and in the section "Making the cut," later in this chapter, you can uncover your role in helping these pros perform at their best.

Lining up the doctors

At least two doctors help set the course for your care after your PD diagnosis — your primary care and PD physician (neurologist or movement disorders specialist). In addition, you may have other specialists (or you may add them at a later date) if you have other chronic conditions, such as arthritis, diabetes, hypertension, and the like. The more doctors you have, the more vital it becomes for one doctor (most likely your primary care physician) to take the role of quarterback to oversee and coordinate the plan to meet all your health needs.

Your primary care physician

Your *primary care physician* (PCP) may be a general practitioner (GP) who focuses on family medicine, or that person may be an internist who treats adults only. Depending on your age, your PCP may be a *geriatrician* who specializes in the care and health of older people. You've probably been seeing this doctor for some time and have built a trust and style of communication that works for both of you. Now that you have PD, you need to talk with your PCP about two things:

>> The PCP's willingness to consult and communicate with your PD doctor (who'll take the lead on treating your PD symptoms)

>> How your PD treatment can integrate with your overall healthcare plan

Your PD doctor (neurologist or movement disorders specialist)

Your PCP probably referred you to a specialist to confirm the PD diagnosis. If so, these two professionals may already have a good working relationship. However, if you went for a second (or even third) opinion and chose another physician to oversee your PD care, be sure that these two doctors meet (at least through an exchange of information) and show a clear willingness to work together. It's also helpful if your PCP and PD doctor are on staff at the same hospital in case you need hospitalization or emergency treatment down the road. (For tips on locating and choosing a PD specialist, see Chapter 4.)

Other specialists

REMEMBER

In the event you need to consult with other specialists (a cardiologist, urologist, or the like) for new medical situations that arise, these physicians must work closely with your PCP and PD doctor so that they're all communicating from the same playbook. Think of these doctors as coming off the bench. When they get into the game, they need to get up to speed on your game plan and their specific roles. As PD progresses and more non-motor symptoms may present, other specialists become as important as your PD doctor to help you navigate the advanced stages of the disease.

Before you go to an appointment with a specialist, ask your PCP (and PD doctor, if appropriate) to send the specialist a copy of your most recent records. After your visit with one of these doctors, ask them to send a copy of the office visit report to your PCP, with a copy sent to you at the same time. With this exchange of information between doctors — and by assembling your own file of reports — you enhance the likelihood that everyone is on the same page, working from the same information.

TIP

If you're not already registered in an online system that healthcare professionals and patients use to share records, ask your PCP how you can sign up. In today's techie world, hospitals and physicians can post lab results, medications, allergies, and other information to an online database known as EHR (electronic health records) or EMR (electronic medical records). Using an EHR or EMR program keeps all of your medical information in one place and makes that information readily available without your needing to transport physical copies of reports between doctors.

Calling up the therapists

Because PD is a movement disorder that affects your ability to perform basic movements, your physical, occupational, and (possibly) speech therapists are important players on your healthcare team. These professionals offer proven methods to enhance and prolong your control of symptoms and improve your overall sense of well-being. Your insurance may or may not cover their services, unless your doctor's prescription notes them as *medically necessary* to treat your PD.

Physical therapist

A *physical therapist* (PT) can teach you how to build muscle strength, increase flexibility, and improve your posture, coordination, and balance to prevent falls and serious fractures. Techniques may include exercise programs (standard programs, as well as alternatives, such as yoga), heat and cold packs, and water therapy (exercises in water).

Your PT can design a program of exercises specific to your individual symptoms and abilities to preserve and even increase your muscle strength and flexibility. Make sure that your PT is aware of the specific needs of patients with PD and neurological conditions. Start by asking whether the PT is certified in the LSVT BIG technique, which is geared to retrain PWPs to perform both small (such as buttoning a shirt) and large (such as walking) movements. The "Speech therapist" section, later in this chapter, offers more information about the LSVT website and programs.

Not only does exercise appear to slow the progression of PD, but recent studies indicate that it may help prevent the orthopedic muscular and skeletal effects of *akinesia* (slowed or impaired ability to move) and lessen *rigidity* (stiff muscles). Exercise helps you maintain balance and prevent falls. Get off that couch!

REMEMBER

Your PT can't work miracles. If you exercise only when you go to a session with your PT, you probably don't see ongoing or long-term benefits. When the physical therapy sessions end (or when the time between sessions stretches to two weeks or more), you need to pursue your own regular program of stretching, strengthening, and aerobic exercises if you want the physical therapy to be successful in the long run. Ideally, you should be able to exercise every day. See Chapter 9 for a suggested program of stretches and exercises. Review these suggestions with your PT to develop a program that fits your needs and abilities.

Occupational therapist

Essentially, the *occupational therapist* (OT) helps preserve your sense of independence and self-confidence by showing you new ways of performing simple and routine tasks (known in the medical profession as *activities of daily living*, or ADLs) that you may now find difficult. One significant benefit of working with an OT is simply knowing that you can preserve your control (with alternative techniques) when the loss of control seems a foregone conclusion. For example, an OT may teach you new techniques (such as a *cueing*, which means using a reminder system) and provide assistive devices (such as a special cane) that help you perform certain movements and tasks.

For more information on ways to adapt to your changing symptoms, check out the information in Part 3 about living with PD.

Speech therapist

Not every PWP needs speech therapy, but if you're experiencing a softened vocal tone, unintentional mispronunciations, or wrong word choices, a speech therapist can help. These professionals can also help if you ever develop swallowing or other throat muscle problems that can come with PD.

TIP

If you can't find a trained speech therapist in your area, consider trying a program especially for PWP called the Lee Silverman Voice Treatment (LSVT) LOUD. For more information about LSVT Global, its programs, and links to other PD groups, check out its website at www.lsvtglobal.com. This site is also a useful resource for PTs certified in the BIG technique (as noted under the section "Physical therapist," earlier in the chapter).

Drafting other team players

As a PWP, you have your front-line defense that consists of your PCP and your neurologist, as well as trained movement, activity, and speech therapists. But, have you considered the number of other professionals that can help you to manage your symptoms and continue living a normal life as long as possible? Be sure that you include the following care professionals and experts when you're assembling the team.

Pharmacist

Pharmacists are in the business of knowing medications and their interactions. They know your current medications, the potential side effects of those medications, and the possible impact of any new medication that your PCP or neurologist may prescribe. And because their area of expertise focuses on medications, a pharmacist is your best resource for answering any questions you have after you carefully read the printed information on your prescriptions. (For more information about prescription medicines, be sure to check out Chapter 10.)

WARNING

Your job is to watch out for unintended clashes among your medications. To help ensure that your supplements and prescribed meds play nicely together, pick one pharmacy (or a chain that shares information among all branches) to fill all your prescriptions and stick with that pharmacy or chain. Also, make sure the pharmacist knows which over-the-counter (OTC) medicines you're taking or considering taking.

REMEMBER

GET IT ALL AT MULTIDISCIPLINARY CLINICS

An increasing awareness of PWP's need for treatment involving physical, occupational, speech, and other therapy led to the creation of one-stop-shop clinics known as *multidisciplinary PD clinics*. Advanced PD programs — such as those at University of Florida in Gainesville or Cedars-Sinai in Los Angeles — offer multidisciplinary day-long clinical experiences that enable your medical team to communicate in real-time and create a comprehensive approach to your care for the following months. You can search for a multidisciplinary clinic in your area on the Parkinson's Foundation website. Go to www.parkinson.org/search and click on the In Your Area link (it's blue) at the top of the screen.

Psychologist or counselor

Anxiety (constant worry, nervousness, or unease) and *depression* (lack of pleasure and energy, and often, reduced appetite and sleep) are part and parcel of having PD. On one hand, they're perfectly normal reactions to hearing a diagnosis of a chronic, progressive condition. On the other hand, they may be a non-motor symptom of the disease, which sometimes precedes the motor symptoms such as tremors or difficulty with movements.

Do not minimize possible symptoms of anxiety or depression and tell your doctor about them. In addition to (or as an alternative for) specific medications for anxiety and depression, a trained and licensed counselor may become a key member of your professional care team. Whether you see this person on a regular basis for talk therapy sessions, or you visit them just now and then for some emotional unburdening, consider choosing a counselor shortly after your doctor confirms your diagnosis. (See Chapter 13 for more about choosing a counselor.)

Support groups

Throughout this book, we tout the benefits of joining a support group — for you and your care partner. You may reject this idea in the early stages. "I don't want to sit around talking to a bunch of strangers or listening to them complain about their PD. I've got my own problems." Wrong! Well, sort of. You definitely have your own problems. But here's the point you're missing: A support group can help you find ways to cope with those problems.

You can find many types of support groups for PWP and their care partners. These days, PD support groups do far more than sit around and talk about it. Some groups take a broader advocacy approach, while other groups focus more on living with PD (exercise and diet programs, social gatherings, and updates on new treatments). All support groups should have a *trained professional* (someone with experience and credentials) who leads or facilitates the discussions. Ask your PD doctor if they are aware of local PD support groups. For more information about finding or creating a support group, see Chapter 13. Here are other resources:

>> **Parkinson's Foundation:** Look for a group in your area on this organization's website at www.parkinson.org/search. After you reach the website, click on the In Your Area link at the top and follow the prompts.

>> **Alliance of Independent Regional Parkinson Organizations (AIRPO):** Connect with this alliance — a collaboration of PD-related nonprofit organizations — through the Parkinson's Foundation website at www.parkinson.org. After you reach the website, search for *airpo*.

Legal and financial advisors

Your PD may eventually affect your ability to make key decisions about finances and legal matters, the future of your family, and your own future. The truth is that working with legal and financial experts as early as possible after your diagnosis makes sense. And putting key documents and plans in order is just smart planning — whether you have PD or not. (For a full discussion of the legal and financial matters that need attention, see Chapter 20.)

TIP

Given the complexities of PD costs, you might want to draft an insurance advisor for your team. This person can guide you and your care partner through the multitude of questions related to disability (short and long term), Medicare, Medicaid, Health Management Organizations (HMOs), Preferred Physician Organizations (PPOs), Health Savings Accounts (HSAs), and any other alphabet-soup plans that will undoubtedly surface in the future.

Spiritual advisor

Taking a holistic approach — caring for yourself physically, mentally, and spiritually — can give you a jump on managing your PD symptoms. Many people focus on the physical and mental but figure the spiritual takes care of itself. *Remember:* Your spiritual wellbeing has just as many levels as your physical and mental health.

If you have a spiritual mentor that you can tap to join your professional care team, do so early on. This person may be your clergy, someone who's mentored you through other passages, a practitioner of alternative or complementary medicine, or even the counselor that we mention in the section "Psychologist or counselor," earlier in this chapter.

Making the cut

REMEMBER

Drafting a team of experts in your battle against PD has benefits well beyond the expertise of each member. When you choose them carefully and treat them with respect, these men and women will go to great lengths for you. They even become some of your most enthusiastic cheerleaders, offering support and encouragement, humor, and affection while you confront the challenges of living with PD.

How do you evaluate each member of the team? The criteria are pretty standard — regardless of the profession. Check out Table 6-1 for questions to ask yourself regarding the suitability of the professionals you're considering for your team.

TABLE 6-1

Selecting PD Care Team Members

Criterion	How to Evaluate It
Qualification	Does this person have the right stuff — the appropriate credentials and experience — to handle the job?
Synergy	Is it a good fit — are you comfortable with this person? Can you talk about anything or ask the silliest question without feeling intimidated?
Thoughtfulness	Does this person really listen? Are they open to ideas that aren't their own?
Patience	Does this person give you the time you need — especially when your PD may slow your movements, thinking, and ability to put thoughts into words?
Collaboration	Is this person willing to admit limits to their knowledge and expertise, and refer you to someone more qualified to handle a specific issue?
Availability	Will this person be there when you need them?

Establishing Game Plans

Once you have your team in place, it's time to consider "what-if" situations and how you and your team will respond to such events. Stuff happens, and worst-case scenarios happen unexpectedly. Maybe you fall or burn yourself while preparing dinner and end up in the emergency room. Or, despite all precautions, you experience an adverse drug interaction that requires a stay in the hospital. Nonmedical emergencies — a fire, a weather event (such as a hurricane or tornado) — can also crop up.

Our advice throughout this book is this: Have a plan in the event something unexpected happens. Preparation doesn't mean you're assuming the worst. You just want to be ready — or as ready as possible.

TIP

Think through possible unexpected event scenarios during the relative calm of your normal routine and prepare for those scenarios when you have a cool head on your shoulders. *Be prepared* — the motto of the Boy Scouts of America — is just as useful for PWP and their care partners. You or your care partner may never need to dial 911, but if you do, you have a plan in place.

Prep for an emergency on the home front

Start your emergency plan with home safety by reviewing the tips for accident-proofing your home in Chapter 21. Then consider what to do in case of a medical emergency, such as an allergic reaction, a dislocated shoulder, or some other emergency beyond your control — a fire, a flood, a blackout. Who do you call? Where do you go? What do you do?

TIP

Your home is unique, just like you, so the best way to prepare for a safety emergency is to contact your local fire department. It may have a program where a firefighter comes out, assesses your home for fire safety, and then offers pointers for handling emergencies. The American Red Cross (www.redcross.org) also offers a checklist for creating your own evacuation plan.

Gather and secure personal records

Take advantage of the following tips for having the information you need in place; these prepared resources put you ahead of the panic if a medical or safety emergency does arise. Start by gathering this vital information:

>> **A list of all prescription and OTC medications** and a list of any allergies and chronic health conditions you have besides your PD

>> **Insurance and/or Medicare** numbers

>> **Your medical history,** including past surgeries or events (such as a stroke)

>> **Names and contact numbers** for your doctors and an emergency contact person other than your care partner if needed (an adult child, a close friend, or a neighbor)

TIP

Prepare a folder specifically for the emergency room. (People administering emergency care don't have time to sift through what are probably lengthy old records.) In your ER folder, include all of the vital personal information (medicines, allergies, insurance numbers, medical history, and care team contacts) listed in this section. In addition, include a copy of your *advance directive* (a living will and a medical power of attorney), even if the hospital and your doctor already have it on file. If you don't want the medical staff to provide certain interventions or extraordinary measures to save your life, you must provide that information. (See Chapter 20 for more info on these and other legal issues.)

Then, secure your gathered information by

>> **Dating and updating** it regularly, especially when you add, change, or discontinue meds.

>> **Keeping copies in your wallet or purse and car(s)** at all times. Both you and your care partner should have a copy readily available to provide any medical personnel especially in an emergency situation.

REMEMBER

» **Let key others know where to find the information** in case you can't direct them during the emergency. These others could include your employer or a trusted neighbor who may respond to an emergency.

Make sure that *anyone* — you, your care partners, your family, or emergency responders — who needs it can readily get your information.

» **Prepare a fireproof box** that contains copies of key documents: insurance and Social Security cards; bank and credit card account numbers; wills, powers of attorney (financial and medical), and photos of valuables in case of a fire or weather catastrophe (such as a tornado or hurricane). This is good advice for anyone . . . with PD or not.

» **Post critical emergency contact numbers** on a wall near your home's entrance or on your refrigerator. Those numbers include the local hospital emergency room, fire department, police department, utility company (for power outages), doctors, pharmacist (in the event of an adverse drug reaction), and a relative or friend to contact.

Facilitate easy access for emergency crew

REMEMBER

You may never need emergency intervention, but you're better off with information that an emergency team can readily access. Take the following measures to prevent glitches when seconds count:

» Distribute duplicate house keys to trusted friends and neighbors.

» Be sure that your care partner or someone you have designated as your financial power of attorney can access financial funds any time you may not be able to take financial actions such as writing checks to pay bills or transferring funds from savings to checking accounts, as needed.

» If you live alone, get a medical alert system, which enables you to call for help if you're unable to get to a telephone. (Yup, we're talking about that classic TV commercial — "Help! I've fallen and can't get up!") But don't worry — these days, you can find much more stylish options.

Act decisively if the unexpected happens

WARNING

In an emergency, don't waste time worrying about whether you should call for help. Risking a little embarrassment rather than your life is always the wise move.

However, if you do need to call for an ambulance or go to the emergency room, be realistic about your expectations. Keep in mind that the United States has nearly 40 million people who don't have health insurance; for these folks, the ER doctor is likely their doctor of choice. *Note:* The Centers for Disease Control estimates the average waiting time in the ER (if you're not critically injured or ill) is three hours; in cold and flu season, the wait can be much longer. Because of possible delays, you need to

>> **Speak up** if you're experiencing symptoms such as extreme pain, trouble breathing, dizziness, and other signs of distress.

>> **Be proactive.** Tell every ER person who examines or assists you that you have PD (and any other chronic conditions, such as diabetes or hypertension), even though someone has taken your history and you know these facts are on your patient information sheet. Make sure that the people who treat you are aware of your medications and allergies.

TIP

If your situation is serious but not life threatening, call your doctor or the nearest urgent-care or walk-in clinic for faster response and care. And if your doctor does advise you to get to the ER, speed up the process by having your doctor call the hospital and tell the ER staff that you're on the way.

More tips for managing the unexpected

Emergencies arise for all kinds of people. But because you have PD, such crises may carry the extra elements of stress and panic. You and your care partner may want to consider taking a basic first-aid course through your local Red Cross or YMCA to better prepare yourselves for unlikely emergencies, such as bleeding, choking, medication reactions, falls, and so on.

REMEMBER

If you need to call 911, be prepared to give the following information:

>> Your name and the phone number you're calling from

>> The address from which you're calling and location specifics (such as "It's a 2-block street between Elm and Maple." Or "It's the house with the dolphin-shaped mailbox on the north side of the street.") to help the ambulance get there quickly

>> Description of your condition (or the condition of the person you're calling about — are they breathing? conscious?)

In addition, follow these steps:

1. **Don't hang up until the emergency operator tells you to.**

2. **Be sure that you (or your care partner) unlock the door and turn on outside lights.**

Even if it's not night, the lit porch light allows first responders to more easily locate the right house.

3. **If possible, have another family member or neighbor wait outside to direct the emergency personnel.**

4. **Have your care partner stay close to you so that they can provide answers to key questions.**

   Although you want your care partner close, they need to let the emergency personnel do their jobs.

5. **Gather the information you've prepared and get ready to go.**

   See the section "Gather and secure personal records," earlier in this chapter, for an idea of the information you should have easily available.

TIP

If you don't have a mobile phone, only a landline, consider having only cordless phones so that you can move around the house (unlocking doors and turning on lights) while you're talking on the phone with the doctor or emergency operator.

Planning for a Hospital Stay

If you need to be admitted to the hospital, your PD probably isn't the cause. The more likely reasons include a serious injury (such as a hip fracture or head trauma from a fall) or another chronic or acute health condition (such as diabetes or a heart attack). Regardless, be prepared with the necessary information (see the section "Gather and secure personal records," earlier in this chapter, for suggestions) to make the stay less stressful for everyone.

TIP

Leave valuables (checkbook, credit cards, jewelry, and the like) at home. If you must bring them because of an emergency and the haste in leaving for the hospital, hand them off to a trusted family member or friend as soon as possible. Or ask a staff member whether the hospital has a safe place to keep the valuables until you can make arrangements for them. As uncomfortable as it is to believe, theft of valuables in the hospital can occur.

Monitoring your PD meds

The same suggestions outlined for an emergency (in the section "Establishing Game Plans," earlier in this chapter) apply for a hospital stay. But, because you probably need to stay in the hospital for days rather than hours, you must monitor the orders for your PD medications. The attending physician and the staff may not realize the importance of your PD meds' strict dosing and timing. For example, the hospital staff may interpret your neurologist's orders for medication at

8 a.m., noon, 4 p.m., and 8 p.m. as four times a day over a 24-hour period (meaning 8 a.m., 2 p.m., 8 p.m., and 2 a.m.). Changing the dosing times can cause flare-ups in your PD symptoms at a time when you are already under stress from whatever brought you to the hospital in the first place.

Sometimes, the doctors have to suspend your PD meds so that new medications for the condition that landed you in the hospital can work. Again, be vigilant about your care. Have your care partner alert your neurologist (or the doctor managing your PD care) as soon as you know you're going to the hospital and insist that the hospital on-call physician (or any doctor who orders the suspension of your PD meds) consults with your neurologist before ordering *any* changes in medication.

WARNING

Often, as a consequence of poor medication timing or contraindicated drugs, PWPs admitted to a hospital suffer avoidable complications at a higher rate, which leads to prolonged lengths of stay. And nobody wants to remain in a hospital bed for days or weeks longer than expected. Anytime that your medications are being administered for you (as in a hospital setting), instead of your doling them out to yourself, be sure that you or your care partner carefully examine the pills you get. If any of the meds look different from those you take at home, question it. Also, because hospital staff is responsible for administering medications to a number of patients who have diverse conditions, you may have a delay in getting your PD meds on time. If necessary, have your neurologist contact the attending physician at the hospital to discuss the correct medication regimen. Also, make sure the attending staff knows which medications may be *contraindicated* (harmful) for PWP.

For a table of red-flag medications from the American Parkinson Disease Association, visit the website at www.apdaparkinson.org, hover over the What Is Parkinson's Disease link, click the Treatment & Medication link on the drop-down that appears, and scroll down to click the Medications to Avoid link on the resulting page.

Making care providers aware of your PD

In addition to monitoring your medications, you may have another battle to wage: The hospital staff, even though they're medical professionals, may have limited or no experience with PD and may misinterpret your PD symptoms — on-off cycles, dyskinesias, confusion from the stress of a hospital environment, and the like. For example, if a nursing assistant sees you up and mobile at 2:00 and comes back at 3:00 because you want assistance getting to the bathroom, they may think you're just looking for extra attention. If you want to provide good information for aides, housekeeping, and other staffers who may be unfamiliar with PD, see the sidebar "I'm not fooling around nor drunk — I have PD," in this chapter.

I'M NOT FOOLING AROUND NOR DRUNK — I HAVE PD

Consider printing out something like the following to post in your room:

HI! I have PARKINSON'S DISEASE, so here's some key info that might help:

- It's really important that I take my meds on a schedule specifically set by my doctors for me rather than on a general schedule you may use for all patients on this unit.

- Sometimes I can do normal stuff like brushing my teeth or walking around on my own all by myself and then — BOOM — I need help. It's not an act — I have Parkinson's.

- Sometimes I may appear confused or disoriented — again — NOT intoxicated or trying to get extra attention. It's the Parkinson's, and I need help and understanding.

- Finally — and this is the BIGGIE — there are certain anti-nausea and anti-psychotic meds that just do not work for me. In fact, they can send me over the edge, so PLEASE check with my doctor before administering any new medication.

THANKS FOR YOUR HELP AND UNDERSTANDING!

A Word for the PD Care Partner

This book has a number of chapters that you may want to read and heed. This is one of them. Putting together a network of professionals that you and the PWP can call upon when issues crop up can make life easier for both of you. Within this group of professionals, you need to find your own experts — three people you can turn to with your concerns of managing and coping:

>> **Primary care physician:** You may have the same general practitioner or internist as the PWP. As long as this physician attends to your needs and concerns when you're the patient, that's fine. However, you may want to consider a PCP who isn't involved in your PWP's care. *Remember:* You need someone to focus on maintaining *your* physical health and well being.

>> **Counselor or therapist:** Being a partner in care can be extremely stressful, especially when the needs escalate. But you can better prepare yourself to cope with the unexpected twists and turns along the way if you take time now to connect with a professional who counsels care partners. Don't be stubborn

about this. You're at risk for episodes of anxiety, panic, and depression as much as the PWP is.

>> **Support group and spiritual advisor:** Okay, so we cheated and lumped two into one. But your spiritual health is a vital piece of your ability to partner in care. A support group can provide a safe place to talk about (and let go of) those bad feelings you may be wrestling with (see Chapter 22 for more on this topic). And it has folks who can laugh and share some of the dark humor that comes with being a care partner — they all know, understand, and feel your pain. As for a spiritual advisor, you know yourself best. Your clergyperson, a trusted mentor, your counselor or therapist, and your support-group leader are all good candidates to fill this role.

IN THIS CHAPTER

» Setting a course with your care partner

» Keeping the story straight with your family

» Sharing with your inner circle of friends

» Determining who else needs to know

» Taking the high road when it comes to unwanted input

Chapter **7**

Choosing How and When to Share Your News

Living with Parkinson's disease (PD) can go well beyond the person diagnosed with PD. Day in and year out, the disease also affects the people who live with, work with, care about, and love the person with PD (PWP). It affects generations — children, grandchildren, and even aging parents (in the case of young onset PD, which we talk about in Chapter 8) — who may be facing their own health challenges.

Everyone has concentric circles of personal contacts. In the closest circles, you have your immediate family (spouse, partner, kids, parents) and perhaps a couple of truly best friends. Next comes a little wider circle — friends you socialize with, extended family, and perhaps a couple of professionals, such as your doctor or clergyperson. Further removed from the core of your life, you have another group — your employer and co-workers, acquaintances, and neighbors. Deciding when and how to tell each person or group about your diagnosis is an individual decision, one that you have to base on the dynamics of your relationships and your comfort level in sharing this kind of news.

Before You Start Spreading the News

Even if you initially share your diagnosis with very few people, you need to plan how you want these people to receive the information. You can't control people's reactions, but you can direct how and when you share the news — both immediately and in the future.

Establishing your ground rules

Start by determining your ground rules for the way you plan to address your life with PD and the level of support you want. The following categories identify some of the more common PWP stances:

>> **Some PWP are fighters.** They go on immediate offense, take charge, and fight this enemy with every ounce of strength and all the resources they can muster.

>> **Other PWP take flight.** In some ways, these PWPs choose to downplay the whole situation. Flight folks use their energy and resources to assure everyone (and, most of all, themselves) that nothing has really changed — life goes on.

>> **A third group of PWP hugs the mid-line.** Combining facets of fight and flight, mid-liners want life to continue as normally as possible, but they realize they have to fight back to keep their PD's progression at bay.

Whichever stance you take, you need to think about your ground rules for living with PD. Consider the kind of meaningful care and support that the groups of people in your life can offer while you face life with PD. Those who care about you — family members, friends, neighbors, co-workers — naturally want to help. In many cases, they're not sure how to offer support. You need to explain the ground rules and indicate what will — and won't — be helpful.

Preparing to state your needs

Think through it now — alone, or preferably with your care partner (the person who will most likely be with you for the whole journey) — how other people can help. Initially, you may need people to listen, to distract you when necessary, and to give you the gift of normalcy just by being themselves and continuing to interact with you like they did before you were diagnosed.

While your needs become more specific and you accept the hands-on help of others, you also discover three really important upshots:

>> **You empower people** by allowing them to contribute something truly meaningful to you. Let your friends take you for coffee or drive you to the doctor or be that extra pair of ears to sit in on an appointment and hear what the doctor tells you.

>> **You ease some of the responsibility** that may have fallen on your care partner's shoulders. Give your care partner regular breaks by insisting they continue to see their friends or get their hair done or attend their weekly poker game.

>> **You prevent yourself from becoming isolated,** and you actually increase your ability to take control of situations when they arise. Enjoy interaction by making sure you give as much attention to what is going on in the lives of others as they put the focus on you and your PD.

REMEMBER

Accepting help is not a sign of weakness; in fact, it's a sign of strength. Acceptance shows you haven't surrendered to the challenges of PD. And when you can't fight the battle alone, you still win because you have people willing to step up to fight this disease with you.

Meeting the challenge with good humor

REMEMBER

We can't say this too often: An upbeat, optimistic attitude is one of your most effective weapons against PD. And right next to it is the ability to laugh — with others, at yourself, and especially at your PD. *We're talking dark humor here, folks.*

For example, a diet-center leader famous for her wonderful sense of humor inspired her feeling-sorry-for-themselves clients with the story of her father, a large, barrel-chested man who had always been bigger than life. Then he got cancer and started fading away — literally. One day toward the very end, when he was but a shadow of his former robust self, he said to his daughter, "You know I want to be cremated." She nodded in agreement. "Well," he added, "if I keep dwindling away like this, I think you'll be able to do the job in the microwave!" His daughter was first stunned and then burst into laughter. That's dark humor, folks — and it works because it helps you keep your perspective while you face the sometimes-tough days of living with PD.

BILL OF RIGHTS FOR PEOPLE WITH PARKINSON'S

Declarations of individual rights are nothing new. Perhaps you've noticed Rights lists posted when you visit a hospital or care facility. But we think it's important that you — the person with PD (PWP) — know your own inalienable rights. Feel free to edit and add your own ideas to the following list. Then bookmark it and reread it regularly.

I have the right to

- Take care of and make decisions for myself for as long as I am capable and to expect my care partners to respect my wishes, should the time come when they speak for me.

- Seek help from others when I recognize limits to my own endurance and strength.

- Maintain those facets of my life that were part of my identity before my PD diagnosis for as long as possible — even if each task takes three times as long.

- Occasionally (and humanly) get angry, be depressed, and work my way through other difficult feelings.

- Reject any attempt by others (either consciously or unconsciously) to limit my independence because it'll make life easier for them.

- Expect and receive consideration, respect, encouragement, affection, and forgiveness as long as I offer these same qualities in return.

- Take joy and pride in my accomplishments — regardless of how small — and provide the effort and courage it takes to achieve them.

- Speak out and demand that new resources and eventually a cure be found — if not for me, then for those who follow.

Discussing the News with Your Care Partner

Your care partner was probably with you when the doctor confirmed the diagnosis of PD. If you got the news together, then you don't have to worry about the telling part. But the two of you still need to spend some time working your way through the questions of how this diagnosis is going to affect your lives — individually and together.

What if your primary care partner wasn't present when you got the word that you have PD or your primary care partner isn't your significant other? (Perhaps your care partner is a sibling or an adult child who works, has a family of their own, and lives in another community.) In that case, give yourself a day or so to digest the diagnosis and think about how you prefer to break the news.

When you're ready (don't wait too long; a day or week at most), try to have the conversation in person and allow enough time to work through the discussion:

TIP

>> **Make it one-on-one.** In-person conversations are best, but if you can't talk face-to-face, choose a time when this person isn't distracted by other activities. And have the discussion by phone or via an online video chat, such as Zoom or Facetime.

If you have to deliver the initial news online or by phone, follow up with an email or text that gives your care partner links to some of the websites in Appendix B. The folks at the Parkinson's Foundation (800-473-4636) have some excellent materials for PWP and their care partners. Check it out at the website www.parkinson.org; hover over the Living with Parkinson's link and click Resources & Support from the drop-down that appears.

>> **Be encouraging.** When you deliver the news, reassure this person that the diagnosis isn't currently life-threatening, and you have no need for immediate action.

>> **Plan an in-depth discussion.** Set a time when the two of you can discuss your present needs, your needs down the road, and that person's willingness and capability for supporting you as you address those needs.

During the initial conversation with your care partner, allow enough time to

>> **Share immediate emotional reactions.** Even if you've had a couple of days or a week since you and your care partner heard the news.

>> **Address each different response.** One of you may react with denial and the other with anger. (Before this discussion, you may both benefit by reading the section on personality differences in Chapter 5.)

>> **Write down a list of steps to take.** Include a tentative timeline for each step based on the tips we offer in the following section.

WARNING

Resist the urge (by you or your care partner) to leap ahead and take dramatic and life-changing actions, such as putting your home up for sale and moving in with your daughter, or assuming that you need to quit your job. You have time. You likely won't need to make these lifestyle changes because of your PD for years — and perhaps decades.

Telling Your Family

When and how you deliver the news to your immediate and extended family is an individual choice that's influenced by

>> The status of individual family relationships

>> Your personal feelings about how soon you want even close relatives to know

When you're ready to talk to family members, the easiest way may be a family gathering (if geography or technology, such as Zoom or Facetime, allows) where you tell all the adult members at the same time. Everyone hears the same version of the story, and details won't get distorted through repetition. However, in the rare case that you just can't coordinate a family meeting, consider writing a letter that you copy and send to all members of the family. That way, at least they still receive the same information. Again, you want to deliver the same news to all the adults at approximately the same time.

TIP

If you have children, find a place and time to share your news with them before that larger meeting, especially if your PD is of the young-onset variety and your children are still living at home. Your children will make this journey with you; they deserve to have the same time and privacy to digest this news as your care partner had.

Give adults the facts

When you deliver the news to the adults in your immediate and extended family, stick to the basics:

>> What PD is and is not

>> Whether others in the family are at risk

>> How PD is treated

>> What your prognosis is

Some family members may have suspected a serious illness of some kind; others may be completely shocked at the news and take it hard. In either case, a good first step is to educate and inform, but keep it simple. This is not the time to dive deep into the science of PD.

TIP

As mentioned in the section "Discussing the News with Your Care Partner," earlier in this chapter, every PD association offers a number of basic educational and informational materials that cover fundamental questions about PD. These excellent materials come in many forms: printed booklets or pamphlets, webinars, online lectures, and so on; you can find the contact information for some great associations that offer these materials in Appendix B. Downloading and handing out printed information at a family meeting (or attaching PDFs of the information to a follow-up e-mail if your family is tech savvy or lives elsewhere) gives the recipients a reference for questions after the initial shock wears off. By selecting the same material for everyone, you lessen the chances of that information becoming distorted.

Set a positive tone

After you share the facts of PD with family members (including young children or grandchildren), consider setting the tone for your emerging new relationships. For example, you can add, "There's a lot I don't know, but I do know I can live a relatively normal life in spite of my symptoms. The tough part is figuring out how to live with PD without people feeling sorry for me or treating me differently." With that simple statement, you offer a solid, straightforward base for continued positive relationships:

>> You have PD, but you're still you.

>> You want other people to continue treating you the same; this is most important. (Okay, so Cousin Fred can let you win a few more poker games, and your mother may finally call someone else to get the cat out of the tree each week.)

How much you say about PD beyond the basics — symptoms, research, no present cures, and such — is strictly up to you and your assessment of how much information this group can handle at the first telling.

When that question of "What can I do to help?" comes up, perhaps the best answer is to make three points. Your family members can help you by

>> **Being themselves** and finding ways to continue your relationship as normally and fully as before.

>> **Supporting your care partner** and making sure that person maintains a life outside of yours.

>> **Understanding that you're still the same person inside.** Tell them not to let your PD symptoms scare them or make them treat you any differently.

Don't sugarcoat the situation for kids

Today's children are bombarded with information from every possible angle. Put another way, this generation is far savvier at a far younger age than most adults can imagine. On some level, even very young children can understand that something has changed in their environment. Don't underestimate their capacity for feeling stress and tension, especially when they can sense the undercurrent in the household but no one's talking with them about it. Approach this discussion based on the child's age (and maturity level):

>> **Teenagers** can usually handle the same information you give the adults. If your teen is especially sensitive or perhaps struggling with other emotional challenges (the break-up of a relationship or not making the sports team, for example), you may want to have the conversation with that teen separately so that you can focus on reassuring and comforting them.

>> **Children in their middle years** (ages 9 to 12) are sometimes mature enough to be included with the adults in the general family meeting. But just because they seem to understand and accept the news, don't assume that they don't have concerns or a gazillion questions about how your lives are going to change. Keep a watch for changes in behavior such as withdrawing from you or moodiness and have a one-on-one conversation to address their concerns.

>> **Younger children (or grandchildren)** need the details to be as simple as possible. A terrific resource for telling young children (under about age 9) about PD is the book entitled *I'll Hold Your Hand So You Won't Fall: A Child's Guide to Parkinson's Disease* (Merit Publishing International), by Rasheda Ali and her father, Muhammad Ali.

If the child is your grandchild, decide with your grandchild's parents the best way to deliver the news.

REMEMBER

Regardless of the ages (or seeming maturity) of the children, never forget that they're children; they haven't lived long enough to pile up the life experiences and tools for coping that an adult has. Check in with your children and grandchildren often through positive techniques, such as

>> Seeking their help with innovative ways that you can cope with certain limits to normal tasks (such as tying your shoes or cleaning your eyeglasses) when your PD symptoms hinder you.

>> Continuing to pursue activities the two of you have always enjoyed — even if you have to find ways to adapt, such as getting a recumbent bicycle rather than riding your old one.

» Providing the opportunity (place and time) for them to raise questions and concerns about what your PD means for the future. Perhaps you can take a regular trip to the ice cream shop and talk there.

Giving Close Friends the News

Soon after you break the news to your family, consider how and when to tell your closest friends. Again, you have several issues at play here, including the fact that friends may have already noticed your symptoms and discussed their concerns with each other. They may not have brought their concerns to you directly because they didn't want to intrude.

Looking at the logistics

How and when you choose to tell your friends depends in part on the nature of the group. If your close friends are also close with each other, then consider inviting everyone over to your house and telling them all at the same time. That way, you have the advantage that everyone hears the same words (although they may process them differently) at the same time directly from you. In addition, they can see your response to the diagnosis — hopefully upbeat and optimistic — at the same time. And they can all hear the ground rules for how you want them to respond to your diagnosis. (To figure out how to set up your ground rules, flip to the section "Before You Start Spreading the News," earlier in this chapter.)

In cases where you have close friends who aren't close with each other or friends who live in other places, you may want to tell each friend individually. If so, try to do it face to face (or at least by phone or virtual video — not e-mail) so that the person can see and/or hear how you're handling the diagnosis.

TIP

Consider providing the same helpful information (a fact sheet and list of websites) that we identify in the section "Give adults the facts," earlier in this chapter, so your friends can pursue questions that may occur after you tell them.

Embracing friends' support

Friendships can be critical to your overall sense of control and well-being when you're living with PD. Unfortunately, a lot of PWP, after they get the diagnosis, make the mistake of pulling away from their friends or denying any need for that support (tangible support such as cutting the lawn or intangible support such as just being there to listen).

When PWPs (or their care partners) react as if the support insults them or makes a statement about the PWP's incapacity, they make matters worse. This reaction can have a snowball effect because the friend who wanted to help feels rejected (even embarrassed) at apparently adding to your stress. Before you know it, those treasured friendships (along with the normalcy and pleasure they bring your life) may disappear.

As soon as you and your care partner are ready to go to your friends with the news, take control and set the tone by doing the following:

>> **State your needs regarding your approach to PD.** For example, tell them that you understand that they may want to rush in and start helping you (preparing meals, handling the household and yard chores, and such), but the best support they can offer is to help you maintain as normal a life (and relationship) as possible for as long as possible.

>> **Appreciate any offer of support and help** (even if you shudder to think that they believe you need that help). If possible be specific about the help you would appreciate rather than relying on the person to come up with something. If the offer feels demeaning, then gently reshape it by saying something like, "You know, so far I'm not having any trouble getting in or out of the car, but I could definitely use a hand when I step on or off the curb."

>> **Be prepared to suggest alternate ways** in which your friends can be a part of your network of support and caring. Perhaps consider asking if they might be available for driving you to an appointment and then stopping for coffee the way the two of you used to do.

When you think of outside help, consider your care partner and their soon-to-be-filled-to-capacity schedule. By maintaining a normal routine with friends and associates, you give your care partner a break to pursue life aside from PD.

REMEMBER

When you respond to your friends' invitations to activities that you enjoyed before PD with "I can't," they may stop offering and gradually get on with their own lives. Instead, try an attitude of "I'd love to [play cards, bike, meet you at the coffeehouse]. Help me figure out how we can make that happen." Then you can brainstorm options for activities together.

Actor Alan Alda had this to say in an interview revealing his diagnosis with PD: "I thought, 'It's probably only a matter of time before somebody does a story about this from a sad turn point of view,' but that's not where I am."

Widening the Circle: Informing Others

On the outer fringes of those concentric circles that we describe in the chapter introduction are those people who play a role in your life but not a daily or intimate one (neighbors, community group associates, professionals you rely on, and so on). Don't feel compelled to break the news to this last circle of contacts right away — or ever (with the possible exception of your boss and co-workers; see Chapter 16 for the specifics on that special group). Basically, your condition's really none of their business.

TIP

Don't underestimate the unexpected support and management of resources that may come from the acquaintances in your outer concentric circles. For example, your barber or beautician may offer to make a house call when your symptoms change. Or your neighbor may be happy to be on call for emergencies when you're alone and your partner's at work.

When the timing seems right during the first months following your diagnosis, let these people know you have PD. Only you can decide how much information they need or what kind of support and response they may provide. But, like with anyone you tell, be prepared to set the tone for their response, to correct misinformation they may have about PD, and to appreciate their concern and support however they express it.

Handling Sticky Conversations

We talk a lot in the preceding sections about informing family, friends, and acquaintances about your diagnosis, but we need to get real here. Some people (and they may be in your closest circles) are more hindrance than help when they hear you have PD. One type simply can't handle bad news of any sort, so you end up spending a lot of time and energy comforting and emotionally supporting their (mostly unfounded) fears and anxieties. Another type believes that they have all the answers, even though they have zero real knowledge about PD. They, too, can use up your resources of energy and good humor while you try to educate them about the realities of living with PD. Consider these tips for handling those sticky situations:

>> **For people who simply can't cope** with difficult news, consider being prepared with a specific request. You can ask, for example, "You're such an avid biker, would you be willing to bike with me once a week? My doctor tells me that exercise, especially now in the early stages, is really important, but I'd rather not go out alone."

If this person is a close friend or family member, you may want to speak with them separately and acknowledge those obvious fears and anxieties. Then let that person know that they can help you the most by remaining upbeat and positive — at least, in your presence.

TIP

If all else fails, allow such people an initial period of mourning over your news. Then insist that they get over it or else you'll have to limit your contact with them. Your condition isn't about these people. You're the one with PD and, bluntly stated, you just don't need other people bringing you down.

>> **For the well-meaning folks** (even strangers!) who see your tremor or some other PD symptom and start telling you the story of their uncle's wife's brother who also had PD, you need a different tactic. No doubt such people mean well, but they'll never be part of your care team. This empathy and advice (or showing off!) is about them, not you.

REMEMBER

Don't allow unwanted advice or comments to upset you. Of the two of you, *you* are the expert about PD. Politely acknowledge their effort to help, and then walk away.

Chapter **8**

Young Onset Parkinson's and Lewy Body Dementia

When it comes to young onset Parkinson's disease (YOPD), or PD in general, for that matter, no one's more famous than the popular actor Michael J. Fox, who had hit movies and TV shows throughout the '80s and '90s. The twinkle in his eye and his legendary self-deprecating humor — even about life with PD — make him less the celebrity and more the national support-group leader for millions of people with Parkinson's (PWP) and their care partners.

In an interview, Fox reported that as many as 40 percent of the 60,000 new PD cases each year involve someone younger than age 50. This figure alone blows holes in the myth that only old people get PD. The fact that Fox was first diagnosed in his 30s shines an even brighter light on the growing numbers of young and active people who face this challenge.

The cause of *young onset Parkinson's disease (YOPD)* is as debatable as the cause of traditional onset PD (see Chapter 2). But you can't debate the fact that it hits people in their prime, plays havoc with their established roles (spouse, parent, adult child of aging parents), derails rising careers, and overrides plans for the future.

Now about Lewy body dementia (LBD): we're not going to sugarcoat this one. Lewy body dementia is an umbrella term for two forms of dementia that can occur with PD:

>> **Parkinson's with dementia** (PDD): When dementia occurs years into the diagnosis of PD.

>> **Dementia with Lewy bodies** (DLB): When dementia is an early and prominent symptom within the first three years of parkinsonism. DLB is usually classified as an *atypical parkinsonism*. (See Chapter 2 for more on this classification.)

Because you're likely to find further information sources about the disease by searching for *Lewy body dementia*, we're going to stick with the umbrella term *LBD* — except in cases where there is a clear need to distinguish between the two forms (PDD and DLB).

In this chapter, we take a look at the specific issues facing people diagnosed with YOPD or LBD. When you receive a diagnosis of YOPD for those not yet 60 or perhaps LBD for those experiencing early cognitive decline or symptoms of dementia later in the progression of the disease, you have significant and specific differences in the progression and the sheer impact of the disease for both you and your care partner. We begin this chapter with information that you need if you've been diagnosed with YOPD, and we then discuss similar information for those dealing with LBD.

Comparing YOPD to Traditional Onset PD

The term *onset age* means when symptoms first appear — not when a doctor diagnoses you. If the onset age is earlier than age 50, the diagnosis is usually YOPD. In very rare cases, PD symptoms appear before a person reaches the age of 21; the term *Juvenile Parkinson's* distinguishes it from traditional PD or YOPD. For more information, visit the website at www.apdaparkinson.org, hover over the What Is Parkinson's Disease link and click the Early Onset Parkinson's Disease link from the drop-down that appears.

Excellent resources for information specially aimed at people with YOPD include

The Parkinson's Foundation's Young Onset Parkinson's page. Access the page by going to www.parkinson.org and clicking this series of links: Understanding Parkinson's/What Is Parkinson's/Young Onset Parkinson's.

The Michael J. Fox Foundation site's YOPD page. Visit the site at www.michaeljfox.org and search for the term *young onset.*

And you can sign up to receive regular e-mail bulletins. These periodic updates cover upcoming foundation activities and provide valuable tips and information for PWP and their care partners.

How they're the same

PD is chronic, progressive, and (at least at the time of this writing) incurable, regardless of your age and when you get it. On the positive side, you can live for many years — in some cases, a regular lifespan — in spite of having PD. You can continue to work, to raise a family, to see children marry and have children of their own, and to enjoy many of the same activities that you enjoyed before you were diagnosed.

How they differ

YOPD and traditional onset PD differ in three basic ways:

>> **Certain symptoms can be milder.** People who have YOPD are less likely to experience the cognitive impairment (such as memory problems) or balance problems that affect people whose PD begins when they're older. Part of the reason for the difference is that older people are more likely to have multiple conditions (such as a series of small strokes or adverse medication interaction) that affect memory and balance.

>> **Dystonia, instead of (or in addition to) tremor, may occur.** People who have YOPD may experience a condition known as *dystonia* (unusual muscle cramping, aches, or abnormal movement in a particular area of the body, such as a foot or shoulder). For reasons that still aren't clear, older patients seldom experience dystonia but tend to have *tremor* (shaking), a symptom that's less common for a person with YOPD.

>> Although the medical community recognizes dystonia as the possible first symptom of YOPD, you may have a delay in your diagnosis if your doctor isn't familiar with such PD symptoms in younger patients.

WARNING

>> **Stronger reactions to medication may happen.** In general, people who have YOPD appear to respond well to antiparkinsonian medications, but they may develop *dyskinesia* (uncontrollable movements) more quickly than older PWP. Specifically, those diagnosed with YOPD may experience two specific medication-related problems more than older PWP: early wearing-off of the medication benefits and *on-off* fluctuations (symptoms reappearing before the next dose is due, either predictably or all of the sudden).

Many people who have YOPD (and their doctors) elect to postpone treatment with antiparkinsonian meds as long as possible and instead, elect to start treatment with an MAO-B inhibitor or a dopaminergic agonist (for more information about these medications, see Chapter 10) to avoid some of these escalated symptoms and side effects. However, recent data — which shows that dyskinesia and other long-term complications of levodopa therapy depend more on disease progression than on length of treatment — does not support this strategy.

>> **Family history and genetic predisposition.** People with YOPD seem to have more frequently a positive family history of PD, suggesting that genetic factors play more of a role when developing PD at a younger age. A study from Cedars-Sinai in Los Angeles, using human induced pluripotent stem cells from people with YOPD, showed that their brain cells have the potential to develop PD even before birth. While this may sound scary, it offers a tremendous window of opportunity (30 to 40 years long!) to possibly prevent the disease.

Faster or slower? What's the prognosis?

The jury's still out on the pace of progression for people who have YOPD. However, more advanced therapies may eventually postpone the progression of symptoms for a longer time — perhaps adding years to the person's relatively normal life.

REMEMBER

PD — regardless of the age of onset — affects each individual differently. Like with any health issue, your physical and mental health at the onset of PD (and your fight to maintain that well-being through a balanced diet and regular exercise program) can have an enormous effect on the prognosis. Nothing is carved in stone regarding the progression of symptoms — no matter how old or young you are when they start.

Facing the Special Challenges of YOPD

If you have YOPD, the most difficult challenge may be the very fact that you're young. You had planned a life packed with many goals, and one of them was *not* living with a chronic and progressive condition. Most people in their young adult years tend to see themselves as invincible. They may take steps to ensure financial security for their family and themselves in the unlikely event that something bad happens, but they really don't consider it a possibility.

And now it appears that the unlikely event has happened: You've been diagnosed with YOPD. And that diagnosis is standing directly in the way of the life you've planned. At first, you can see no way around it. But you know better.

Stop for a moment and consider other times when you faced what seemed like an impossible challenge and conquered it. Whatever the situation, recognize that you took action to beat the challenge. In this case, you picked up this book, seeking the information and resources you need to deal with your PD.

In the following sections, we advise you on an approach to life that can help you get through this diagnosis and come out on top — again.

Getting an accurate diagnosis

The doctor bases a diagnosis of YOPD on the same cardinal signs used to diagnose PD at any age:

>> **Bradykinesia:** Slowed or impaired ability to perform fine movements

>> **Tremor at rest:** Trembling when you aren't engaging the body part in activity

>> **Rigidity:** Muscle stiffness, sometimes causing painful cramps

>> **Postural instability:** Impaired balance (less frequent at a young age)

REMEMBER

Patients who present with YOPD less often experience tremor and more often experience bradykinesia and rigidity, presenting at times as abnormal muscle cramps *(dystonia)*. Frequently dystonia affects one foot on the same side affected by bradykinesia. You and your doctor might at first attribute such symptoms to other causes: a sports injury or arthritis, for example.

As noted in the section "How they differ, earlier in the chapter, the genetic element (see also Chapter 2) seems to be more prevalent in YOPD patients than older PD patients. Therefore, your doctor may order a test to rule out one of the known genetic variants associated with PD. If you agree to have this DNA test, be sure you ask to see a certified genetic consultant in order to discuss all the implications (emotional and practical) of this test for you and your family.

Handling the diagnosis: A positive attitude is the best offense

Get ready for a ride on the emotional roller coaster after you get the diagnosis. Your initial reaction may range from disbelief, to denial, to anger, to all of the above, and then some. Your mind may rocket from image to image. Will you see your kids grow up, graduate school, and marry? Will you be able to work and support yourself and your family? What about the dreams you had of traveling, starting your own business, running that marathon? What about those words *no cure*?

Give yourself some time to mourn the fact that your life doesn't — for the moment — seem to be headed in the direction you had hoped. And then get on with it. This is the life you have. Everyone has to deal with challenges and tough choices at some point in life. PD is yours.

REMEMBER

Because you're under 50 (even under 40), you have young onset PD, which has no cure — yet. However, take heart from these thoughts:

>> **Treatments exist.** Researchers have already developed proven techniques and therapies for managing and treating symptoms.

>> **You have time.** You can maintain function and a relatively normal lifestyle over a period of years and — in your case — possibly decades.

>> **PD isn't considered fatal.** You won't die from Parkinson's disease.

>> **You can flourish.** Much of the life you imagined is still within your reach. The odds are very good that you can

- See your children (or your nieces and nephews, or your best friend's kids) grow up to become amazing adults.

- Continue working for years to come and even realize the dream of starting a second career.

- Travel. Why not (see Chapter 17 for travel tips)? Running the marathon may be a little trickier, but not completely out of the question.

- Get very good at finding ways to adapt PD to goals that are really important to you. If your goal is to leave a lower carbon footprint, you may travel by bike whenever possible. But when traditional biking becomes a problem, why not consider an electric bike?

And the best defense is a good offense

Okay, so you've taken time to digest the diagnosis, and you have the attitude thing going. (Check out the preceding section for guidance on these aspects of handling a YOPD diagnosis.) Now what? Take a look at the following sections to keep moving in the right direction.

Brain power

Mark Twain said there are three kinds of lies — lies, damned lies, and statistics. You can choose to believe the statistics and project them onto the rest of your life, or you can refuse to be a statistic. You probably already realize that you're unique, and therefore you should custom design your PD management for you as an individual (with your care team — see Chapter 6). But first, get to work educating yourself (and your family and friends) about this diagnosis.

REMEMBER

You've already taken a positive step by picking up this book. It's chock-full of chapters that offer information for anyone living with PD — young or not-so-young. After you read it (or parts of it) — and, of course, share it with people close to you, including your doctor(s) — keep it handy. While you make this journey with PD, use this book as a guide to the resources you need along the way.

Carpe diem: Seize the day!

The overriding emotion you may feel early on is a sense that you've totally lost control of your life. But you can only lose control if you surrender your life — if you choose to hand it over to someone else and simply follow other people's orders. You can follow a better approach to PD for you and your care partner — one that gives you the best chance of living the life you planned before the diagnosis.

Without going all the way to Pollyanna levels, consider the advantages of a can-do and optimistic outlook:

>> **Time becomes more precious** and can trigger the determination not to waste an hour or a day. Nothing can make you get off your butt, take that trip, write that novel, or go back to school like a progressive illness can.

>> **Close relationships can strengthen** — marriages, parent-child connections (yours as a parent and yours as the child of aging parents), and friendships can all find new depth. Genuine and dedicated friends stick; hangers-on don't (and you may be surprised by who's who in the bunch).

>> **New people come into your life,** and they're interesting and stimulating, understanding and fun. You may find the opportunity to work with other people to make a real difference in the lives of millions. How many people do you know who can say that? (See the section "Your role in the community," later in this chapter.)

>> **You're getting a fresh start** and the real chance to change yourself. Suddenly, you understand — in a very real way — that life *is* finite.

Staying on track in your career

A question that's bound to be at the top of your mind is whether you can continue working. On so many levels, your ability to pursue a career, run a business, or maintain financial security is integral to living the life you envisioned. Be sure to read Chapter 16 for a full discussion of PD in the workplace.

One of the key messages you want to send to your employer, coworkers, and yourself is that *the prognosis of YOPD is good.* With proper management of PD symptoms through exercise, diet, and medications, your career can be good to go for years to come. When your PD doctor, physical therapist, and nutritionist fully understand your job's requirements, they can structure your care plan (and timing of meds when you begin taking them) to provide optimal function when you need it most.

WARNING

Stress can pack a double whammy when it comes to maintaining your job and career. Stress comes with the territory in many (make that *most*) jobs, and it can do a real number on your YOPD symptoms. Take a look at Chapter 16 for ways to manage stressful situations in the workplace — a huge step toward successfully maintaining your position or even advancing your place at work for years to come.

Dealing with YOPD's impact on relationships

REMEMBER

Make sure that the people in your life remember that you're still you! Now that you have PD, your diagnosis can become the two-ton gorilla in the room, sitting squarely between you and other people — if you let it. When you fear that your lover, child, best friend, or coworker can't see you because PD's in the way, then take the initiative. By addressing PD issues that may affect your most important relationships, you can remove that gorilla from the room.

Your role as a spouse or significant other

The roles you and your partner have settled into may undergo quite a makeover while your PD progresses. Fortunately, this progression usually occurs over a period of years with ample time to adjust. But that delay doesn't mean you can't or shouldn't prepare for necessary changes. In other words, begin communicating now. Communication and patience are your best resources for adapting later to these inevitable changes. See Chapters 5 and 6 for information about next steps and creating a game plan.

TIP

Don't rush into changes before you need them. But do take time to plan with your partner the ways that you can adjust certain tasks or roles before you give them up.

While your symptoms progress and your medication timing unexpectedly switches into on-off mode, your spouse or significant other may find it tough to believe that you're suddenly struggling with a task that you managed fine just a minute earlier. Be honest about what's going on. Acknowledge that it looks like you don't want to do this task, but — for now — you really can't. Communication and patience are paramount here!

Another common concern when you have YOPD is the question of intimacy. Okay, to put it bluntly — you're wondering about its impact on your ability to perform sexually. The answer: If you experience a change in your sexual desire, performance, or pleasure, a host of underlying causes are possible.

REMEMBER

PD may cause sexual dysfunction, but this symptom usually occurs several years into the progression of the disease, and other symptoms (side effects of meds, stress, anxiety, and the like) can play a role. Don't simply assume that a change in your desire for intimacy or ability to make love is a normal part of PD. Solutions are available, so talk to your doctor and look at Chapter 15 for more information on sexual dysfunction.

TIP

Maintain a sense of humor. Surely, even at your healthiest, you had those moments — embarrassing, silly, laugh-out-loud times when it all went haywire at a critical moment. Plan to roll with them. Shared laughter can be incredibly sexy.

Your role as a parent

How life may change for you and your kids depends on their ages when you're diagnosed. If they're very young, you can keep the news simple and guide your children while they grow up and your symptoms progress. By the time they reach their middle or high school years, living with a parent who has PD will seem so normal that it'll be their friends' parents who seem different.

If your children are older (middle or high school) when you're diagnosed, you may have more trouble communicating with them. At this age, your children are dealing with a lot already. They're trying to locate their own sense of identity among their peers and within the family unit, they're trying to live up to adult expectations, and they're facing ever-escalating pressure to make the right choices. No wonder they shut down sometimes!

Now you come along and deliver the news that you have PD — a disease that they may have heard of, but they may know only some real misinformation about it. Depending on their age and your relationship, your children may or may not ask questions, but don't assume that they have none. On the other hand, dole out information carefully. You may hear "TMI!" (too much information) from your teen when you start throwing around terms such as *bradykinesia*, *substantia nigra*, and such. See Chapter 7 for ideas about sharing information with children of various ages.

TIP

If you have teens or middle-schoolers, you may want to ask them for help in researching information. They're undoubtedly proficient on the computer. Give them a focused PD topic to research and guidelines for differentiating information from misinformation; then ask them to share their findings with the family. For example, you could put them to work locating and bookmarking the best PD websites for the family. What organizations can they find? What are the strengths of each site? By proactively including your children in a management plan for your PD, you take away a lot of their fear and distress that can come from being left out of key discussions and decisions.

Your role as a friend

If you're fortunate enough to have a network of close friends — even if that network is only two or three people — you have a fabulous resource for coping with your PD. Friends can listen when you really don't want to burden your spouse or significant other. And they can take your focus off PD to get you back on the track of living the life you'd planned. Friends can make you laugh and let you cry. They can push, shove, and irritate you until you'll do anything to get them off your case. They can admire your courage, wonder at your ability to contain this beast, and celebrate each passage — just like they did when you didn't have PD, and just like you've done for them.

Friendship is a two-way street. Your friends can only be there if you let them, and they'll be there for the long term only if you let them know you'll do the same for them. For more ideas on PD and friendships, see Chapter 15.

Your role as a coworker/employee/employer

By some estimates, up to one-third of PWP (at any age) are actively employed. While the news of your diagnosis spreads at work, your coworkers probably take one of two positions: Some immediately come forward, express their concern, and ask what they can do to help; others pull back, taking a let's-see-how-this-goes position.

Like with all your relationships, this one is yours to manage. Frankly, to make sure you are the one driving the conversation, let people know that you have PD (after you tell your employer). Otherwise, your messenger becomes the rumor mill. Consider sitting down with members of your department (with your supervisor's approval) to give them some brief, basic facts about YOPD. You can then ask these coworkers to use these facts to squelch rumors they may hear around the business.

If you're the employer (or department head), be aware of immediate employee concerns for you *and* for themselves. What does your PD mean for the future of the business and their job security? Again, carefully prepare by anticipating questions and concerns (from good employees seeking other positions or ambitious staffers eyeing your position), about both you and your business.

Whatever you do, you need to realistically assess (and reassess regularly and frequently) your ability to handle the job.

Your role in the community

You get much more from maintaining (or instigating) community relationships than just the personal returns. When you volunteer at your child's school or join in for a charity walk or bike event, you're making a better world for others — and that's empowering. You're not this poor PWP; you're someone who chooses to take advantage of an opportunity to make a real difference for yourself and the community around you.

TIP

Speaking of community action, get involved with the well-organized Parkinson community — at the national, regional, and local levels. By taking an active role in advocating for more research dollars, better therapies, and eventually a cure, you empower yourself and other PWP. Not a marcher or the outspoken sort? Not a problem. Check out www.parkinson.org/get-involved or any of the national organizations listed in Appendix B of this book for ways you can get involved behind the scenes.

The Dollars and Cents of YOPD Financial Planning

Definition of *terrifying*: The experience of persons in the prime of life getting news that they have a chronic and progressively debilitating illness. Although people who have YOPD can hope for a cure in their lifetime, unfortunately, they can't realistically base their financial futures on such a pipedream.

You'll live with PD for many years to come; years that may include getting married, raising a family, developing a successful business, traveling the world, securing the future for your partner, caring for aging parents — a host of situations that can create emotional and financial challenges. Our suggestion? Regardless of your economic status, take your partner to a financial planner *now* (see Chapter 21 for tips on choosing one) to help you plan for the future.

TIP

With financial planning, you're wise to prepare for the worst scenario. You may ask, "But what if I never need to put the plans in action?" The best answer is a different, more challenging question: What if you *do* need to?

If you haven't already done so, take time to ask the big questions:

» What benefits do I get through my current health insurance plan?

» What hospitalization, disability benefits, and programs can I get through my work?

>> What are the benefits and limitations of the COBRA program if I have to stop working?

>> What long-term care insurance program can I (or my partner) benefit from?

>> Am I eligible for that program?

WARNING

If you have no health insurance, talk to your financial planner immediately about options that you may qualify for in your state or through federal programs. If the financial planner can't answer your questions or provide information in a timely manner, find another planner.

For a more detailed discussion of legal and financial concerns that need your attention sooner rather than later, turn to Chapter 20.

CONNECTING WITH OTHER YOPDers

"I have plenty of friends," you say, "so I don't need to connect." Oh, but you do. You have a condition that usually strikes people decades older than you. You have a chronic, progressive condition that's going to impact every facet of your life. On top of that, you have this life — of work, and relationships, and social events, and community functions, and so on. So, over the coming months and years, you're going to have times when the very person you need to talk with is someone who understands what it means to have YOPD, someone who's been there, who's still there — someone who can tell you to knock it off, stop wasting precious time, and get on with your life when you start feeling sorry for yourself.

So where can you find these people? If you're really fortunate, a YOPD support group is close enough for you to conveniently attend meetings. If you can't find a support group near you, then check with the facilitator of any PD support group that meets in your area to see how many of the participants have YOPD. If that fails, ask your PD doctor whether they treat other YOPD patients. If they do, perhaps your doctor can ask these other patients whether they're comfortable exchanging names and contact information with you.

Your best resource may be the Internet:

The Michael J. Fox Foundation at www/michaeljfox.org is a great place to start.

The National Parkinson's Foundation at www.parkinson.org can lead you to a number of good resources. Go to the site, hover over the Living with Parkinson's link, and click the Blog link in the drop-down that appears. On the resulting page, choose Tips for Daily Living from the Category drop-down menu and type young-onset tips in the Keywords text box.

Healthline Media at www.healthline.com is a good source for information about finding a support group that meets your needs. Go to the website, click the Search icon, and type *Parkinson's support group* in the search text box.

The point is that you (and your care partner) can connect with others your age who understand and have experienced or are experiencing many of the same frustrations you are. Your friends and family members may be terrific — supportive and concerned — but how can they possibly understand the full impact of YOPD? Not even your PD doctor can fully appreciate what it means to have PD in the prime of your life.

When you connect with YOPDers, you don't have to give up on friendships that have sustained you (and that still sustain you). But connecting with other YOPDers can lessen your sense of isolation and provide you with resources and news to manage your symptoms in a variety of situations. Another person who has YOPD may not become your new best friend — but then again, don't rule out the possibility.

A Word for the YOPD Care Partner

When you discover that someone you love has a condition that compromises that person's functions and abilities, your instinct may be to go into full caregiver-mode and take charge. Please resist that urge! The person you love is exactly the same person that they were before the diagnosis. PD doesn't change a person overnight. In fact, the changes are gradual enough for the two of you to take the time to adapt, prepare, and plan.

REMEMBER

But you don't want to run away from care partnering, either. Throughout this book, we talk about the fight-or-flight response to tough situations. If you're a person who takes flight (backs away and finds reasons to become disengaged), then you need to reassess that instinct. The person you love and are devoted to needs you — your support and understanding — in the early going, and they may eventually need you to act as their spokesperson and advocate.

If you're a fighter (a person who takes charge or refuses to lose), you may need to dial it down a notch or two. Although you're the care partner, the operative word is *partner*. You're not in charge; you don't have YOPD. Contribute and discuss options — yes. Coax and encourage — absolutely. Defend your right to a life beyond your partner's PD — positively. But in the final analysis, the person with YOPD has the right (as well as the ability) to decide how they want to face this challenge, even should the day come when the person with YOPD relies on you to speak for them. It's called *patient autonomy,* and it's the very foundation of medical ethics.

Comparing LBD to Traditional Onset PD

Actor and comedian Robin Williams and his wife, Susan, thought that he was developing PD, and they set about preparing for that journey. But early on, the motor function symptoms (slowed mobility, muscle stiffness, and the like) were overshadowed by troubling mental disturbances, such as bouts of significant deficits in executive functions (such as problem-solving or judgment).

According to the Lewy Body Dementia Association (www.lbda.org), Robin certainly was not alone. By LBDA estimates, as many as 1.4 million Americans currently suffer from LBD. Like with YOPD, scientists don't yet know the cause of LBD; and furthermore, like with Alzheimer's Disease, doctors can't make a definitive diagnosis until the person dies and they can perform an autopsy. What we do know is that this disease takes an enormous toll on the person who has LBD, and also on their care partner. But researchers are making progress, so even when dementia becomes a part of the diagnosis, there is hope for PWP and their care partners to continue to enjoy quality of life.

REMEMBER

In the early stage of PD, *Lewy bodies* (abnormal clumps of the protein alpha-synuclein) are present in the parts of the brain that control motor/movement functions. In later stages, parts of the brain that control things such as memory, problem-solving, and the like may become affected in a condition defined as *Parkinson disease dementia* (PDD). As described in the chapter introductory paragraphs, in dementia with Lewy bodies (DLB), the Lewy bodies attack the parts of the brain that deal with cognitive function much earlier, even before the more common movement signs of PD. Both disorders share the same underlying changes in the brain and present with similar symptoms, but the symptoms appear in a different order depending on where the Lewy bodies first form.

How do you get an accurate diagnosis of LBD?

Doctors have no easy way to diagnose LBD. Your best option is to find a specialist — a neurologist or movement disorders physician — who most likely will

>> Take a full medical history, focusing on your (and your care partner's) detailed descriptions of the troubling symptoms that caused you to seek help.

>> Conduct extensive physical and neurological exams, including a neuropsychological screening test called MoCA (for Montreal Cognitive Assessment).

>> Use bloodwork and brain imaging to rule out other possible causes, such as clinical depression, a tumor, or some other reversible issue.

If everything points to some form of Parkinson-related dementia, the doctor then wants to distinguish between dementia with Lewy bodies (DLB) and the Parkinson disease dementia (PDD) that can come in the later stages of the disease. One key element in making that distinction involves the timing of when symptoms begin:

>> If cognitive symptoms appear at the same time or even before movement symptoms, the doctor will likely diagnose dementia with Lewy bodies

>> If cognitive problems come later — more than three to five years after you notice impairment to your motor skills — the doctor will probably diagnose Parkinson's disease dementia

In either case, to deal with the diagnosis, you need to work with a team of experts who will help you plan for the future. Fortunately, across the U.S., a network of medical/academic/research institutions, known as Research Centers of Excellence, provide people diagnosed with LBD and their care partners the latest updates on care, treatment, and research. To find the Research Center nearest to you, go to www.lbda.org/research/research-centers-of-excellence and use the map. Clicking on a location on this map pulls up the contact information for that location.

What are the symptoms of LBD?

An onset of problems with mental acuity — including loss of executive function (planning and processing information); memory; the ability to understand visual information; or fluctuations in cognition, attention, or alertness — can signal LBD. A person dealing with LBD may exhibit some of the following additional symptoms:

>> **Visual hallucinations:** Seeing things that aren't present

>> **Sleep disorders:** Such as acting out one's dreams while asleep

>> **Behavioral and mood indicators:** Including depression, apathy, anxiety, agitation, delusions, or paranoia

>> **Changes in normal body functions:** Including blood pressure control, temperature regulation, and bladder and bowel habits.

REMEMBER

Not all symptoms present at the same time, and notably, symptoms may come and go. The person seems fine one minute, and then they become agitated or paranoid seemingly out of the blue.

How do you treat LBD?

Like with traditional PD, doctors don't yet have a cure for LBD. Even so, people who have LBD can benefit from and even improve with treatments that may include a combination of medications and therapies that target the specific behavioral symptoms. Some medicines developed for people who have Alzheimer's disease can help those who have LBD, as well, by improving cognition and mental alertness. These meds can also help reduce the occurrence of hallucinations and sleep disturbances.

If you've begun to experience the loss of motor function (muscle stiffness, tremor, and the like), medicines meant to treat the movement issues of PD may be part of your LBD regimen, as well. But you and your doctor will need to find a balance because the meds for PD can sometimes contribute to problems with confusion and hallucinations for people who have either form of LBD.

REMEMBER

Research has found that traditional antipsychotic drugs doctors often prescribe to patients for depression or anxiety can actually backfire when used by a person who has LBD, making the condition worse. Be sure your primary care doctor (and any specialist treating you for a separate condition such as arthritis or a lung condition) is aware of the danger of these drugs for PWP. That said, antipsychotics that are safe for PWPs, including quetiapine (*Seroquel*), pimavanserin (*Nuplazid*), and clozapine (*Clozaril*), do exist.

WARNING

Like with any medication, side effects can occur with whatever regimen your doctor prescribes, especially if you're taking prescription meds for other conditions, such as a heart issue or diabetes. In addition, if you're struggling with sleep or urinary urgency issues, you must avoid any over-the-counter aids promising to help unless your doctor suggests adding them.

What therapies can help people with LBD?

Because your doctor and you can find it tricky to get the balance of drug therapy just right, the Mayo Clinic recommends trying targeted therapies, such as

>> **Beginning with your surroundings:** Get rid of the clutter and make use of labels on drawers and cabinets that can serve as cues when memory lapses occur.

>> **Sticking to simple routines:** Post a list of daily tasks that you need to complete (grooming, dressing, eating, taking meds, and such). Work with your care partner to break each task into simple steps that you perform at approximately the same time each day.

>> **Sharing the work:** Remember how when you were in school, you might have someone check your homework? That's not a bad habit to adopt now. Keep doing the things you managed before LBD, but have your care partner check your results — and celebrate any success.

>> **Accepting the illogical or odd behavior:** Share this idea with anyone who's likely to travel this road with you. Many care partners make the classic mistake of trying to apply reason to or correct the behavior of a person dealing with dementia. *Note:* Unless the person who has LBD is in danger of harming themselves or someone else, the best response is reassurance — and even validation. You can tell them that you believe they see the purple polka-dotted cow.

A Word for the LBD Care Partner

You may feel like you and the person whom you love — the one who has some form of Lewy body dementia (LBD) — drew the short straw on this one. But the good news is that you are both still here, and while the life you planned may not be the life you are living, find the blessings and joy in what you have. Keep in mind that, like with any chronic disease, you don't get an absolute road map to follow. You'll undoubtedly make a few wrong turns, but you can do this.

Tools and tips for dealing with LBD

Basic techniques and activities available for making life more pleasant and productive while caring for someone suffering from LBD include

>> **Getting physical:** Exercise is good for anyone, but for the person dealing with any form of dementia, a walk outdoors, a swim, or a bike ride can calm anxiety and perhaps even slow the progression of mental decline.

>> **Puzzling it out:** Whether you go with a jigsaw or crossword puzzle, a simple card game, or some other mind game, activities that require basic skills in thinking can help the person with LBD focus and find much-needed moments of success.

>> **Creating a masterpiece:** Do something artsy. Make music. Organize a singalong.

>> **Socializing:** Invite friends to join the two of you for an evening out, a walk, or a cup of coffee. Continue to attend group gatherings, such as book club discussions, concerts, or religious services.

REMEMBER

>> **Keeping it simple and direct:** When communicating with your partner who has LBD, take your time and focus. Any negative sign from you, such as impatience or dismissal, can trigger even more anxiety in the person who has LBD. This anxiety, in turn, can trigger resistance to the very engagement that you're trying to accomplish.

TIP

Find out how to deal with *sundowning*. Simply put, when the sun starts to set, symptoms such as anxiety and confusion may escalate for people who have dementia, including people who have LBD. While currently there is no identified cause, the same habits that apply for anyone wanting a good night's sleep can work here:

>> Limit naps and caffeine during the day. Replace them with exercise and activity.

>> Turn off the TV (at least in the bedroom) but leave a nightlight on.

>> Take a cue from the way you might calm an overactive child at bedtime — read them a story, play some soothing music, or lie with them until they fall asleep.

And don't forget yourself

Two people are in this fight — the person who has LBD and *you*. The plain truth is that you can't give care unless you take care — of yourself. Over time, while you deal with the day-to-day roller coaster of caring for someone who has dementia, you're bound to have moments when the frustration and downright anger (often followed by guilt) seem overwhelming.

Recognize that you're doing your best, but you can't do it all (or all the time) without help. Take a moment to check out the Caregiver's Bill of Rights found in Chapter 19. Then, start looking for ways you can continue to care — for both of you:

>> **Asking for help:** Friends and family may want to step up but don't know exactly how to do that. Or in their absence, consider paying for occasional help to give you a break.

>> **Caring for your physical needs:** You need exercise and a healthy diet as much as the person who has LBD does.

>> **Finding a support group:** Take advantage of the comradery and understanding that you can find in such a group. If you don't have a specific group for LBD in your area, consider joining a group for Alzheimer's disease care partners.

At times, you may feel like you're alone in this fight to secure a quality of life for the PWP—and for yourself, but you don't have to let that be the case. You have resources that you can draw upon. Check out Appendix B for some great places to start.

3

Crafting a Treatment Plan Just for You

Keep yourself healthy through good sleep, diet, and exercise to slow the disease's progress.

Discover prescription medications to help you manage your Parkinson's disease.

Weigh the risks and benefits of surgery.

Treat your PD with complementary and alternative therapies.

Address any anxiety and depression that you experience.

Help find a cure (or improve treatments) by taking part in clinical trials.

IN THIS CHAPTER

» **Eating to live versus living to eat**

» **Treating night sleep like your best friend**

» **Improving mobility and mood through exercise and activity**

» **Focusing on maintaining flexibility**

» **Stabilizing through strengthening exercises**

» **Getting (and staying) physical**

» **Empowering the mind and spirit**

Chapter **9**

Eat Well, Sleep Well, and Exercise

You got the bad news, but you're determined to fight Parkinson's disease (PD) tooth and nail. You fielded your A-team and chose your medical professionals (see Chapter 6). And you're probably ready to take medications for the rest of your life. Now consider this: Although no cure for PD exists at the time of this writing and medications only alleviate the symptoms of the disease, we know that lifestyle modifications can significantly influence the inevitable progression of PD. Before you review the medical strategies for treating PD, take a thorough look at your lifestyle — and make positive changes. Doing this can go a long way toward keeping PD from adversely affecting your quality of life. And most importantly, it helps get you back in control!

You've heard it since you were a child — *go to bed early, eat right, and exercise!* But, for people with Parkinson's (PWP) and their care partners, we can't overemphasize the importance of eating a proper diet, getting a full night of uninterrupted sleep (consistently), and establishing a regular program of exercise. The resulting benefits go well beyond physical fitness to bring relief from the general stresses of living with a chronic, progressive disease. In addition, a good diet, proper night rest, and regular exercise help fight off the anxiety and depression that can so often accompany PD. With or without PD, you owe it to yourself to be as rested and fit — physically, mentally, and spiritually — as possible. How else are you going to participate fully in life?

In this chapter, you can find out how good health isn't about training for a marathon or depriving yourself of the social life or foods that you love. It's about making the choices that give you the best chance of living well and pursuing the pleasures of your life for many years — in spite of PD.

The Joy of Good Food — Diet and Nutrition

According to the National Institute of Aging, the combined effects of not making the right food choices and not being physically active make up the second largest underlying cause of death (behind smoking) in the United States. Often, the element most absent from the diets of Americans is *nutrition*, foods that provide the proteins, carbohydrates, vitamins, minerals, hydration, fiber, and — yes — fats that the body needs to operate at its best. Add to that the fact that PD medications and symptoms can significantly reduce the pleasures of eating, and you have a situation ripe for disaster.

The following sections don't focus on losing those extra 20 pounds; they discuss making the best food and nutrition choices to maintain optimal health while you fight the progression of PD.

Balance is the key

As a PWP, you have to perform a real balancing act when it comes to your diet. Along with the ready-made factors that impact nutrition and diet (such as age, gender, and physical fitness), you have to deal with the nutritional sideshows of PD. For example, side effects of medications may include loss of appetite or even nausea. While your PD progresses, swallowing and constipation can become issues. And you may have side effects from medications for other chronic conditions, such as high blood pressure, diabetes, or arthritis.

Finding the proper balance between a healthy diet and these PD issues may require the help of a professional, so your PD doctor may prescribe a consultation with a nutritionist or dietician as part of your treatment plan. If not, in Appendix B, we include links to additional resources for diet and exercise advice that you may find helpful.

WARNING

Be sure that you and your PD doctor discuss the timing of meals and medications to offset potential problems with their interactions. Timing the dosing of your medications (see Chapter 10) with meals is always important, but especially so for meals that include significant servings of protein. Protein — although essential for a balanced diet — can compete with the absorption of your antiparkinsonian meds. The usual recommendation is to take medication at least 30 minutes before meals. But if you experience nausea or *dyskinesia* (uncontrolled twisting, writhing motions) after taking your medications, you may need to consider these adjustments to your routine:

>> **If nausea is the problem,** your doctor may recommend you have a low-protein snack with your meds, such as crackers or some other carbohydrate-based snack such as yogurt, fresh or dried fruit, or pretzels.

>> **If dyskinesia occurs,** ask your PD doctor about timing of meals and medications to offset this problem.

Banishing the bad and embracing the good-for-you foods

No doubt you've seen the food pyramid recommended by the U.S. Department of Agriculture. But now you can create a plan tailored to your specific gender, age, weight, and height. (See www.myplate.gov/myplate-plan.) You probably know you should keep your intake of fats and oils (not to mention desserts) to a minimum and spend most of your calories on fruits, veggies, whole grains, and dairy. (By the way, a banana split doesn't count in your fruit and dairy allowance!). But your normal food habits, coupled with having PD, may call for reinforcements. Presumably, you're prepared to fight this PD that's parked like a tank in your designated space. And your diet can be a formidable weapon, if properly understood and used. See the sidebar "Questions and answers for your PD diet" (in this chapter) for more diet information.

With that said, a nutritionist or dietician can really help show you how to adapt your needs to your lifestyle when you follow steps like these:

1. **Tell your dietician or nutritionist how you normally eat.**

   Are you on the run, in your car, standing at the kitchen counter, or seated with the family at the table? Do you eat at home with meals you prepare, in fine restaurants, or at fast-food joints?

2. **Reveal your food weaknesses to the chosen professional.**

   Let them know that you hate veggies, love bread, and so on.

3. **Work with the professional to build a food plan that fits your lifestyle and your likes and dislikes.**

Before choosing a nutritionist, make sure you investigate their level of expertise as it relates to PD. If you can't meet with a nutritionist, you can find the diets most commonly recommended for PWP, listed in Table 9-1, through the Mayo Clinic (www.mayoclinic.org).

TABLE 9-1   **Healthy Diets for PWP**

Name	Benefits	Search Term to Use at www.mayoclinic.org
Mediterranean Diet	Heart health	Mediterranean diet
MIND Diet	Brain health	MIND diet

TECHNICAL STUFF

QUESTIONS AND ANSWERS FOR YOUR PD DIET

Ask (and answer) a few simple questions to establish an approach to diet that supports your PD lifestyle efforts:

What is a good diet for PD, and why is it good?

Can foods affect the progression of PD, and what are they?

What is the microbiome, and why is it important?

When it comes to PD, in addition to general guidance from the government recommended food pyramid, other — more specific — dietary information may be useful. For example, several large population studies show that a diet rich in vitamin E may be beneficial to brain aging in general and abnormal brain aging (such as Parkinson's and Alzheimer's diseases) by association. We don't mean vitamin E pills, mind you, but we do mean a diet rich in vitamin E, which includes foods such as vegetable oils, nuts, avocados, and some fish.

Can diet have a role in the progression of PD? Apparently yes. According to a study by Dr. Mischley at Bastyr University, two to four servings per week of certain foods are consistently associated with slower than average progression of PD, while other foods seem to somehow make PD progression worse.

The good foods: Fresh herbs, vegetable oils, nuts and seeds, fresh fruits and vegetables, fish, and wine appear to be good for PD.

The bad foods (some of which are the usual suspects): Canned fruit and vegetables, frozen and fried foods, soda, and of course, ice cream. Others that make the bad list may surprise you, for example, milk and yogurt, pork, chicken, and beef.

When you eat, you not only feed your body, but you also feed some trillions of bacteria living in your guts. These bacteria are collectively known as the *microbiome,* and they serve many good purposes in our life, including helping to digest food, regulating the immune system, protecting against other bacteria that may cause disease, and producing key vitamins such as B12 and K.

As an integral part of the *gut-brain axis* (a bidirectional communication between the central and the enteric nervous systems), the microbiome can also affect the brain, playing a role in brain diseases like PD. And sure enough, PD seems to be associated with microbiome alterations, resulting in too many bacteria fed by milk products and animal proteins and too few of those fed by dietary fibers from fruits, vegetables, and nuts. Got the point? Make sure to feed your friends and starve your enemies!

Focus on these key issues when you start filling your plate (or glass):

» **Water, water, water:** Flavor it with a slice of lemon or a little fruit juice if you can't take it straight, but drink six to eight big glasses every day. (And, no — soda, coffee, and tea don't count.) Caffeine beverages may increase *diuresis* (your amount of urine output) and, as a result, cancel your efforts to hydrate your body. *Note:* Some studies have shown that caffeine may reduce the risk of PD for some people, so caffeine in moderation probably won't hurt — and may help.

» **Fiber:** Whole-grain breads (not the mushy white stuff), brown rice, and whole-wheat pasta. In fact, stay away from white foods, in general. Green leafy vegetables, whole grains, and nuts are rich natural sources of fiber that may have a protective effect against PD (see Chapter 12 for more info on diet as therapy).

TIP

According to the National Institutes of Health (NIH), whole grains are not only a form of healthy carbohydrates for your heart, but they are also a primary energy source for your brain because they contain vital nutrients essential for cognitive function, such as zinc and B vitamins.

>> **Bone-strengthening nutrients:** Calcium, magnesium, and vitamins D and K. Think dairy products and, believe it or not, exposure to sunlight (which actually triggers your body to produce vitamin D).

Also, regular exercise (which we discuss in the section "Use It or Lose It — The Healing Power of Exercise and Activity," later in this chapter) can help you keep bones strong, maintain balance, and prevent the falls so devastating for PWP.

REMEMBER

Although your doctor may recommend adding supplements (such as a daily mul-tivitamin, iron, vitamin D, or calcium pill) to your regular diet, the key word here is *supplement*. Such products can't substitute for a nutritionally balanced diet.

But you may find that you can prepare delicious, good-for-you foods more easily than you imagine. One example is the fabulous fruit smoothie: Throw berries, half a banana, a cup of fat-free yogurt, and some ice cubes in a blender. Add a teaspoon of ground flax seed for fiber, turn the blender on high, pour the milkshake–like concoction into your car mug, and you're good to go. Smoothies that contain foods rich in probiotics (yogurt, for example) can also help prevent the constipation associated with PD medications.

Food as celebration

If, like millions of Americans, you find yourself stuck in a rut when it comes to when, what, and where you eat, think about spicing those meals up. The following list includes ideas for making meals more of a celebration than an afterthought:

>> **Choose your setting to match the menu, the mood, and the season** — dining room, kitchen table; inside, outside; at home or at a sidewalk café.

>> **Set the table,** even if it's just for one.

>> **Think *S.H.E.*—** simple, healthy, and engaging — when cooking at home.

>> **Try adding special (non-salt) seasonings and flavorings** to spice up your food and make it more enjoyable.

>> **Be adventurous** when eating out or cooking at home; try new dishes you've never tasted.

TIP

Request a spoon when you order items such as rice or small veggies (peas, corn, and such) in a restaurant. A spoon may make these foods easier to manage if you have a tremor.

>> **Savor food with all your senses** — the vision of healthy food presented well; the smells, tastes, and textures; even the sounds of laughter and conversation interspersed with clinking dishes and glasses.

Food is essential for life — and as a PWP, you understand the importance of celebrating every moment.

Stoking Your Brain Health with Consistent Night Sleep

Who doesn't appreciate a full night of sleep? I'm sure you love a refreshed morning feeling that leads to a positive mood and a productive day. Unfortunately, experiencing that feeling may occur less and less as you grow older. According to the National Institute of Aging, older individuals tend to go to sleep and wake up earlier than they did at a younger age. Although older people may not get enough night sleep for a variety of reasons — some of which apply specifically to PD — the idea that older adults need less night sleep than younger individuals is a myth.

The fact that you may have difficulty getting the sleep you need doesn't mean that you need the sleep any less. In fact, the National Sleep Foundation guidelines recommend that people over 65, just like younger adults, should get seven to eight hours of sleep every night.

REMEMBER

So why do older folks tend to sleep less? Like hair thinning and turning grey or skin losing that youthful smoothness, people's natural sleep architecture tends to deteriorate with age. In particular, the proportion of two fundamental pillars of sleep — *slow-wave* (deep stage) and *REM sleep* (when you dream) — decreases with age. (You don't need to be an architect to imagine that having your house pillars begin to creak is bad news.) In addition, the production of sleep-related hormones changes with age. For example, melatonin levels decline gradually with aging, and this decline relates to decreased sleep efficacy. Ask your doctor if supplementing melatonin may be a good idea.

Examining sleep disorders

Unfortunately, the deterioration of sleep quality with aging is more often due to a series of mental and physical health problems that could include depression, anxiety, heart disease, diabetes, or conditions that cause pain, such as arthritis and back troubles. Abnormalities that are specific to sleep, such as restless leg syndrome, REM sleep behavior disorder, or sleep apnea are also possible causes of sleep deterioration. These conditions deserve extra attention because they happen frequently in PD and have predictable (but treatable) negative effects on the quality of PWPs' sleep.

>> **Restless leg syndrome (RLS)** can be a condition separate from PD but is a common problem for PWPs. The syndrome causes tingling sensations that result in an irresistible urge to move your legs, particularly when lying in bed at night. RLS can cause more than a sleepless night if not properly addressed and treated. The good news is that it usually responds very well to the same dopaminergic drugs used to relieve PD symptoms (see Chapter 10).

>> **REM sleep behavior disorder (RBD),** a condition in which you talk in your sleep or seem to act out your dreams, is intimately connected to PD. As we discuss in Chapter 3, RBD can be an important early indicator of PD because it usually occurs before the typical neurological symptoms of PD develop.

>> **Sleep apnea** is also very common in PD, to the point that sleep apnea is considered one of the possible risk factors of PD. If you snore loudly and feel tired even after a full night of sleep, you might have sleep apnea, a condition in which your breathing repeatedly stops and starts.

WARNING

Sleep apnea is a serious sleep disorder. In fact, it has been (sardonically) defined as a *silent killer*. Patients with severe sleep apnea die, on average, ten years sooner than those with normal sleep. Up to 85 percent of those who suffer from sleep apnea don't know that they have it. If you snore loudly or your bed partner notices that you stop breathing (for more than a few seconds) during the night, you should consult your doctor and have a sleep study test (called a *polysomnography*).

Results of sleep loss

So what's the big deal about losing a few hours of sleep? After all, don't *they* say that the early bird catches the worm? One scenario is to wake up early in the morning after a full eight-hour, uninterrupted night of sleep; another is to wake up several times during the night and log in only four or five hours. The recognized consequences of chronic sleep deprivation are multiple and scary, as shown in Table 9-2.

The consequences in Table 9-2 may sound familiar because many of the symptoms of PD overlap with those of sleep deprivation. In fact, a good Parkinson's specialist may often spend more time discussing your nighttime problems than your daytime problems.

TIP

Be aware of the so-called *sleep stealers* and try to avoid them. For example, avoid caffeinated beverages in the afternoon or evening, and excessive screen time (whether in front of the TV or your laptop) before bedtime. Lack of exercise is another known sleep stealer (see the next section for more about the benefits of exercise). Also, certain medications taken too close to bedtime — including some of the dopaminergic drugs used to control PD symptoms (see Chapter 10) — can adversely affect your sleep.

TABLE 9-2

Consequences of Sleep Deprivation

Increased Health Risks	Nagging Daily Symptoms
Chronic depression	Anxiety
Diabetes	Depression
Heart attack	Difficulty concentrating
Hypertension	Fatigue
Obesity	Irritability
Stroke	Memory Loss

REMEMBER

Take any sleep problems seriously, discuss them with your doctor, and adopt appropriate lifestyle changes. This one thing is certain: Your brain cannot function properly without a consistent, restful night of sleep. You'd better hit that sack and sleep like a log every night!

Use It or Lose It — The Real Healing Power of Exercise and Activity

Plenty of research backs up the fact that regular exercise can do wonders for your health, and in the case of PD, regular exercise can actually *slow* the progression of the disease! Consider that exercising regularly

» **Boosts the power of neurotransmitters** in your brain to enhance your mood and your ability to see life in a more positive light.

» **Can relieve the muscle tension** from your body's natural instinct to lock up in the face of challenges or battles.

» **Can enhance your self-image,** which can lead to greater self-assurance and confidence, which can lead to a greater ability to deal with life's stresses.

Talk about a win-win-win!

REMEMBER

Many PWP who exercise regularly experience a milder and less-progressive disease process. In fact, exercise can be as good for brain function as it is for heart and weight factors. Recent studies have shown that physical exercise can potentially reduce the rate at which brain cells die.

Many exercise programs can benefit PWP. A combination of aerobic (walking is a good one), strength-building, and stretching (which we talk about in the following section) is the way to go. You might also add a dose of some activity that promotes agility and balance, such as yoga or tai chi (also outlined as a form of alternative medicine therapy in Chapter 12), or dancing. In any case, experts recommend 150–200 minutes of moderate exercise per week. Okay, don't freak out. That breaks down to about 20–30 minutes a day. You can do that!

The guidelines of a stretching/flexibility exercise program for PD are the same as those for sports-medicine rehabilitation:

» Listen to your body.

» Avoid joint pain during exercise.

» STOP if you experience significant pain, dizziness, or excessive sweating.

» Remember, for mild to moderate joint or other pain following exercise, "Ice is nice; hot is not."

WARNING

Because PD frequently develops in a person's later years, you may already have other bone and joint conditions, such as *osteoarthritis* (wearing of joints) and *osteoporosis* (thinning of the bones). So before you begin any exercise therapy, get the approval of your doctor (preferably your movement disorders specialist) and a prescription to work with a trained, experienced physical therapist.

Dr. Gary Guten — an orthopedic surgeon and one of the original authors of this book's first edition — lived with PD for over 20 years before his death in 2018. A lifelong athlete and marathon runner, Gary knew the benefits of regular exercise long before he received the PD diagnosis. Working with a team of professionals at the Performance Centers of Wheaton Franciscan Healthcare in Milwaukee, Wisconsin, he designed the exercises that we describe and illustrate in the following sections of this chapter. As a PWP, Gary worked to make sure that this exercise routine supplies a program aimed at PWP and specifically addresses the need to stretch and strengthen the key muscle groups for optimal flexibility and balance.

TIP

Begin your exercise routine with the stretching exercises and repeat them during the cool-down period after the strengthening exercises. Your doctor and physical therapist may fine-tune these exercises to match your specific needs, but this program gives you a good starting point.

Stretching to Enhance Flexibility

Always with your movement disorders specialist's or physical therapist's approval, guidance, and ongoing monitoring, do these flexibility exercises every day, even twice a day.

TIP

If you also do strengthening exercises (such as the ones in the section "Strengthening to Build Muscle and Stabilize Joints," later in this chapter) or an aerobic activity, such as walking, bicycling, swimming, or working out on a treadmill, use these stretching exercises to warm up and cool down.

REMEMBER

Stretch your muscles slowly, smoothly, and gently. No bouncing allowed! And if a stretch starts to hurt, listen to your body and ease up.

Neck stretches

Begin your routine by gently stretching the muscles in your neck, head, and shoulders.

To perform the Chin Tuck (5 to 10 reps), follow these steps:

1. **Looking forward, tuck your chin by pulling it in.**

   You should look a little like a turtle (see Figure 9-1).

2. **Hold your chin in the tucked position for five seconds.**

3. **Untuck your chin and relax.**

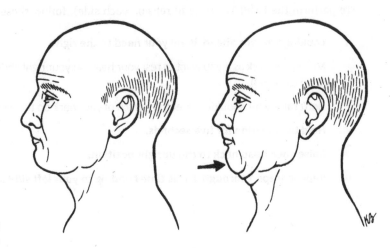

FIGURE 9-1:
The Chin Tuck.

To perform the Head Turn (5 to 10 reps on each side), follow these steps:

1. **Looking straight ahead, slowly turn your head to the right until you're looking at the view to your right (see Figure 9-2).**

   Don't force the movement; at first, you may only be able to turn your head slightly to the right or left; with practice, you can become more flexible.

REMEMBER

2. **Hold the position for five seconds.**

3. **Return your head to center.**

4. **Repeat Steps 1 through 3, this time turning to your left.**

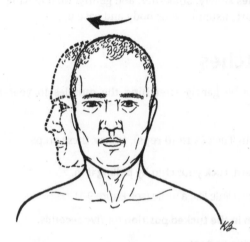

FIGURE 9-2:
The Head Turn.

To perform the Head Tilt (5 to 10 reps on each side), follow these steps:

1. **Looking straight ahead, bend your head to the right.**

   Move your neck as if you want to rest your head on your right shoulder (see Figure 9-3).

   Don't raise your shoulder — let the stretch of your neck do the work.

2. **Hold the position for five seconds.**

3. **Raise your head back to the upright position.**

4. **Repeat Steps 1 through 3, this time bending to your left side.**

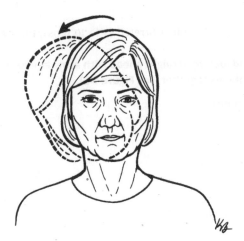

FIGURE 9-3:
The Head Tilt.

To perform the Shoulder Roll (5 to 10 reps each direction), follow these steps:

1. **Standing tall and looking straight ahead, lift and roll both shoulders backward in a circular motion (see Figure 9-4).**

2. **Relax.**

3. **Lift and roll your shoulders forward in a circular motion.**

4. **Relax your shoulders and arms, shaking them out a bit.**

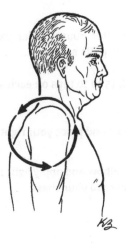

FIGURE 9-4:
The Shoulder
Roll.

To perform the Chest and Shoulder Stretch (5 to 10 reps), follow these steps:

1. **Standing tall and looking straight ahead with arms at your sides, pull your shoulder blades together (see Figure 9-5).**

2. **Hold for five seconds.**

3. **Relax.**

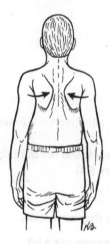

FIGURE 9-5:
The Chest and
Shoulder Stretch.

Upper body stretches

Use the following stretches before and after your regular exercise routine to lengthen your muscles and prevent muscle pulls and tears.

To perform the Posterior Shoulder Stretch (5 to 10 reps on each side), follow these steps:

1. **Reach your right arm across your chest and place your right hand over your left shoulder (see Figure 9-6).**

2. **With your left hand, grasp your right elbow and apply light pressure to the elbow, moving your right arm closer to your chest.**

3. **Hold for five seconds.**

4. **Return your arms to your sides.**

5. **Repeat Steps 1 through 4, this time stretching your left shoulder.**

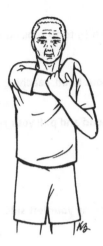

FIGURE 9-6:
The Posterior
Shoulder Stretch.

To perform the Anterior Shoulder Stretch (5 to 10 reps), follow these steps:

1. Reach behind your back and clasp your hands, interlocking your fingers and keeping your arms straight, with elbows turned in (see Figure 9-7).

2. Lift up your arms until you feel a stretch (not pain) in your shoulders and across your chest.

3. Hold your arms in the elevated position for five seconds.

4. Lower your hands and relax.

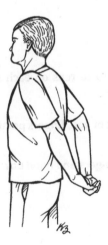

FIGURE 9-7:
The Anterior
Shoulder Stretch.

To perform the Posterior Shoulder Side Stretch (5 to 10 reps on each side), follow these steps:

1. **Raise your right arm above and behind your head, reaching toward your left shoulder (see Figure 9-8).**

2. **With your left hand, reach behind your head and pull your right elbow gently in toward your head.**

3. **Hold for five seconds.**

4. **Relax, returning your arms to your sides.**

5. **Repeat Steps 1 through 4, this time stretching your left side.**

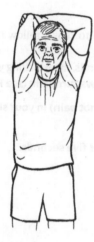

FIGURE 9-8:
The Posterior Shoulder Side Stretch.

To perform the Wrist/Forearm Stretch (5 to 10 reps on each side), follow these steps:

1. **Extend your right arm straight in front of you, fingers pointing toward the floor.**

2. **With your left hand, gently pull your fingers and hand down (see Figure 9-9a).**

   Your arm should remain extended.

3. **Hold for five seconds.**

4. **Release your fingers.**

5. **Flex your right wrist back so that your fingers point to the ceiling.**

6. With your left hand, gently press your fingers and palm back toward your forearm (see Figure 9-9b).

7. Hold for five seconds.

8. Release your fingers.

9. Repeat Steps 1 through 8 five to ten times.

10. Repeat Steps 1 through 9, this time extending your left arm and stretching your left wrist and forearm.

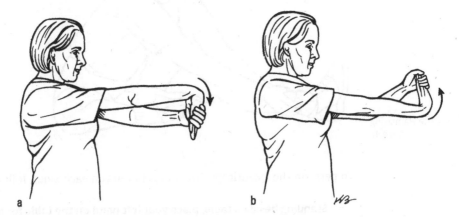

FIGURE 9-9:
The Wrist/
Forearm Stretch.

a   b

Leg stretches

These stretches work on the hips, legs, knees, and ankles. Like with any stretch exercise, they're good before and after your strengthening or aerobic routine to prevent muscle-strain tears and pulls.

To perform the Hamstring Stretch (5–10 reps on each side), follow these steps:

1. Sitting on the floor or a stable raised hard surface with your right leg straight out in front of you, bend your left leg so the bottom of your left foot rests on the inner thigh of your extended right leg (see Figure 9-10).

2. With your hands on your outstretched calf or ankle, slowly bend forward from the waist, keeping your back straight.

   Don't bounce. Stretch only until you feel a mild (non-painful) stretching sensation in the back of your thigh.

3. Hold the stretch for five seconds, and then relax, releasing your calf or ankle and returning to the upright position.

4. Repeat Steps 1 through 3 five to ten times.

5. Repeat Steps 1 through 4, this time extending your left leg and tucking your right leg.

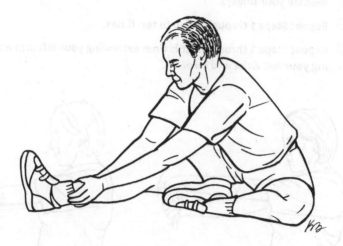

FIGURE 9-10:
The Hamstring
Stretch.

To perform the Quadriceps Stretch (5–10 reps on each side), follow these steps:

1. Standing beside a table, place your left hand on the table for balance.

2. Bending your right knee, grasp your ankle with your right hand and pull your foot backward toward your buttocks (see Figure 9-11).

You can also place a belt or long scarf or beach towel around your ankle and grasp it.

Don't lean forward. Feel the stretch in the front of your thigh.

TIP

3. Hold the stretch for five seconds.

4. Relax, returning your right foot to the floor.

5. Repeat Steps 1 through 4 five to ten times.

6. Turn around (or move to the opposite side of the table) and repeat Steps 1 through 5, this time bending your left knee.

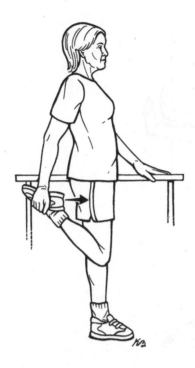

FIGURE 9-11:
The Quadriceps
Stretch.

To perform the Standing Gastroc Stretch (5 to 10 reps on each side), follow these steps:

1. **Standing about 2 feet from the wall, lean forward so that your flattened palms are against the wall.**

2. **Keeping your left foot planted, bend your left knee while you step backward with your right leg.**

3. **Lean forward into the wall until you feel a stretch in your right calf (see Figure 9-12).**

   Your right leg should remain straight, with your heel on the floor and your toes turned slightly outward.

4. **Hold for five seconds.**

5. **Relax, bringing your feet together.**

6. **Repeat Steps 1 through 5 five to ten times.**

7. **Repeat Steps 1 through 6, this time bending your right knee and stepping backward with your left leg.**

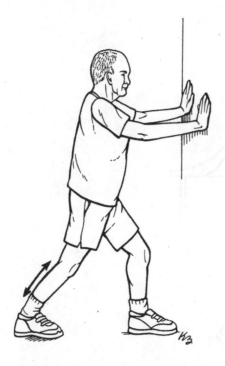

FIGURE 9-12:
The Standing
Gastroc Stretch.

To perform the Inner Thigh (Groin) Stretch (5 to 10 reps), follow these steps:

1. **Sitting on the floor, bend your knees so the soles of your feet face each other (see Figure 9-13).**

2. **Cup your hands around your toes, and gently press down on your thighs with your forearms until you feel a gentle stretch in your inner thighs.**

   Don't bounce your knees — stretch only until you feel a slight pulling sensation in your inner thigh.

3. **Hold for five seconds, and then relax.**

Lower back stretches

The following stretches can protect your back from injury and help you maintain flexibility.

To perform Knees to Chest Stretch (5 to 10 reps on each side), follow these steps:

1. **Lying on your back, slowly raise your right knee to your chest (see Figure 9-14).**

2. Use your hands to hold your knee to your chest; you should feel the stretch in your lower back.

3. Hold this position for five seconds.

4. Relax, returning your right leg to the floor.

5. Repeat Steps 1 through 4 five to ten times.

6. Repeat Steps 1 through 5, this time bringing your left knee to your chest.

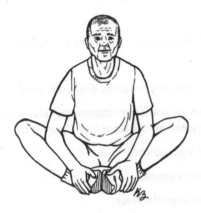

FIGURE 9-13:
The Inner Thigh (Groin) Stretch.

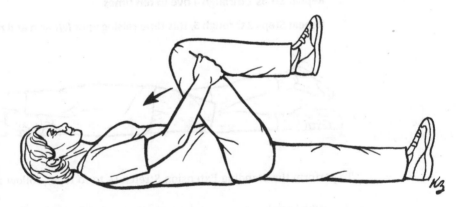

FIGURE 9-14:
The Knees to Chest Stretch.

To perform the Bridging Stretch (5 to 10 reps), follow these steps:

1. Lying on your back with your arms at your sides, bend your knees so that your feet are flat on the floor (see Figure 9-15).

2. Tightening your stomach muscles, slowly raise your buttocks until they're even with your knees.

3. Hold this position for five seconds.

4. Relax, lowering your buttocks to the floor.

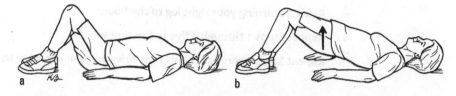

FIGURE 9-15:
The Bridging
Stretch.

To perform the Alternate Arm and Leg Lifts (5 to 10 reps on each side), follow these steps:

1. Lying on your stomach, extend your arms over your head.

2. Tightening your stomach muscles, simultaneously raise your *right* arm and your *left* leg 3 to 6 inches off the floor (see Figure 9-16).

Keep both arms and both legs straight.

3. Hold this position for five seconds.

4. Relax, returning both limbs to the floor.

5. Repeat Steps 2 through 4 five to ten times.

6. Repeat Steps 2 through 5, this time raising your *left* arm and *right* leg.

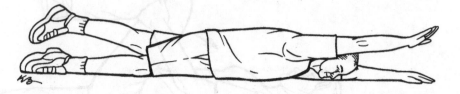

FIGURE 9-16:
The Alternate
Arm and Leg Lifts.

To perform the Standing Extension Stretch (5 to 10 reps), follow these steps:

1. With both hands on your lower back, bend as far back as is comfortable (see Figure 9-17).

2. Hold this position for five seconds.

3. Relax, straightening to the upright position.

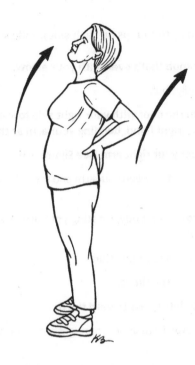

FIGURE 9-17:
The Standing
Extension Stretch.

Strengthening to Build Muscle and Stabilize Joints

Although stretching can help you maintain flexibility, don't ignore the benefits of strengthening your muscles — especially the muscles that you need for maintaining balance and postural stability. You can perform the shoulder and leg exercises in the following sections three to five times a week to help maintain strength in these key areas.

Shoulder strengthening

The following exercises strengthen the shoulder area, especially the rotator cuff muscles (where your shoulder and arm connect). Your physical therapist can provide the stretchy exercise bands, as well as help you adjust the tension and size to your needs. Or you can purchase a five-foot length of rubber tubing at a hardware store or athletic supply shop (they call it a *sports cord*). For some of the exercises, you also need a large bath towel to stabilize your arm.

To perform Internal Rotation (5 to 10 reps on each side), follow these steps:

1. **Attach a band to a doorknob that's even with your elbow.**

   Make sure the door is solidly shut.

2. **Standing three feet from the door with your right side toward the door, grasp the band with your right hand, bending your arm at the elbow.**

3. **Place a rolled towel under your right arm (see Figure 9-18a).**

   You want the towel positioned between your arm and the right side of your body to stabilize your arm.

4. **Pull the band slowly across your body, rotating your arm and shoulder inward (see Figure 9-18b).**

5. **Slowly return your arm to its start position.**

6. **Repeat Steps 4 and 5 five to ten times.**

7. **Turn around so that your left side is toward the door.**

   Don't forget to move the towel from under your right arm to under your left arm.

8. **Repeat Steps 2 through 6, this time pulling with your left arm.**

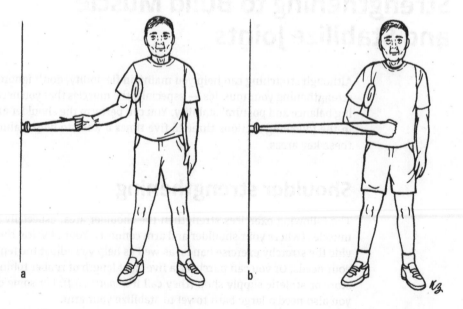

FIGURE 9-18: a   b
Internal Rotation.

To perform External Rotation (5 to 10 reps on each side), follow these steps:

1. **Wrap the ends of a sports band around each hand.**

2. **Place a rolled towel under your right arm and place your left hand on your left hip, keeping your right hand close by (see Figure 9-19a).**

   Position the towel between your arm and chest to stabilize your arm.

3. **With your right hand, slowly pull the band across your body, rotating your arm and shoulder outward (see Figure 9-19b).**

4. **Slowly return your arm to its start position.**

5. **Repeat Steps 3 and 4 five to ten times.**

6. **Repeat Steps 2 through 5, this time pulling with your left hand.**

   Don't forget to place the towel under your left arm.

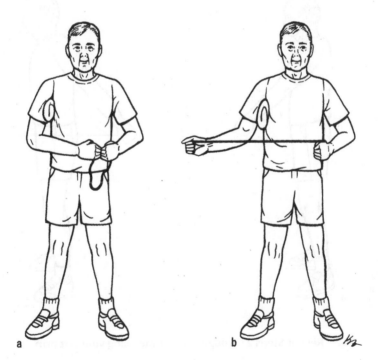

FIGURE 9-19:
External Rotation.   a   b

To perform the Extension Pull (5 to 10 reps on each side), follow these steps:

1. **Attach a band to a doorknob that's even with your elbow.**

   Make sure the door is solidly shut.

2. **Stand facing the door (about 3 feet from the door) with the band in your right hand (see Figure 9-20a).**

3. **Starting with your arm straight and forward, pull the band back by slowly lowering your straightened arm until it's at your side (see Figure 9-20b).**

4. **Slowly return your arm to its start position.**

5. **Repeat Steps 3 and 4 five to ten times.**

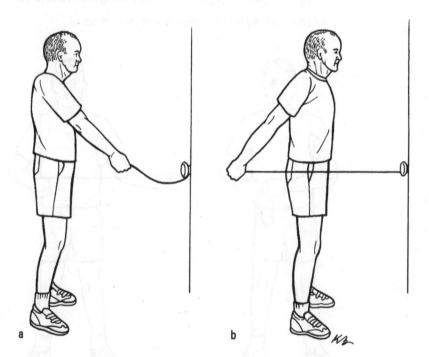

FIGURE 9-20: The Extension Pull.

a   b

6. **Repeat Steps 2 through 5, this time using your left arm.**

To perform Flexion (5 to 10 reps on each side), follow these steps:

1. **Place one end of an exercise band under your right foot and hold the other end in your right hand (see Figure 9-21a).**

2. With your thumb on top of the band and your elbow straight, raise your right arm forward until it's level with your shoulder (see Figure 9-21b).

3. Slowly return your right arm to its start position.

4. Repeat Steps 2 and 3 five to ten times.

5. Repeat Steps 1 through 4, this time having the band under your left foot and raising your left arm.

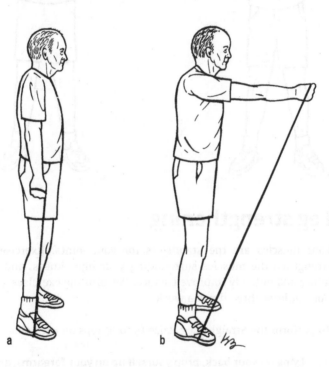

FIGURE 9-21:
Flexion.

a   b

To perform Horizontal Pull (5 to 10 reps), follow these steps:

1. Hold the band with both hands at shoulder height (see Figure 9-22a).

2. With your hands close together, extend your arms out in front of you and slowly stretch the band out until your arms are wide open (see Figure 9-22b).

3. Slowly bring your arms back together.

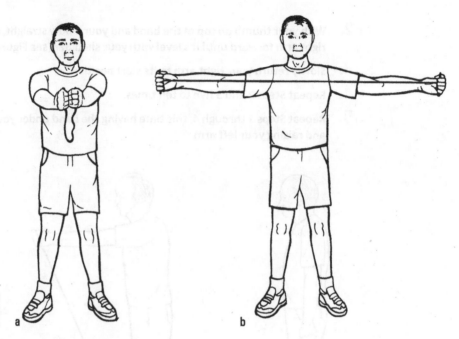

FIGURE 9-22:
The Horizontal
Pull.

a   b

Leg strengthening

Your muscles are the stabilizers for your joints. Exercises that stretch and strengthen the muscles surrounding your hips, knees, and ankles can prevent injury and possibly improve balance. Perform the exercises in the following sections at least three times a week.

To perform the Straight Leg Raise (5 to 10 reps on each side), follow these steps:

1. **Lying on your back, prop yourself up on your forearms, and slightly bend your left knee; keep your left foot flat on the floor.**

2. **Tightening your right leg's front thigh muscle, raise your right leg 8 to 10 inches from the floor (see Figure 9-23).**

   Keep the extended leg straight and knee locked while you perform the exercise.

3. **Slowly return your right leg to the start position.**

4. **Repeat Steps 2 and 3 five to ten times.**

5. **Repeat Steps 1 through 4, this time bending your right knee and raising your left leg.**

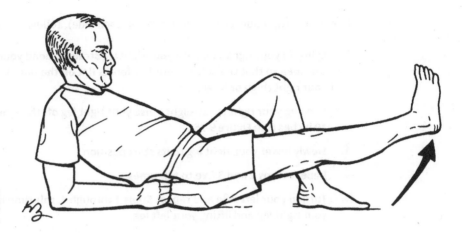

FIGURE 9-23:
The Straight Leg
Raise.

To perform Hip Abduction (5 to 10 reps on each side), follow these steps:

1. **Lie on your left side with both legs straight.**

2. **Slowly lift your right leg toward the ceiling to a comfortable height (at least 5 to 10 inches).**

   Keep both legs straight (see Figure 9-24).

3. **Slowly lower your right leg.**

4. **Repeat Steps 2 and 3 five to ten times.**

5. **Turn to your right side and repeat Steps 1 through 4, this time lifting your left leg.**

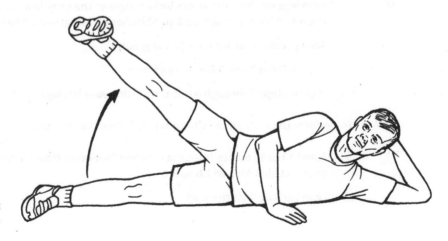

FIGURE 9-24:
Hip Abduction.

To perform Hip Adduction (5 to 10 reps on each side), follow these steps:

1. Lying on your right side with your right leg straight, bend your left leg at the knee so that the sole of your left foot is flat on the floor in front of your right thigh or knee.

2. Keeping your right leg straight, raise your right leg off the ground 5 to 10 inches (see Figure 9-25).

3. Slowly lower your right leg to its start position.

4. Repeat Steps 2 and 3 five to ten times.

5. Turn to your left side and repeat Steps 1 through 4, this time bending your right leg and lifting your left leg.

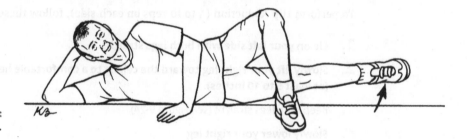

FIGURE 9-25:
Hip Adduction.

To perform Hip Extension (5 to 10 reps on each side), follow these steps:

1. Lie on your stomach with both arms bent and under your chest.

2. With legs straight and knees locked, tighten the muscle in your right thigh and lift your right leg 8 to 10 inches off the ground (see Figure 9-26).

3. Slowly lower your leg back to the ground.

4. Repeat Steps 2 and 3 five to ten times.

5. Repeat Steps 2 through 4 this time lifting your left leg.

To perform the Wall Slide (5 to 10 reps), follow these steps:

1. Stand 12 to 16 inches from the wall and face away from the wall with your feet shoulder-width apart.

2. Lean back against the wall.

3. Slowly lower your buttocks toward the floor as far as you can.

Don't go lower than your thighs being parallel to the floor (see Figure 9-27).

4. Hold this position for five to ten seconds.

5. Tighten your thigh muscles and slide back up to a standing/leaning position.

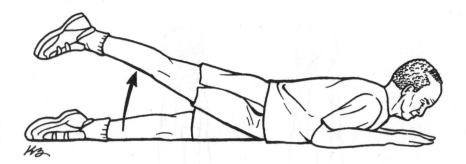

FIGURE 9-26:
Hip Extension.

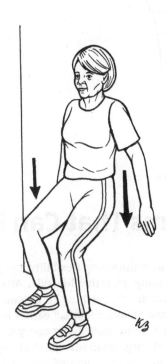

FIGURE 9-27:
The Wall Slide.

To perform the Toe Raise (5 to 10 reps), follow these steps:

1. **Stand with both feet flat on the floor.**

2. **Lift your heels and rise up on your toes (see Figure 9-28).**

3. **Hold this position for five seconds.**

4. **Lower your heels back to the floor.**

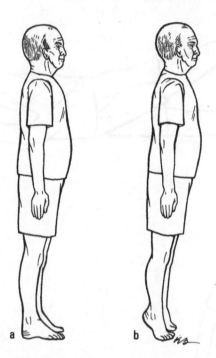

FIGURE 9-28:
The Toe Raise.

Other Exercise Programs That Can Help

Structured exercise is important in maintaining flexibility and physical function, but equally important is maintaining an active lifestyle. After you master the stretches and exercises in the sections "Stretching to Enhance Flexibility" and "Strengthening to Build Muscle and Stabilize Joints," earlier in this chapter, you may be ready for a program that's more challenging and yet specifically structured for PWP. Many national PD organizations consider regular exercise so essential that they've created a variety of programs and tools to help you get started.

Some resources that you may find helpful are

>> **Rock Steady Boxing (RSB)** (www.rocksteadyboxing.org) is the first gym in the country dedicated to the fight against Parkinson's disease. The gym's program bases its exercises on boxing drills because boxers condition for optimal agility, speed, muscular endurance, accuracy, hand-eye coordination, footwork, and overall strength. This conditioning helps boxers defend against and overcome opponents. In an RBS affiliate program, PD is the opponent.

>> **Motivating Moves for People with Parkinson's:** In this program, developed by movement specialist Janet Hamburg, participants sit while doing the exercises. The program is available in DVD format through many local libraries; go to www.worldcat.org, click the DVD tab above the search text box, and use the search term *title motivating moves for people with parkinsons*. You can also purchase the DVD from Amazon; go to www.amazon.com and search for the term *DVD motivating moves for people with parkinsons*.

>> **What Types of Exercise Are Best for People with Parkinson's Disease?:** Dr. Rebecca Gilbert's blog on the American Parkinson Disease Association (APDA) website (www.apdaparkinson.org/article/what-exercise-to-do-with-parkinsons) provides suggestions, advice, and even some videos.

The APDA also has free online exercise programs. (Check out www.apdaparkinson.org/upcoming-events.)

Beyond a Structured Exercise Program — PD and Physical Activity

We imagine you've had to find ways to redefine yourself following life-changing events, such as a career change, retirement, the end of a relationship — or a diagnosis of PD. When circumstances change the way you define your satisfaction and happiness, you can either adapt or choose a less-than-satisfactory mindset, which may include depression and self-pity. Far better to work at rediscovering your identity by using new resources for pleasure and purpose.

Enjoying recreation

Physical activity, or recreation (see how that word is really *re-creation?*), differs from exercise because *recreation* usually provides an element of immediate pleasure, accomplishment, or revitalization that structured exercise may not. For example, if you garden, think about the pleasure of seeing the results of your hard work. In a similar way, biking and canoeing allow you to be physically active while taking in the fresh air and scenery.

REMEMBER

Recreation goes beyond simple physical endeavors; it includes contact with other people and opening yourself to new experiences and information. When you were a kid, you called it *playing*. Well, adults can still play, even when they're facing grown-up stuff like PD.

Keeping up with routine roles and activities

You probably played multiple roles before getting the diagnosis of PD. Take a moment to list them: son/daughter, spouse/lover, friend/companion, parent/grandparent, employee/employer/coworker, community leader/volunteer. How about the roles you played at home? Cook, gardener, decorator, financial manager, handyman/woman.

Don't assume you can't

Ask yourself whether you think you can no longer handle some of these roles. For example, do you think you can't keep up with your current job (see Chapter 16), or do you withdraw from social functions because you don't want pity from friends and family (see Chapter 15)? Maybe you don't cook anymore because the tremors make a mess. Or maybe you're afraid of making a mistake in keeping track of the bills, so you've handed over the finances to your significant other.

Now, take a good look at Chapters 2 and 3 to see whether you find a cause or symptom of PD that says you have to start peeling away pieces of your life and abandoning vital relationships. We'll wait . . . . Did you see it? Aha! We knew you wouldn't! (Okay, so we know because we wrote the book. But we also know because no such cause or symptom of PD exists, period.)

Re-evaluate those activities that you may have assumed you could no longer do — employment, volunteer work, and social activities, such as card playing, sports, and the like. The harder you work to maintain your normal routine and activities, the less likely you are to allow your PD to dominate your life.

Make adjustments so you can

True, you may need to make some adjustments in physical activities to accommodate your PD. For example, you may find that sports that require more lateral (side-to-side) movement, such as golf and ping pong, are easier for you. Or, if you were a marathon runner before your diagnosis, think about race-walking — or just plain walking. One PWP, Jim "Parky" Wetherell, biked over 50,000 miles in a ten-year period by switching to a recumbent three-wheel trike. His motto: "Let's take the PARK out of Parkinson's."

You do have choices, and you can take charge instead of allowing assumptions to dictate your routine. Work with your doctor and other members of your professional health team to determine the right physical activities for you.

Exercises for the Mind and Spirit

Okay, you're exercising regularly and maintaining an active and productive lifestyle. Caring for the physical body is huge for you and for those people who make this journey with you. But be sure you give attention to the mind and spirit. What's happening inside your head? For that matter, what's going on with your care partner (or partners) — that person (or persons) that you have had with you from the moment you got the diagnosis of PD?

In fact, many PWP develop apathy, a condition defined by

>> Reduced interest and participation in routine activities

>> Lack of initiative

>> Difficulties in starting or sustaining an activity

>> Lack of concern for events and people around them

In other words, the mind and spirit seem to simply give up.

REMEMBER

Apathy in PD is more likely a direct consequence of *physiological* changes in the brain than a *psychological* reaction to the disability. As a result, this condition is different from the other psychiatric symptoms and personality changes associated with the disease (such as depression and anxiety — see Chapter 13). In addition, PD apathy can trigger major frustration for that person's care partner, especially when the care partner knows that they're working harder at keeping the PWP active and involved than the PWP is.

Basically, you can approach your life's uncertainties in two ways: Devote your efforts to worrying and trying to change the situation, or devote your energy toward living the most fulfilling life you can. Although you can't control the progression of your PD, you can control your choices. You decide whether you

>> Exercise

>> Remain engaged in the community

>> Set a tone for your friends and family — that you may have PD, but it doesn't have you

>> Wake up every morning and make good choices all over again

Choices for the person with PD

Just like proper diet and exercise are the best choices for maintaining your physical health, they're also your best weapons for maintaining the health of your mind and spirit. People who walk, bike, or run often report that they do their best thinking then; they're working out mental and emotional issues, as well as physical ones.

Here are some exercises you can make a part of your daily (or at least weekly) routine:

>> **Practice daily spiritual renewal.** (See Chapter 12.) Meditate, pray, read inspirational books or poetry, take a walk in a beautiful setting, or attend religious services — whatever gives you a sense of calm and renewal.

>> **Challenge your mind.** Work a crossword or Sudoku puzzle, play along with a TV game show (preferably one that actually requires some mental effort), or read a book.

>> **Learn something new.** Take a class online or at the local college or community center, ask a friend to teach you a craft or new sport, attend a lecture, or watch a documentary. Then share what you've discovered with someone else.

>> **Get involved in your community.** Take an active role in a cause or organization that you think is important: the local library, a museum or historical site, or national projects that have local chapters (such as Habitat for Humanity).

>> **Create a legacy for your children and grandchildren.** Write or record your family history, research the family tree, or organize photo collections into albums or onto digital devices that truly tell the story of your family's past.

>> **Seek activities with your partner.** Find activities you both can participate in, and maintain the activities you both enjoyed before your diagnosis. Go to that play, that ballgame, or that festival.

>> **Join a support group** — preferably one for PWP — where you can interact with other people who fully understand the problems you and your care partner are facing.

Choices for the PD care partner

As the care partner to someone living with PD, you also live with it. It affects your daily life in ways you had never imagined or planned for. A person in your shoes may want to abandon pieces of their own life to take care of the partner. And the most likely piece to fall by the wayside is your own physical health. You eat (or maybe don't eat!) as a reaction to your worries, rather than as a source of nourishment. And when you add the responsibilities of caring for someone with PD to your full calendar, something's gotta give; the most likely candidate is your own regular exercise. *Stop!*

Before you go any further down that rabbit hole of self-defeating behavior, take a moment to consider the following:

>> Someone you care about has PD and will *eventually* need help.

>> Your partner is managing fine with their present treatment plan. This plan can last for years if your partner and their medical team monitor the disease and use appropriate medications.

>> You have choices to make about how you respond to your partner with PD's disease progression. You could

- *Project the worst* while you try to control the future by making life-changing decisions that you don't need to make right now, or

- *Make reasonable plans and preparations* by educating yourself about options, and then live your life, which still remains relatively normal.

If you elect the second option for dealing with your PWP's PD, congratulations! Plan to familiarize yourself with the information in other sections of this book, especially Parts 4 and 5.

We haven't forgotten about *your* body, mind, and spirit. Start by following the guidelines we suggest in the section "Exercises for the Mind and Spirit," earlier in this chapter. Then read Chapter 19 for more information about caring for yourself, as well as your PWP.

REMEMBER

You don't have PD. You have a life beyond caring for this person — just like your PWP has a life beyond living with it. Mental and spiritual well-being for each of you depends on maintaining normalcy as long as possible. The greatest danger is surrendering your potentially good and happy years to anxiety and depression, which can be a major factor with PD. Check out Chapter 13, where we address that concern in depth.

Chapter 10

Managing PD Symptoms with Prescription Medicines

Your Parkinson's disease (PD) diagnosis will include treatment options for managing your symptoms. If you aren't really troubled by any symptoms of functional disability at the time of your diagnosis (in other words, if the PD doesn't interfere with your ability to live your normal life), then your doctor will most likely prescribe programs such as exercise and nutrition counseling, good sleeping habits, a support group, and, of course, regular appointments to monitor symptoms and any signs of progression.

When your symptoms begin to affect your work, social, and routine activities, your doctor will likely add *pharmacologic* therapy (prescription medications) to the treatment plan. In this chapter, we look at the most common medications for managing symptoms, some that have been around for decades and others that are relatively new to the scene. We also pass along some suggestions for staying on top of your medication regimen.

REMEMBER

Because PD has no cure at this time and you can't prevent its progression, the treatment goal is to manage the symptoms, postpone their progression, and minimize the onset of new symptoms for as long as possible.

Managing Motor Symptoms with Proven Prescription Medications

In managing PD symptoms, your doctor may prescribe a variety of medications to help prolong your current level of function. The medication may be available only as a brand-name drug (meaning it's still under patent protection), or it may be available in the generic form (meaning the patent has expired). Brand-name drugs are usually newer, more expensive, and usually targeting specific problems not resolved by available medications. The main categories of drugs most used for managing the motor symptoms of PD are:

>> **Levodopa:** A drug that's converted into dopamine in the brain

>> **Dopamine agonists:** Drugs that mimic the effects of dopamine

>> **Monoamine oxidase B (MAO-B) inhibitors:** Drugs that prevent an enzyme called MAO-B from breaking down dopamine

>> **Non-dopaminergic medications:** Drugs mainly used as add-on treatments for motor control in PD

REMEMBER

Most medications that treat PD have the goal to restore the concentration of dopamine in the brain to near-normal levels. To achieve this goal, your doctor may prescribe one or more medications that in your case may be more beneficial than taking a single medication. That said, the number of pills you take doesn't necessarily correlate to the gravity of the disease!

Your care team will craft your medication regimen to achieve the best possible outcome, given your age, the severity of your symptoms, the possible side effects, and the fit with your work and social life. You and your doctor have access to an always growing arsenal of medications that you can use to treat your PD symptoms.

TIP

To stay current on what meds are available and scope out any recent additions, see the Full List of Medications Approved for the Treatment of Parkinson's Disease in the USA table at www.apdaparkinson.org. Go to the website, hover over the What is Parkinson's Disease link, click the Treatment & Medication link from the drop-down list that appears, and then click the Read More on Parkinson's Medications link.

L-dopa and carbidopa: A dynamic duo

Over 50 years after its introduction, the combination of *levodopa* and *carbidopa* (also known as Sinemet, its original brand name) is still the preferred treatment for most people with Parkinson's (PWP).

Levodopa — The gold standard

Levodopa (often abbreviated to *L-dopa*), which brain cells use to produce more *dopamine* (the neurotransmitter that PD reduces), remains the first line of defense for controlling PD symptoms as it is the most effective and best tolerated. Producing more dopamine permits relief for PD symptoms such as slow movements (*bradykinesia*), stiffness, *tremor* (shaking), facial mask, cramped handwriting, and impaired *gait* (walking).

Historically, L-dopa was administered alone, which caused a whole list of side effects, including nausea, loss of appetite, vomiting, lowered blood pressure (leading to dizziness and possible falls), and rapid heart rate. Because these side effects were so significant, researchers almost dropped L-dopa from the regimen before they discovered the advantages of prescribing it with its now-conventional partner, *carbidopa*. Coupled with carbidopa, L-dopa can almost completely control PD symptoms for a honeymoon period that may last for several years.

WARNING

Unfortunately, 50 percent of PWP develop motor complications after 5 years of levodopa therapy; virtually all of them experience a decline in the benefit of levodopa after 10 to 15 years of therapy. PWP who take this drug over the long term commonly notice diminished effectiveness (commonly defined as *wearing off*) before the next scheduled dose. You definitely need to schedule regular visits with your doctor to assess how well your current medication routine is working.

Carbidopa — L-dopa's companion

Any time the treatment seems worse than the condition, researchers look for ways to make the treatment more tolerable for the patient. Carbidopa's main purpose is to prevent the body from transforming L-dopa into dopamine before it gets to the brain — and therefore offset the serious and uncomfortable side effects of levodopa — hopefully without causing side effects of its own. In addition, carbidopa

>> Allows your system to absorb the essential vitamin B_6

>> Lessens the amount of levodopa that you need to take in order to control symptoms

When your symptoms do require medication, your doctor will probably prescribe a low dose of carbidopa/levodopa. In the United States, there are several formulations of carbidopa-levodopa, so get familiar with a few brand names.

The most common brand name for carbidopa/levodopa in the United States is *Sinemet*, which is a pill that is swallowed. Alternatively, there is *Parcopa*, a tablet that dissolves on the tongue. Another option is a carbidopa/levodopa medication in an extended release or *controlled release* (CR) form. More recent additions include another extended-release carbidopa/levodopa medication, *Rytary*. According to the Michael J. Fox foundation, in addition to lessening motor symptoms, Rytary may decrease total daily *off-time* (periods when symptoms are not controlled).

The prescription includes two numbers — usually 25/100. The first number refers to the amount of carbidopa (25 milligrams [mg]), and the second is the amount of levodopa (100 mg). Your doctor monitors your symptoms on this low dose (usually taken at regular intervals three to four times a day). If you experience side effects, your doctor may double the amount of carbidopa in your prescription. While the symptoms of PD progress, your doctor may increase the dosage and shorten the periods between doses.

TIP

Rytary has different number combinations (for example, 23.75/95 or 36.25/145) for the carbidopa and levodopa, which can be confusing at times. Make sure to ask your doctor if the prescription numbers don't make sense to you.

Recent innovations in drug delivery offer alternative forms of levodopa, including *Inbrija*, a levodopa powder that can be inhaled or *Duopa*, a levodopa gel that can be continuously pumped into the intestines through a tube surgically inserted in the stomach (see the related sidebar "New delivery systems"). And researchers in advanced centers are testing even more levodopa formulations, including subcutaneous pumps and transdermal patches. Stay tuned . . .

Dopamine agonists (DAs)

Unlike levodopa, which is transformed into dopamine, *dopamine agonists (DAs)* imitate the characteristics of dopamine. Your doctor may recommend that you try a DA before prescribing Sinemet. A DA can provide a first-line treatment trying to delay the complications associated with the use of levodopa over the long haul. (See the section "L-dopa and carbidopa: A dynamic duo," earlier in this chapter, for more about Sinemet.) DAs have been in use for decades and have proven effectiveness in treating PD symptoms. But DAs do come with troubling side effects, such as daytime sleepiness, low blood pressure, *edema* (swollen feet), vivid dreams, and (on occasion) visual hallucinations.

A number of dopamine agonists are available. Older-generation drugs (such as bromocriptine and pergolide) have been virtually discontinued because of possible cardiac side effects. Newer generations of DAs (including pramipexole and ropinirole) offer effective management of symptoms and have relatively fewer side effects.

Like levodopa, DAs have alternative delivery modes, including a transdermal patch rotigotine or *Neupro*, (noted in the sidebar "New delivery systems"), and subcutaneous injections (*Apokyn*) or sublingual strips (*Kynmobi*) of apomorphine. Apomorphine is the oldest new drug available for PD; it was originally used (more than 100 years ago) as an *emetic* (a drug to cause vomiting) in cases of food poisoning. Because of the emetic effect, apomorphine cannot be taken as a pill but needs to be either injected or absorbed under the tongue. Apomorphine is extremely effective and quickly active (within 5-10 minutes!), but its benefits are short-lasting and often limited by the same side effects (for example, low blood pressure and visual hallucinations) as the other DAs. And so, its use is limited to rescuing situations of wearing-off, creating a bridge between two doses of carbidopa/levodopa.

TIP

If you have an unfavorable response to one DA, ask your doctor about trying a different one to see whether it's more successful. Of the several DA medications available, studies haven't proven one to be more effective than another.

Monoamine oxidase B inhibitors (MAO-B inhibitors)

The monoamine oxidase inhibitor (MAOI) class of drugs works by interacting with *monoamines*, chemicals in the brain that transmit messages between nerve cells. Of the three monoamines (dopamine, serotonin, and norepinephrine), dopamine is the main focus for PWP because it controls messages related to movement.

The fundamental task of MAO-B inhibitors is to inhibit or block the *oxidation* (burning) of dopamine, which clears the dopamine from the *synaptic space* (the tiny space between brain cells where chemical messages are exchanged). With less dopamine oxidation, more dopamine is available in the brain, which improves PD symptoms. Interestingly, MAO-B inhibitors may provide an additional benefit by acting as a kind of neuroprotector (see Chapter 2), possibly slowing the progression of PD and delaying the need for carbidopa/levodopa therapy.

The original drug from this group is *selegiline*, which doctors still prescribe for the early stages of PD because it provides some control of PD symptoms. A formula of orally disintegrating (ODT) selegiline (*Zelapar*) has the added advantage of a once-a-day dosing schedule. Or your doctor may prescribe rasagiline (brand name *Azilect*), another MAO-B inhibitor that you take once a day for the treatment of early PD. For PWP in the moderate to advanced stages, a combination of selegiline and L-dopa can improve symptoms. And finally, the FDA has approved a new MAO-B inhibitor safinamide (*Xadago*) for PWP experiencing off episodes. Safinamide's unique feature is its effectiveness in improving off symptoms while maintaining stable doses of carbidopa/levodopa.

WARNING

The downside to MAO-B inhibitors is their potentially serious effect on blood pressure, especially if you're taking other medicines that also affect blood pressure. Take these precautions to avoid serious problems:

>> **Watch for potential medication clashes.** Be sure all of your doctors know that you're on an MAO-B inhibitor. Always check with your pharmacist before using

- *Certain over-the-counter (OTC) products:* Such as cold-cough remedies (especially those including dextromethorphan) and diet supplements

- *Some prescription medicines:* Such as antidepressants that increase serotonin levels (SSRIs)

>> **Inform specialists before surgery:** If you're scheduled for surgery, be sure the anesthesiologist knows that you're taking an MAO-B inhibitor because that, in combination with anesthesia, can cause a dangerous drop in blood pressure.

>> **Take care when eating foods that affect blood pressure.** Be aware that MAO-B inhibitors can cause abnormalities of blood pressure if you eat or drink something that contains the compound tyramine. Food and drink containing tyramine include aged cheese (so this blood pressure issue is sometimes called the *cheese effect*) and red wine.

Consult your doctor if you have additional questions about the serious side effects of MAO-B inhibitors.

Dopamine action extenders - COMT inhibitors

PD therapy options have expanded to include a class of drugs called *catechol-O-methyl transferase inhibitors* (COMT inhibitors). COMT inhibitors block the enzyme 3-O-methyldopa, allowing even more levodopa to reach the brain. Imagine levodopa with two bodyguards — carbidopa and a COMT inhibitor — to shelter it from dangerous enzymes on its journey toward the brain.

Other advantages of adding a COMT inhibitor to L-dopa include

>> Longer duration of L-dopa effectiveness

>> Potential for reducing the needed amounts of carbidopa/levodopa

>> The possibility of managing medication off times more effectively (See the section "Tracking the on-off fluctuations of your meds," later in this chapter.)

These brand-name COMT medications may be prescribed for PWP:

>> **Comtan** (a brand name for entacapone) is the most widely used COMT inhibitor, due to its benefit and tolerability. It can consistently add 20-30 minutes to every dose of carbidopa/levodopa, reducing or eliminating wearing-off periods. Entacapone may give urine an unusual dark orange color, which is not dangerous. In other cases, it may cause diarrhea, which may be severe enough to require discontinuation.

>> **Stalevo** combines the COMT inhibitor entacapone with carbidopa and levodopa. This three-in-one combination makes dosing easier because you take one pill, not two (or more) at the same time.

>> **Tasmar** (a brand name of tolcapone), is another available COMT inhibitor, but has some limitations associated with liver toxicity.

>> **Ongentys** (a brand-name of opicapone) is a recently approved COMT inhibitor prescribed for PWP with wearing-off episodes that complicate levodopa/carbidopa therapy. The PWP needs to take opicapone only once per day, which is a possible advantage over entacapone and tolcapone. The PWP always takes entacapone or tolcapone in association with levodopa, which means three to four (or more) times per day.

Amantadine — one more tool in the Rx toolbox

Amantadine may also be used to treat the symptoms of Parkinson's disease, especially the movement problems (*dyskinesias*) that complicate the use of other PD medications. An extended-release formulation (*Gocovri*) has been developed, similar to the combination of levodopa and carbidopa (such as Rytary or Sinemet CR), to treat *off-time episodes* (times between medication doses in which symptoms return as dopamine levels drop) in PWP. The use of amantadine can be limited by side effects like cognitive decline, visual hallucinations, and an unusual skin discoloration called *livedo reticularis*.

Exactly how amantadine helps relieve symptoms isn't clear. In fact, it was originally (and continues to be) a treatment for the flu, but scientists serendipitously stumbled on its potential benefits for PD treatment.

The new kid on the block: adenosine receptor antagonist

Researchers are always on the hunt for new ways to control or offset medications' side effects that may occur over time. In 2019, the FDA approved a new drug — the adenosine receptor antagonist *istradefylline* (brand name *Nourianz*). This medicine is prescribed in tandem with levodopa and carbidopa to treat adults with PD who experience off-time episodes.

NEW DELIVERY SYSTEMS

In most cases, prescribed medications come in a tablet or capsule form. But researchers have discovered other ways to get the drugs into your system with improved effectiveness, fewer side effects, and a shorter waiting period before the drug takes effect.

A transdermal patch (Neupro patch) applied daily delivers the dopamine agonist *rotigotine* through the skin, directly into the bloodstream. You apply the patch to your skin (back, shoulder, or abdomen) once a day. The advantage of the patch is its consistent delivery of medication throughout the day. Consistent delivery of the dopamine agonist helps smooth out the amount of medicine you receive unlike the peaks and valleys that occur when taking tablets or capsules multiple times each day.

A second unique delivery system is Duopa therapy, a form of carbidopa/levodopa delivered via a gel (enteral suspension) rather than a pill. A surgeon makes a small incision (called a *stoma*) in your stomach wall and places a tube in your intestine. A pump then delivers Duopa directly to your intestine through this tube. Duopa uses the same active ingredients as orally administered carbidopa/levodopa but is designed to improve absorption and reduce medication off times by delivering the drug directly to the small intestine.

Other delivery modes, approved by the FDA, are recent introductions to the market. *Inbrija* is a new powder formulation of levodopa (without carbidopa) that can be inhaled, similar to asthma medications. While dosing may require a little training, Inbrija can be quickly absorbed through the lungs and rescue a period of worsening symptoms (wearing-off). As mentioned in the section "Dopamine agonists (DAs)" also in this chapter, sublingual delivery (*Kynmobi*) and subcutaneous injections (*Apokyn*) are available for apomorphine, a powerful dopamine agonist that would not be tolerated if taken by mouth.

Flagging Non-Motor PD Symptoms

PWP must deal with a whole range of symptoms — only some of which involve movement. Non-motor symptoms can be equally as, or more disruptive to a PWP's daily routine. Learn to recognize and report non-motor symptoms to your doctor; they may need specific attention and do not normally respond to changes in levodopa (or similar medications) dosage. Non-motor symptoms may include

>> **Dizziness or changes in blood pressure when you stand after lying down or sitting:** Report this symptom to your doctor! Treatment may include changes in habits (such as increasing fluid intake or wearing support stockings), change in PD medications or adding specific medications to support falling blood pressure.

>> **Increased saliva in your mouth or difficulty swallowing:** Again, your doctor needs to know about this because it may be either a side effect of a medication or the progression of your PD. Either way, don't ignore it!

>> **Sleep disturbances:** The disease itself and some of your antiparkinsonian meds can cause sleep disturbance. Ask your doctor whether you may benefit from a sleep aid. *Note:* Don't start taking a sleep aid until you ask your doctor. If you have especially troublesome sleep disturbances, your doctor may recommend you participate in a more specific sleep study.

>> **Pain, cramping, or uncomfortable tingling and numbness:** These symptoms can be extremely disabling and sometimes worse at night or bedtime (think *restless leg syndrome*). A change in your evening dose of L-dopa (higher or lower) may solve the problem. You can also ask your doctor whether anti-inflammatories (such as ibuprofen), muscle relaxants, or dopamine agonists may help. In other situations, deficiency in specific vitamins like B6, B12, or folate can cause these symptoms.

>> **Nausea, stomach upset, constipation, and heartburn:** These symptoms may be part and parcel of your medication routine but can be an unresolved symptom of the disease (particularly constipation). Talk to your doctor about when, how often, and to what degree of discomfort these symptoms occur.

>> **Urinary frequency or urgency:** Conditions other than your PD — such as prostate hypertrophy or a urinary tract infection (UTI) — may affect urinary issues. Talk to your doctor if you experience any change in urinary habits, especially if you experience pain or any sort of unusual discharge when you urinate.

REMEMBER

If you're seeing more than one doctor or taking medication for high blood pressure or another chronic condition, be sure your PD doctor and all the doctors you're seeing consult with each other before prescribing new meds for you.

WARNING

Don't self-medicate — even with over-the-counter (OTC) meds or supplements you've routinely taken in the past. OTCs can have adverse interactions with your prescription medications. In particular, overdosing vitamins (like B6) can cause unpleasant symptoms like *neuropathy* (weakness, numbness, and pain, usually in the hands and feet). Check with your doctor before adding anything to your medication regimen.

Using Your Medication Safely and Effectively

As a person with PD, you need to pay close attention to your medication timing and dosing. You also need to make note of changes in performance and function (mental or physical), especially if such changes seem to relate to your medication routine. In short, you need to

>> **Take an active role** in monitoring your medications and the results you get (or don't get) from them.

>> **Inform your doctor and pharmacist** of any side effects, new symptoms, or worsening of current symptoms.

The following sections cover the important ways you can work with your doctors and pharmacist to maintain a healthy regimen with your meds. We also pass along some advice for keeping track of your meds and their effectiveness with your PD symptoms.

TIP

KEEPING THE COSTS OF MEDS UNDER CONTROL

If the cost of your medications is overwhelming, you may be eligible to receive some of your prescription medications for a reduced cost or even for free. The American Parkinson Disease Association (APDA; www.apdaparkinson.org) partners with a coalition of health providers, pharmaceutical companies, patient advocacy groups, and other organizations to help you get the medicine you need. Start by calling the member benefits number on the back of your insurance card and ask the representative you speak with for a full explanation of your pharmacy benefits. You can also check out PhRMA's Medicine Assistance Tool (571-350-8643; http://medicineassistancetool.org) and the National Council on Aging's BenefitsCheckUp (800-503-6897; https://benefitscheckup.org) for information about what benefits programs you may be eligible for.

Partnering with your doctor and pharmacist

Work with your PD doctor to review *all* your medications from time to time. Be sure to include any OTC products you take regularly. And remember to pay special attention to any dosing changes or new prescription meds another doctor may have ordered.

When your PD doctor and other doctors write a new prescription for you, ask the following questions:

>> Why are you prescribing this medication at this time?

>> What results should I expect after I begin taking this medication?

>> How soon should I expect positive results?

>> How should I take the medication? (Find out about timing, dosing, whether to take it with or without food, and so on.)

>> What side effects might I experience?

>> What side effects should I notify my doctor about immediately?

>> What side effects would require me to get to an emergency room or call 911?

>> What does the medication cost?

>> Can I get the same benefits in a less expensive way?

>> Do I need to watch out for any interactions between the new medication and other prescription or OTC meds that I'm already taking?

When you get a medication for the first time, be sure the pharmacist prints out and reviews the prescribing information sheet with you. (If you don't have a regular pharmacist, ask your PD doctor to recommend pharmacies in your area.)

TIP

Before you leave the pharmacy

>> **Ask questions if anything the pharmacist mentions raises a red flag for you.** For example, if a side effect of the new med is low blood pressure and you're taking medication to manage high blood pressure, how will the new drug affect it?

>> **Check the label to be sure you can read it and that you received the right medication according to your doctor's instructions.** If a substitution has been made (a generic for the brand your doctor prescribed, for example), ask the pharmacist to call the doctor to be sure the switch is okay.

>> **Open the package and look at the medicine, especially if it's a refill.** If the pill or tablet doesn't look like the med you've been taking, immediately bring that question to your pharmacist's attention.

Mixing prescription and OTC medications

Turn on the TV, engage with social media, or pick up any magazine these days, and you probably see an ad or article touting the advantages of some herbal supplement or vitamin. Or maybe a friend recommends some OTC product for your heartburn, headache, or cold symptoms. The question is: How will these commonly used products interact with your prescription meds — especially your anti-parkinsonian meds?

WARNING

Anyone who takes a prescription medication in order to manage or treat a chronic illness needs to vigilantly read labels on all OTC medications, as well as prescription products, for potential interactions. Call your primary care physician or PD doctor and talk to the pharmacist before taking any new meds or supplements. Let these professionals help you decide whether you can benefit from taking this med or supplement, or whether it might cause problems.

Common signs of potentially dangerous drug interactions include accelerated or slower heart rate, diarrhea or constipation, heartburn, nausea, stomach cramping, fever, skin rashes, unusual bruising, dizziness, confusion, loss of appetite, or abnormal fatigue. If you experience any such side effects, contact your doctor. If you experience severe side effects — or your doctor is unavailable — call 911 or get to an urgent care clinic or emergency room.

Note: Ask your doctor whether grapefruit juice can have an effect on your medications. Studies have shown that grapefruit juice can interfere with the liver's ability to break down some medicines — especially prescription drugs.

REMEMBER

Balancing the benefits of medications against their potential side effects is delicate. In partnership with your doctor, determine what combination works best for your lifestyle and quality of life. The goal is to keep you *in* control — as opposed to *under* the control — of your meds and your PD.

Setting up a routine for managing your meds

Humans have a tendency to ignore or bend the rules, especially when it comes to faithfully following a medication regimen. Sometimes, they skip doses, miss the timing by a couple of hours, cut the dose to save money, and even share prescription meds with other people (because it did so much good for them). We really do have to say it: do NOT do any of these things!

If you have PD, taking medicine and taking it in the prescribed and timely manner is critical. And, because you probably take more than one medication for PD (not to mention the meds you may take for other conditions, such as high blood pressure), timing is indeed everything.

While your PD progresses, you may experience memory problems, so you absolutely must figure out now how you're going to remember to take your meds.

Here are three keys to avoid problems with your medications:

>> **Designate an overseer.** Make sure that one (and only one) doctor — your PD doctor is the best choice — oversees all your medications, including OTC vitamins, supplements, or herbal remedies.

>> **Choose one pharmacy.** Select one pharmacy (or pharmacy chain that maintains your records regardless of where you are) to fill all your prescriptions.

>> **Document your meds.** Take a list — if not the actual meds — to every doctor's appointment (including dentists, podiatrists, and so on) and to the hospital or emergency room if you need to go there.

Managing meds at the hospital

Hospitals use several medications to combat nausea following anesthetic exposure that are *contraindicated* (meaning not to be used) for PWP. These drugs not only worsen PD symptoms but can actually produce Parkinson-like symptoms in people who have no diagnosis of PD.

In general, being *admitted to the hospital*, usually for reasons other than PD can expose PWP to unexpected problems. As the focus of care is geared toward the admitting diagnosis (maybe a needed surgery, maybe those painful kidney stones), many important aspects of PD management — including timing of medications and possible contraindications — may be overlooked. This situation affects your quality of care and ultimately the length of stay in the hospital. Be prepared and let nurses know what medication you need and at what time.

Managing meds at home

You also need to get organized at home — where you most likely take your meds. You've probably seen or even used those plastic pill containers that organize meds by day (or even by dose throughout the day). Some of these containers come with a beeper that signals the time for a dose. Alternatively, you can set reminder alarms on your phone or watch.

TIP

Consult with your pharmacist on the best choice in medication organizers for your purposes. Think about your daily activities:

>> **Are you home all the time?** One large, multi-sectioned container may be a good choice for having everything in one place.

>> **Are you at work when one dose comes due?** A smaller pocket container or one that has a reminder alarm can help you keep track of that dose.

Establish a regular time (the same time and day every week) for loading the meds into the proper container. Then place the container(s) in the most obvious place to remind you. (For example, you may want to put your morning and bedtime meds next to your toothbrush.)

Tracking the on-off fluctuations of your meds

As if multiple motor, cognitive, and other symptoms of PD aren't enough, the common PD medications can also affect the course of the disease. Read any PD article or get into a discussion with any PD patient or care partner, and sooner or later, you hear the terms *wearing off*, *on-off*, and *dyskinesia*. We talk about these issues in the following sections.

The wearing-off effect

The *wearing-off* effect may appear when the PWP has been on the same dosage for some time. Over time, the positive effect of the med simply wears off before the next dose. In that window — between the end-of-dose benefit and the delivery of the next dose — the PWP may experience heightened symptoms of PD, such as tremors, difficulties with balance and coordination, and so on.

Incidents of heightened symptoms commonly occur after a relatively long *honeymoon*, the time during which the antiparkinsonian meds seamlessly control the symptoms from dose to dose. In response to *wearing-off* your doctor may recommend shortening the time between doses, increasing the dose, and/or adding other meds.

The on-off phenomenon

The *on-off* phenomenon (which is fairly unique to PD) refers to the PWP's ability to perform common physical activities one minute and then be totally incapable the next minute, all within the same dosing cycle. Another way of looking at this phenomenon is that the wearing-off effect loses its predictability, so PD symptoms emerge fairly quickly and without warning. Some PWP actually refer to the sensation as someone flipping a switch. Usually, this effect occurs in the advanced stages of PD.

We recommend that you track your on-off fluctuations after they begin by noting the following and reporting your findings to your doctor:

>> The time the symptoms reappear in relation to your next scheduled dose of medicine.

>> The exact symptoms that reappear.

>> The frequency of the off period. Is it every dose or just now and then? If it's now and then, can you determine a recurring pattern?

REMEMBER

For friends and family, this seemingly random ability of the PWP to act normal one minute and need help the next minute may appear calculated, to gather sympathy or manipulate other people. Although we don't know the cause, the on-off phenomenon is a verified symptom of PD. Recent theories link the continued loss of dopamine-producing cells and years of drug therapy as a possible cause. The PWP, as well as family and friends, must understand that the PWP has no control over this on-off effect, and this effect may not respond to a change in the medication routine.

Seemingly random actions

Dyskinesia (involuntary movements) can involve one body part, such as an arm or leg, or the entire body and often looks like fidgeting, head bobbing or a dancelike movement. Dyskinesia tends to occur most often when PD symptoms such as tremor, slowness, and stiffness, are well controlled. In fact, dyskinesia are usually attributed to some form of over medication and can be controlled by reducing the dose of levodopa or other dopaminergic medications. Other remedies include amantadine and, in more advanced cases, deep brain stimulation (DBS) (see Chapter 11).

Chapter **11**

When Surgery Is an Option

s Parkinson's disease (PD) progresses, medications often lose their effectiveness; sometimes they cause, rather than alleviate, problems for the patient. In these instances, surgery may bring much-needed relief and even restore some level of normalcy to the patient's functions and life for many years. In this chapter, we explore current surgical procedures and raise the important questions for you to ask before deciding to proceed with a surgical option.

Deciding Your Candidacy for Surgery

First things first: Of the many people with Parkinson's (PWP), which ones are more likely candidates for surgery? The following questions are a general guide to help you understand your chances for a successful outcome from surgery:

» Have you successfully used antiparkinsonian medications (primarily L-dopa therapy) for four or more years?

>> In spite of an optimal medication regimen, are you experiencing increasing *motor fluctuations* (PD motor symptoms reappear before the next dose is due), *dyskinesia* (abnormal involuntary movements — a major side effect of taking the antiparkinsonian meds), and *freezing episodes* (sudden difficulty in moving)?

>> Is your tremor so severe that medication can't control it?

>> Are the side effects of your anti-PD meds interfering with your daily life in a way that's becoming intolerable?

Of course, your age, past medical history, and general health are always considerations before deciding to undergo surgery, but you're more likely to benefit from surgery if you answered yes to two or more of the above questions.

Note: Unfortunately, PWP whose main issues involve cognitive loss, impaired balance that doesn't respond to L-dopa, *dysarthria* (difficulties with speech), or *dysphagia* (swallowing problems) are less likely to be helped by DBS surgery. In such cases, Duopa therapy (see Chapter 10 and this chapter's "Also an implant: Duopa therapy" section) may be an option.

REMEMBER

Even if you appear to be a prime candidate, you have a great deal to consider before deciding whether surgery's right for you. Most importantly, remember that you may experience relief — even significant relief — of some symptoms, but your PD will still progress. In particular, symptoms that surgery can't address (such as non-movement-related dysfunction or cognitive decline) may still be a factor in the progression of your PD.

On the other hand, if certain symptoms such as tremor and other movement issues have begun to rule your life, surgery may buy you some much-needed relief and time to enjoy a higher quality of life. You and your doctor shouldn't make this choice lightly.

Weighing Your Surgical Options

At the time of this writing, surgical options for treating PD are limited to *deep brain stimulation* (DBS), *focused ultrasound* (FUS), and *intraduodenal levodopa gel* (Duopa) therapy. As scientists continue to seek new procedures that may prove more effective in controlling symptoms or stopping them altogether, allowing the patient to remain symptom-free for a period of time, more advanced options may become available in the near future. (See the sidebar "Stem cell research: The Future," in this chapter.)

Taking the most traveled road: DBS

The established standard of care for surgical treatment of PD-related motor symptoms is a process called deep brain stimulation (DBS). Since the FDA approved DBS for treatment of PD in 2002, over 150,000 PWP have had the procedure done. DBS can also effectively treat other neurological conditions, such as essential tremor and *dystonia* (muscle contractions or spasms that result in involuntary movement and posture). In all cases, doctors should consider DBS surgery only for people whose medication regimen no longer works effectively to control their symptoms.

During the DBS procedure, a specially trained surgeon implants an *electrode* (a long wire with 4 or more electrical contacts at its tip) deep in the brain and then connects it to a *neurostimulator* (a battery-operated device similar to a pacemaker). The neurostimulator is then programmed to deliver electrical pulses — through the implanted electrode — to those brain areas that control movement.

WARNING

Before deciding to move forward with DBS, you must go through a proper screening with a medical team experienced in the treatment of movement disorders and DBS. These professionals must discuss with you, the PWP, the potential benefits, as well as the risks, of surgery.

Considering the pros and cons of DBS

Some of the advantages of DBS include

>> **Customization:** The procedure includes programming the neurostimulator to the individual PWP in order to maximize benefits and minimize side effects.

>> **Less medication:** DBS can substantially reduce the amount of medication you need.

>> **Diminished side effects:** DBS can result in significant relief from the troublesome side effects (such as dyskinesia) of the medicines that you take by reducing your needed dose sizes.

>> **Reversal:** Your doctor can reverse the DBS procedure in the future if a new, more promising procedure becomes available.

Here are some of the downsides of DBS:

>> **It comes with surgical risks.** This is still brain surgery with potentially severe — though rare when DBS experts perform the surgery — complications, including brain *hemorrhage* (bleeding).

>> **It's not a cure.** DBS can't stop the progression of your PD.

>> **You have to make a substantial time commitment.** A significant factor you must consider is your proximity to the center where experts perform the procedure, although modern technology has recently developed the option of programming the electrodes remotely via telemedicine.

Tool-specific therapy: Focused ultrasound

Magnetic resonance-guided *focused ultrasound* (FUS) therapy is a technique for targeting brain lesions in PWPs. In FUS therapy, a machine uses powerful, focused beams of non-ionizing ultrasonic waves to precisely target specific areas of the brain (the same areas targeted by DBS). Similar to when we used a magnifying lens to burn a hole in a dry leaf as children, FUS can heat the target and produce a small lesion in the thalamus (*thalamotomy*), the globus pallidum (*pallidotomy*) and other key structures in the brain. These small lesions can effectively treat tremor (in the case of thalamotomy) or other symptoms of PD (in the case of pallidotomy or subthalamotomy).

The advantages of FUS (it has basically the same indications as DBS) are the non-invasive nature of the procedure and no need for general anesthesia. *Non-invasive* implies no skin incisions, no skull drilling, no brain penetration, and no implanted electrodes or pacemaker. The procedure usually occurs on an outpatient basis and takes under an hour. While published FUS outcomes have been comparable to DBS, the procedure (approved by the FDA in 2018 for PD tremor and in 2021 for other PD symptoms) can only be performed on one side of the brain, due to safety concerns with bilateral lesions. Other possible disadvantages, as compared to DBS, are the permanent, irreversible, and nonadjustable nature of the brain lesions and the relative novelty of the technology, which means that fewer surgeons currently have an advanced level of expertise.

Also an implant: Duopa therapy

As described in Chapter 10, *Duopa therapy* is a system for delivering carbidopa/levodopa in gel form directly into the small intestine. To receive this therapy, you need surgery to create a small opening (a *stoma*) in the wall of your stomach, through which your doctor inserts a tube into your intestine. The tube is connected to a pump that allows you to deliver your dose of L-dopa directly to your small intestine, rather than ingesting the medication orally.

You could be a candidate for Duopa therapy if

>> Your PD is fairly advanced and you continue to respond to L-dopa.

>> Your doctor has tried adding additional medications, such as dopamine agonists or MAO-B inhibitors, with no results.

>> Your off-time motor fluctuations have escalated.

REMEMBER

Like with any surgery, Duopa therapy comes with risks (bleeding, infection, the possible dislocation of the tube), and the gel form of L-dopa shares the same potential side effects (nausea, dyskinesia, dry mouth, constipation) as its orally delivered sibling.

Looking to future surgical possibilities

Scientists are constantly working on improvements to DBS, focusing on such details as a smaller and longer-lasting battery pack or a battery pack in the electrode so that everything operates as one unit in the scalp. Another possibility involves providing branch leads or connectors in the stimulator that network to various parts of the brain that control movements.

Beyond DBS, researchers hope to prevent, stop, or even reverse the death of dopamine-producing cells through advances in gene therapy and cell regeneration. For example, research on stem cells and Parkinson's is ongoing in a number of clinical trials as researchers seek to learn more about how stem cell therapy might offer improved treatment or perhaps provide the path to a cure. That said, understand that a great deal of work is yet to come before clear answers emerge about the safety and benefit of such treatment.

Undergoing Deep Brain Stimulation

Of all the surgical interventions mentioned in the section "Weighing Your Surgical Options," earlier in this chapter, the one most often pursued is DBS. Brain surgery is pretty scary, but it certainly places a whole new light on managing PD's symptoms and living a full and functional life for as long as possible. Keep in mind that this surgery is elective — it's *your* call, not the doctor's.

Note: Because, with the possible exception of FUS, DBS has replaced all previous types of surgeries to treat PD, we focus on DBS in the following sections.

Asking the right questions before DBS

Regardless of what your doctor tells you, this decision is yours to make. So, take time to educate yourself (and your family), and consider this surgery from all points of view. Before making a decision, take advantage of the following suggestions:

>> **Inform yourself thoroughly.** Read the literature your doctor offers and educate yourself fully about the procedure, the benefits, and the risks. Get written information about possible complications and risks. A primary question to ask is, "Can DBS make my PD worse?" (*Spoiler alert:* the answer to this primary question is no, barring the worst-case scenario complications described below.)

>> **Get the scoop on risks.** Meet with your PD doctor and the neurosurgeon. Like with any potential surgery, ask questions, and expect definitive answers about the risks and worst-case scenario. (For example, less than 3 percent of patients experience serious complications, such as stroke or bleeding, from DBS surgery performed by an experienced neurosurgeon; but a slightly higher percentage may develop an infection at the implantation sites.)

>> **Question your neurosurgeon.** Ask about

- What percentage of their total practice involves DBS procedures, and how many DBS procedures have they performed
- Whether the surgeon has ever been sued for malpractice related to a DBS procedure
- Who will follow up with you after the implant
- Whether your neurosurgeon collaborates with an experienced implant programmer and movement disorder specialist to manage the settings on your neurostimulator
- Whether your neurosurgeon is part of an established DBS program or works independently

>> **Seek out DBS surgery patients.** Ask your PD doctor (or your support-group facilitator) to introduce you to at least two other patients who have had the procedure — at least one of whom is a few years post-surgery. Talk to those patients about their experiences before, during, and after the surgery.

If you decide to go forward after weighing all the pros and cons of surgery, the following sections can help you and your family know what to expect.

Passing the presurgical tests

Before you can schedule your procedure, you need to pass several presurgical tests. These tests are fairly standardized and usually include a general medical examination to confirm that you're healthy enough to endure the stresses of surgery; neuropsychological testing to confirm that you don't have dementia and are emotionally and mentally prepared for the surgery; routine blood tests, an electrocardiogram, chest X-rays, and brain imaging tests (such as an MRI) that the surgeon uses to calculate the trajectory of the implant.

Ironing out the details

After successful preliminary testing (see the preceding section), you're ready to schedule the procedure. DBS is never an emergency, so timing will likely be based on your surgeon's schedule and availability, as well as your (and your family's) convenience.

Use the time (could be days or even weeks) before the doctors get to work on your brain to

>> **Outline a medication plan.** Make everyone involved in your surgery and postsurgical care needs aware of your medications (for PD and anything else). Make sure that your care team has a clear plan in place for managing all your medications (including those for other conditions, such as high blood pressure or diabetes) during postsurgical care and throughout your recovery.

Some drugs (such as an anti-anxiety medication) commonly used in the postsurgical recovery period can really cause problems for PWP. Make sure your post-surgical team has a plan in place to prevent some well-intentioned hospitalist or resident from inadvertently prescribing one of these meds.

>> **Set up a post-surgery meeting.** Make sure your family knows when and where they can expect to see your neurosurgeon following the surgery.

What to expect during and after surgery

For three to six hours, you'll be under local (or possibly no) anesthetic, off your medication, aware of your surroundings and the doctors, and experiencing the full range of your PD symptoms. The good news is that you'll be so integrally involved in the procedure — answering questions from the surgeon and other people while they work — that you'll probably be less aware of the discomfort than you imagine.

Prior to surgery, your doctor can provide printed information and a full description of the procedure so that you have some idea about what's going on. Here's a big picture look at the initial surgery and subsequent procedures:

>> **During your initial DBS surgery,** the surgeon drills a small hole in the skull and then inserts an electrode (a thin wire, called a *lead*), positioning it in a targeted area of the brain. This is the scary portion of DBS surgery; after you're done with the implant, the road gets a lot smoother.

>> **In a subsequent procedure** (two to four weeks after the implant of the lead), the surgeon inserts an implantable neurostimulator (sometimes called a pulse generator or IPG), or battery pack, under the skin in the area of your collarbone. Finally, they will connect a thin, insulated wire (called the extension) from the battery pack to the lead.

After this connection, your neurostimulator can be programmed to send signals appropriate to your individual condition and symptoms; this programming may take several sessions to complete.

Gearing up for the precise procedure

Because DBS requires precise work, your surgery team places your head in a helmet-like contraption that attaches to both your skull and the operating table to ensure that your head remains still throughout the procedure. (Sounds like something out of a sci-fi or horror movie, but in most cases, the only complaint is a post-surgery headache.)

Your neurosurgeon must follow precise and demanding steps to implant the neurostimulator. Fortunately, modern technology has special brain-imaging equipment that permits your surgeon to calculate the precise coordinates of the targeted area deep in the brain. In addition, most surgical centers *map* your brain activity during the initial DBS surgery by recording the electrical activity of different groups of cells encountered during the journey from the surface of your brain to the depth where the surgeon places the lead.

In fact, every area of the brain has a distinctive electrical *language*, which allows the surgeon to match the initial coordinates for implanting the lead with the proper area of electrical activity. (This process was once compared to a tourist traveling blindfolded through Europe trying to identify their position based on the local language.)

Alternatively, some centers use an approach called *interventional MRI-guided* DBS implant, which uses real-time MRI images to guide the placement without having to map the electrical activity of the brain. As a consequence, the procedure can be performed under general anesthesia, which is often desirable for PWP who may not be eager to spend one or more hours awake while a surgeon drills a hole in their skull.

Connecting the implantable pulse generator (IPG)

After your surgeon gets the lead in place (see the preceding section), they may implant the battery and extension wire at the same time, or they may wait up to a week or two before connecting the system. Compared to implanting the electrode (lead) in the initial DBS surgery, connecting the system is child's play:

1. Your surgery team places you under general anesthesia.

2. Your surgeon makes a small incision near your collarbone and forms a pocket under the skin.

3. They insert the implantable pulse generator (IPG) in that pocket.

4. Your surgeon runs a small wire from the IPG up your neck and behind your ear.

5. They connect the IPG to the DBS lead in your scalp.

6. Your surgeon closes the incision with stitches or staples.

The hospital stay and recovery

Hospitalization for DBS surgery is usually two days, with one overnight stay. For more complicated surgeries (when post-surgery confusion, infections, or other complications occur), you may have to stay longer. In most cases, however, you can recover simply by resting. This rest is important for a number of reasons: to get past the emotional and physical exhaustion that can be a part of any surgery; to rest after the possible slight headache (because of the helmet apparatus); and, in some cases, to reduce the mild confusion experienced immediately after surgery. Most DBS patients are able to leave the hospital the morning following the procedure.

Most routine postoperative conditions clear up after the first day. Your doctor will remove the stitches or staples in your scalp a week or so after your discharge. You can see the IPG (battery pack), which is usually implanted two to four weeks after your initial DBS surgery, as a slight bump in your chest (especially if you're slender), but you don't feel the wires or apparatus while they work.

Programming DBS into Your Life

Surgery of any type takes a lot out of you. You have to deal with stress and anxiety from anticipating the procedure, exhaustion from the procedure itself, and suspense and concern about whether it worked, whether it was worth the trouble. The following sections can help you anticipate your life after your DBS surgery.

Changes you can expect

Following DBS surgery, your PD doctor determines the best time to begin reducing your medication. But first, your neurostimulator must be programmed. This process may take one long initial programming session, as well as a few outpatient visits. In the same way that you have unique responses to medication, you may have unique responses to the stimulator.

REMEMBER

You may not realize the full benefits of DBS for weeks or even months, although most people experience some effects the same day the unit is programmed. Tremors and dyskinesias are usually the first symptoms to respond. Be patient while your doctor works with you to balance the settings on your stimulator with your medication regimen.

During this sometimes-exasperating trial-and-error process, you may have some temporary discomfort, such as minor shocks or muscle spasms. These symptoms are related to adjusting and programming the neurostimulator and should be brief. Before you leave the office after a programming/adjustment session, your doctor may want you to wait around with them for an hour or so, just to be sure you're okay with the new settings.

Warning signs you need to heed

Although you may experience some discomfort and unusual symptoms while your doctor programs your neurostimulator, let them know if you experience any of the following symptoms or signs that the transmitter may not be functioning accurately after implantation or between programming sessions:

» Shocks or tingling sensations

» Numbness or spasms, especially in the face or hands; dyskinesia-like movement

» Impaired balance or dizziness

>> Sensory effects such as slurred speech, or blurred or double vision

>> Depression

Precautions you need to take

TIP

The patient-information manual you receive post-surgery provides common warnings about possible problems associated with the implanted device. Review these warnings in detail with your treating physician or programming nurse. And while you go about your normal routines after surgery, take these precautions:

>> **Be careful around airport security.** Ask for a hand-check when you go through security while traveling because the electromagnetic field of the security equipment can cause your neurostimulator to shut down. (If that happens, you can turn it back on with a handheld remote.) Not to worry: Airport security personnel are accustomed to travelers who have implants, such as a defibrillator or pacemaker.

>> **Rethink contact sports.** If you play sports, carefully rethink any high-level contact sports, such as basketball or soccer. Repeated direct blows to the implant or its connectors can cause the device to malfunction. The last thing you want or need is to have to go through another surgery to replace or repair them.

>> **Watch for neurostimulator interference.** At home, try to stay away from microwave ovens (while they're in use) and be aware of the magnetic strip that keeps the refrigerator door shut. Swinging the fridge door near your chest may inadvertently turn off your neurostimulator.

>> **Double-check before medical imaging tests.** Check with your PD doctor before fulfilling any doctor's orders for imaging tests, particularly an MRI. The test may be perfectly safe for you, but it doesn't hurt to be sure. CT scans are generally safer.

IN THIS CHAPTER

» Noting the distinctions: Alternative versus complementary therapies

» Grasping options for your mind and body

» Choosing the right CAM professional

» Facing life with PD with a positive attitude

Chapter **12**

Considering Complementary and Alternative Medicine Therapies

M edication and surgical procedures are only two of the options for treatment of your Parkinson's disease (PD) symptoms. Increasingly, the healthcare profession is embracing the benefits of some complementary and alternative medical treatments. While these therapies may not always be covered by insurance, they are worth discussing with your doctor. The good news is that in some cases, CAM treatments can be considered medically necessary, and your insurance will cover at least part of the cost.

This chapter helps you understand the differences between complementary and alternative therapies so that you can sort through the various options and weigh the potential benefits of each. It also helps put you in touch with reputable practitioners if you decide to expand your treatment plan.

REMEMBER

Don't underestimate the importance of diet and exercise to your success in managing your PD symptoms. These topics are so vital that they get their own discussion (see Chapter 9). In this chapter, though, we look at therapies you may have heard of but never considered as viable complements or alternatives to the conventional plan that you expect your doctor to recommend.

What's in a Name? CAM Therapies Defined

Techniques, medicines, and therapies that take a holistic (mind, body, and spirit) and unconventional approach to the treatment of disease are often called *complementary* or *alternative medicine* (CAM) therapies. See Table 12-1 for a high-level look at these therapies.

TABLE 12-1   **CAM Therapies**

Category	Description	Examples	Usual Usage
Alternative medicine	Approaches to well-being not standard in Western society but common in Eastern societies	Yoga, tai chi, acupuncture, herbal remedies	May replace or accompany conventional treatments
Complementary therapy	Techniques and approaches to healthy living more familiar to Western societies	Physical, occupational, and speech therapies; modifications to diet (more veggies and less meat for example); regular exercise regimens	Augments conventional treatments

REMEMBER

Although alternative and complementary treatments may work in tandem with more traditional medical treatment, they usually haven't passed (or even been required to pass) the rigorous, scientific, evidence-based tests that conventional medicines and treatments must navigate for the Food and Drug Administration's (FDA) approval.

However, in 1998, the National Institutes of Health (NIH) established what's now known as the National Center for Complementary and Integrative Health (NCCIH). The NIH created this center because it recognized the growing popularity of alternative and complementary therapies, and thus the need for

>> Establishing standards for practitioners

>> A respected resource for validating information and conducting research on the therapies' benefits

NCCIH focuses on four key areas:

>> Research

>> Training and career development for researchers working on projects related to alternative or complementary treatments

>> Public outreach and education

>> Integration of CAM treatments with conventional medicine

You can find information about specific therapies on the NCCIH website at www. nccih.nih.gov.

WARNING

Before you consider any alternative or complementary therapy, make sure the therapy is from a licensed, certified practitioner. (See the section "Finding the Best Practitioner," later in this chapter, for tips on determining the right profes-, sional for the job.) Also, talking about the CAM therapy you're considering with the doctor(s) managing your PD treatment plan is not a bad idea.

DEBUNKING THE MYTHS ABOUT TREATING PD

PD treatment has a number of urban myths that surface from time to time about what does and doesn't work. Often, these falsehoods are from credible sources (such as members of your support group or even articles in respected, usually trustworthy publications). The Internet is another prime source for such rumors. For these reasons, remember to seek and confirm information by asking questions of your doctor or other trusted healthcare professionals (such as your pharmacist). And use only reliable PD information resources, such as those listed in Appendix B.

The following are some of the more prevalent myths floating around:

• **Levodopa is toxic.** Actually, it's been working for PWP for over half a century.

• **Levodopa will stop working after a while.** No, but symptoms may escalate, causing you to need stronger, more frequent dosing.

• **You die from PD.** How you're going to die is as much a mystery now as it was before you were diagnosed — could be a car accident, lightning, a heart attack, and so on.

(continued)

(continued)

- **You're definitely going to be in a wheelchair.** Keep in mind that PD is unique to every person. Your chances of being in a wheelchair are probably higher than some PWPs and far lower than others'.

- **You're definitely going to be demented or a vegetable.** PD has no definite outcomes. As for being a vegetable? Just focus on eating vegetables and stop predicting the future.

- **Your children will have PD.** Go back and read Chapter 3 right now — and discover the possible genetic correlation with PD.

- **You can't eat proteins while taking levodopa.** Ah, the protein myth — see the section "The protein factor," in this chapter, for the role of protein in the life of a PWP. Meanwhile, eat your protein.

- **Surgery doesn't work for PD.** It may not work for some people. But it does work in combination with prescription medications for most others, and you may be one of them.

- **You can cure PD by using alternative therapies.** Such "miracle" therapies include special combinations of herbs and vitamins. We've said it before, and we'll say it again — PD doesn't have a cure yet.

- **You can cure PD by having your feet massaged.** This is our personal favorite PD myth; we're not even going to comment any further.

Somewhere along the path that your life has taken, someone told you: If something sounds too good to be true, it's probably not true. So when someone tries to sell you the snake-oil-of-a-cure, or a concoction that reverses symptoms, or a plan that halts PD's progression, just walk away. Your best weapons against this web of half-truths? Be informed, keep up with new research, and ask questions.

Introducing Your CAM Options

The concept of any therapy other than traditional medical methods (medications and surgery) may be new to you. And one of the beauties of reading up on these various CAM options is that you can do so in the privacy of your own home before you talk to your doctor about them.

In the following sections, we introduce you to several of the more prevalent therapies. Before taking any action, though, be sure you discuss with your PD doctor the potential of such therapies for helping your PD symptoms. (Then again, maybe your PD doctor has suggested one or more of these techniques, and you're reading this section because you — wisely — want to get a better idea of just what you're in for.)

East treats West: Acupuncture and other traditional Chinese medicine

For centuries, Western medical experts considered Eastern medical techniques to be experimental at best and quackery at worst. But these days, that attitude has changed dramatically. Traditional Chinese medicine (TCM) is founded on the concept of *qi* (or *chi*), when the person's natural flow of energy is in balance. This system includes forms (such as exercise, herbal remedies, acupuncture, and massage) that work with energy points that TCM practitioners have identified in the body.

Perhaps the most familiar TCM is *acupuncture*. This therapy usually requires a series of appointments by a trained and licensed therapist who inserts sterile needles (about the size of a human hair) into a part of the body believed to affect the area needing treatment. Although acupuncture hasn't been shown to relieve PD symptoms, it may help persons with Parkinson's (PWPs) who experience cramping, stiffness, pain, or non-motor symptoms such as sleep disturbances or anxiety. (For more information, check out the American Society of Acupuncturists website at www.asacu.org.)

Ohhh! Ahhh! Experiencing body-based CAM therapies

Treatments that manipulate or move various parts of the body (such as muscles and joints) are considered *body-based CAM therapies*. Major examples of this category are chiropractic and osteopathic therapy and body massages.

Chiropractic and osteopathic therapy

Chiropractors focus on the structure of the body as it relates to the function, preservation, or restoration of various parts. *Note:* In chiropractic literature, you may find some poorly defined theories that relate PD to previous head and neck traumas, which then suggest neck manipulations to treat (and cure!) the disease. *Remember:* PD currently has no cure. While trauma may be one of the environmental triggers of PD (see Chapter 2), these assumptions are criticized even within the chiropractic profession. The exact role of chiropractic therapy in PD is unknown at this time.

Osteopathic medicine is a more holistic medical approach based on the principle that all the body's systems work together. When one system is affected, then other systems are likely to be affected, as well. The hands-on techniques of some osteopaths to manipulate various body parts are considered a CAM therapy. Doctors of osteopathic medicine (DOs) are licensed doctors and can perform surgery and prescribe medications. Some DOs are the primary care physicians for those who live in small towns and rural areas, but many are accomplished movement disorders specialists and take great care of PWPs in major medical centers. An MD studies *allopathic* (conventional medicine that focuses on drugs and surgery) medicine, and a DO studies *osteopathic* (holistic medicine that considers environmental and lifestyle factors) medicine.

Massage

Many people associate massages with a ritzy spa or salon. But many medical professionals view regular massage therapy by a trained and certified therapist an important complement to conventional medical care. Massage can help relieve some of the stiffness and muscle contractions common in PD by

>> Increasing blood supply to the muscles

>> Increasing range of motion

>> Stretching the muscles for greater flexibility

REMEMBER

You may find that massage sometimes feels uncomfortable. Although you may experience some discomfort especially at the start of your session, you shouldn't ever feel pain. If you do, ask the therapist to stop and take a moment to discuss adjustments to the treatment before continuing.

TIP

A bonus to the physical benefits of massage is the mental payoff: reduced stress and anxiety. You and your care partner may find that regular sessions with a massage therapist can relieve stress and build a sense of well-being and calm.

Massage is also a good form of relaxation. Under the right circumstances, it offers an environment conducive to meditation and centering. See the following section for more about these benefits.

REMEMBER

Your insurance may cover therapeutic massage and other CAM therapies if your doctor prescribes them as medically necessary.

WARNING

If you're taking a blood thinner such as Warfarin, or you have osteoporosis or deep vein thrombosis, the pressure applied during massage can actually cause harm and therefore may be contraindicated. As always, check with your doctor.

Exploring mind and body options to relieve tension, stress, and anxiety

Mind and body therapies rely on the mind's ability to influence physical function and symptoms. These therapies include meditation, creative outlets (meaning music, art, or dance), and so on.

Employing relaxation techniques

Living with a chronic and progressive illness takes a lot out of you. Combine that reality with life's thousand other pressures (such as work, relationships, financial security, crime, the weather, and such) and you have a prescription for stress. So when you have PD, finding ways to eliminate tension from your mind and body makes especially good sense.

You can have planned relaxation without going anywhere, hiring anyone, or paying any money. You simply need to find a quiet place to focus totally on *you* for at least 15 minutes twice a day. Follow these steps:

1. **Find a comfortable, quiet place, and then take a seat and close your eyes.**

   In this position, let yourself become aware of your *physical* tensions.

2. **Breathe in and out, slowly and softly, while you relax each muscle group one at a time.**

   Go literally from head to toe. Consciously relax your forehead, neck, shoulders, arms, hands, fingers, torso, hips, thighs, calves, ankles, feet, and finally toes.

3. **Feel your body relaxing and take note of where you tend to store stress and tension.**

   For example, you may hold tension in your neck and shoulders, your fingers, or perhaps your jaw. Using the process outlined above, you will eventually be able to relax those areas beyond your planned relaxation sessions.

Trying out meditation

You can also use meditation when your tension is not only physical, but also mental and emotional. It can take many forms; consider the mantra-chanting practice of Zen meditation or the visualization techniques that follow recorded prompts to imagine (visualize) a calm, peaceful setting. Check out the apps for your phone (some are actually free) that are available for guided meditation by searching online with the term *apps for meditation.*

TIP

If you've never tried meditation, the Mayo Clinic recommends these tips to help you get started:

>> **Select a fitting form of meditation.** The practice should fit your lifestyle and daily routine, and work with your fundamental beliefs.

>> **Set aside the time.** If 15 minutes twice a day seems too much, start with 5 minutes and work your way up to longer sessions.

>> **Forgive your slips.** If your mind wanders, recognize it. Then come back to your focus on relaxing and calming your mind, body, and spirit.

>> **Experiment.** It may take some time to find the timing and method that works best for you.

REMEMBER

In combination with relaxation, meditation can reduce stress for mind and body. But, like all complementary and alternative practices, meditation should supplement — not replace — your doctor's traditional therapies.

Getting in touch with your creative side

Quilting. Woodworking. Gardening. Knitting. Playing an instrument. Dancing — by yourself or in a group. Writing poetry or stories. Journaling. Everyone has a creative side. And, like G.K. Chesterton sagely said, "If a thing is worth doing, it is worth doing badly." You may not be Picasso or Mozart, but you can find pleasure in creating something unique, which doubles as good therapy because making art in any form (music, painting, writing, crafting) stimulates the mind and provides a welcome break from the stress of living with chronic illness.

Several regional Parkinson's organizations have added regular art classes and exhibitions to their programming. The Parkinson's Community of Los Angeles offers an exhibit they call *Living Artistically with Parkinson's*. An online search for the term *Parkinson's and art* can turn up some interesting and inspiring sites.

Based in the United Kingdom, the Parkinson's Art — Centre of Creativity (https://parkinsons.art) is a non-profit dedicated to showcasing and supporting creative projects produced by PWP through art, writing, and poetry. They offer these projects on their website and through traveling exhibits.

Here are some tips to get your creative side in gear:

>> **Find a new or return to a former hobby, art, or craft that appeals to you.** Establish a regular time to pursue it — an hour every evening, or once or twice a week if time is tight.

>> **Consider taking lessons at a local art center, community center, or shop.** You can enjoy the dual therapy of creativity plus socialization.

TIP

Can't draw? Try dancing! Dancing is maybe the highest form of creativity because it works on all levels: mental, emotional — and physical! Plus, you and your partner can enjoy it together. Check out the Dance for PD website at https://danceforparkinsons.org.

Letting those creative juices flow isn't about being accomplished. It's about finding pleasure, escape, and relief from the daily grind of managing your PD symptoms. Just say "Ahhh!"

Staying active via alternative exercise

Postural instability (the loss or impairment of your natural ability to hold yourself upright and maintain balance) can be a major problem for PWP. The greatest danger, of course, is falling. But a close second is the fear of falling that causes you to overcompensate for these off-balance positions, further jeopardizing your stability. One of the benefits of regular physical activity involves fostering the alignment, stability, and balance that are vital to your overall well-being and independence.

For PWP, Eastern exercise programs may be as beneficial, if not more so, than the traditional, strenuous Western types. Eastern exercise therapies tend to be performed slowly and focus on stretching motions that can enhance flexibility rather than rely on strength or speed. These therapies require no special equipment, and you can practice them when and where you choose. That said, Eastern methods aren't for everyone because some people find the slow movements and unusual poses difficult to conquer. But if you haven't been off the couch and gotten real exercise in a while, you may want to consider this variation.

Check with your doctor before beginning any exercise program — conventional or alternative.

Tai chi

This ancient, low-impact Chinese exercise combines measured breathing with slow, dance-like movements that develop flexibility, enhance cardiovascular health, and improve balance. Although you can find books and instructional visual aids, the best way to get started is by working with a trained professional to understand the proper moves and breathing combinations. Check with your local community center, senior center, or health club for classes in your area.

Yoga

Yoga incorporates stretching and balancing exercises in a slow, rhythmic pattern of movement. Forget the painful-looking, pretzel-like positions you may have seen on television or in movies. Yoga — properly done — combines stretching with breathing and meditation to achieve a greater sense of physical, mental, and spiritual balance.

Like with tai chi, yoga classes have levels from beginner to advanced and different styles of teaching. For example, some instructors focus more on the physical movement; others distribute the focus between the physical, breathing, and mind exercises.

If possible, find an instructor who can and will modify the traditional yoga positions and movements to accommodate your limitations. For example, if getting up and down from a mat is difficult, perhaps you can do a modified version of the movements while sitting in a chair.

REMEMBER

Adding one or more of these CAM therapies to your treatment plan means you're taking a more holistic approach to your wellness. Just be sure that you talk over any such addition with your doctor first.

Delving into dietary, protein, enzyme, and vitamin options

Although Chapter 9 has a detailed discussion of diet and exercise, the subject of complementary therapies also involves dietary issues. Because each person's individual physical make-up and PD plays a unique, participatory role in such therapies, the following sections provide information about CAM diets and diet supplements.

Diet — The usual rules apply

You know the drill. With or without PD, a healthy lifestyle includes a diet rich in fruits and vegetables but low in sugar, fats, and highly processed foods (*white foods* like white bread, white flour, white rice, and such).

WARNING

You also want to avoid foods that have been exposed to pesticides and other toxins. (Stick with organic fruits and vegetables, even though they're more expensive — you're worth it!) As we mention in Chapter 2, overexposure to pesticides and herbicides (common in nonorganic farming) may be one contributing factor in the onset of PD.

For additional help with dietary concerns, consider asking your doctor to recommend a trained nutritionist. A dietary professional may suggest a diet containing foods high in antioxidants (green leafy vegetables and the like) because ongoing studies indicate that such a diet may benefit PWPs. Another diet-specific concern is getting enough calcium because the lack of it may foster osteoporosis, which leads to softer bones and a greater chance of breaks from falls. Finally, studies have shown that the intake of protein in combination with antiparkinsonian meds can be an issue for some PWP. For more on the protein factor, see the following section.

The protein factor

A common PD myth is that protein in a PWP's diet can cause problems. Levodopa is an *amino acid* (the building block of every protein). While time goes by and you've been taking your L-dopa meds for years, if you eat a lot of dietary protein at the same time that you take your L-dopa medication, all that protein may compete with the absorption of your precious medications. Although you certainly don't want to remove protein from your diet, your doctor or nutritionist may recommend that you limit protein intake to particular meals and take your anti-PD meds (in particular, your carbidopa/levodopa) on an empty stomach.

CoQ10, CREATINE, TURMERIC, AND OTHER OTC SUPPLEMENTS

The federal government and medical community continue to sponsor studies involving the use of dietary supplements along with proven PD medications. This trend gives a clear indication of their willingness to consider the possibility that you may be able to better manage PD by using a combination of therapies (including supplements), rather than a single magic bullet (your PD meds). Here are some supplements whose benefits are being studied:

CoQ10 (coenzyme Q10): An antioxidant that is naturally produced by the body, which uses it for growth and maintenance. Levels of CoQ10 decrease with age and in people who have certain chronic conditions such as PD. Available as a dietary supplement, researchers once thought this enzyme might slow the progression of PD for some PWP. However, in 2011, a large clinical trial to assess the potential benefits of CoQ10 was terminated when researchers decided that continuing the trial (using the supplement CoQ10) was unlikely to demonstrate a resulting slowing of PD progression.

Creatine: A natural source of energy for muscle contraction, creatine comes from your diet and is also produced by the liver and kidneys. It is also found OTC as an energy-boosting dietary supplement. A study of creatine's use as a supplement was halted when early results showed no significant benefit.

Turmeric: A common spice that contains a chemical called curcumin. Turmeric is taken to treat pain and inflammation in certain conditions, for example, osteoarthritis. It has also shown some success in reducing symptoms of hay fever (such as sneezing) and depression. According to the website at www.parkinsonsresource. org, a study published in *Experimental and Therapeutic Medicine* found that turmeric may protect the nervous system from the toxins involved in causing the system's degeneration in Parkinson's disease.

No reputable source has created a standard diet for PWPs, but working with a nutritionist can help you adapt food choices to your symptoms and medications.

Vitamin supplements

As a PWP, you can take vitamins to help you maintain your recommended daily vitamin levels. Doing so is particularly helpful when you take levodopa for many years, because chronic treatment with levodopa can literally consume a number of key vitamins, such as B6, B12, and folate (B9). You may consider taking a good multivitamin — one that includes the key B vitamins that you need for brain and nerve health — but first ask your doctor to check the levels of these key vitamins in your blood. You don't want to overload your system either.

Taking calcium along with vitamin D helps prevent osteoporosis, a common concern for PWP, and taking calcium with magnesium can play a role in relieving muscle cramps. Be sure to ask your doctor about whether you should continue the vitamins and supplements you used before your diagnosis and whether you should add new ones.

Too much of a good thing may become a bad thing. Back in the 1980s, several studies looked at vitamin E as a way to prevent the onset of PD or slow its progression, but their results showed not only no benefit for PWP, but also that high-dosage vitamin E supplementation may actually increase mortality. A similar case can be made for vitamin B6, which is frequently contained in high doses in common multivitamin formulations. An excess of vitamin B6 has been associated with symptoms like tingling, numbness, and pain (neuropathy), which can be very disabling. On the other hand, eating a diet rich in natural sources of calcium, as well as vitamin E and C, can always boost your overall health.

In general, no studies have shown that a specific regimen of vitamin supplements can reduce or control PD symptoms. Certainly, because PWP can have a higher risk of bone loss than people of the same age without PD, your doctor may prescribe (especially for women patients) a calcium supplement or a prescription medication for preserving bone mass.

Finding the Best Practitioner

Keeping in mind that managing PD over the long haul is a team effort, be sure you talk to your PD doctor about the potential benefits and pitfalls of any alternative or complementary therapies you're considering. Your doctor(s) may take a "no harm, no foul" attitude without actually supporting the idea. Or they may suggest specific therapies for you to try or to avoid.

Adding CAM therapy to your PD management plan requires you to carefully choose the person who'll administer that therapy. The following tips can help you in that search:

TIP

>> If your PD doctor endorses the idea, ask for recommendations.

>> Confirm that this new addition to your care team has received training from a respected source and, if required, has passed the exams necessary to earn the appropriate degree or license.

In the United States, check the National Certification Commission for Acupuncture and Oriental Medicine to learn what the guidelines are for practicing in your state.

>> Consider adapting the checklist for finding a PD doctor (which we provide in Chapter 4) to guide your choice of alternative medicine practitioners.

After you select a practitioner, on your first visit to them, you still have a number of questions to ask:

>> What benefits can I expect from this therapy?

>> What are the risks associated with the treatment?

>> Does this therapy have any special benefits or risks related to my PD?

>> What are the side effects?

>> How many sessions or how long will I need to have the treatment to achieve the expected results?

>> Is this treatment *contraindicated* (to be avoided) if I have any particular conditions?

>> What do you charge per session?

>> Will my insurance pay for this therapy?

REMEMBER

You're not married to a specific practitioner. If you're uncomfortable with the treatment or the practitioner while the sessions proceed, then stop and talk the problem out. If you aren't satisfied with the response, move on.

Considering How Your Approach to Life Can Help — or Hinder

You know the difference between the eternal *pessimist* (who always expects the worst) and the forever *optimist* (who's over the top, always anticipating the best). Somewhere in the middle is the *realist* (as well as a bit of an idealist, philosopher, and activist) who accepts that bad things do indeed happen to good people. This person faces adversity and then looks for ways to get life back on track.

Celebrities such as Michael J. Fox, Linda Ronstadt, Alan Alda, Neil Diamond, and others are role models for how to make lemonade when life hands you lemons. But chances are good that you also know people within your circle of family, friends, and coworkers who also fit this positive profile. As a PWP, you're going to benefit most from this glass-half-full-and-things-could-be-a-lot-worse philosophy.

Three characteristics that most survivor-types have in common are

>> A positive attitude

>> The ability to laugh, even at the unfairness of life

>> A spiritual core that's as well-tended as their physical or mental health

The way you approach life — and all its joys and adversities — can play an enormous role in how successfully you live that life. The very fact that you're reading this book tells us that you're a survivor and a fighter. We're right here with information and ideas that can help you successfully find ways to live a full and fulfilling life in spite of having PD.

The therapeutic power of positive thinking

Life has no guarantees. But a lot of people live life more fully by rolling with the punches and taking a positive, can-do approach.

TIP

So, how do you deal with a diagnosis like PD? How do you face the progressive symptoms and side effects of the medicines? Believe it or not, the one factor that remains in your control throughout this journey is your attitude. You can't always maintain an upbeat attitude, and an occasional down period is normal. But instead of expecting the worst, you can fight back by choosing to live life fully and positively — as if you had never heard that diagnosis.

As a matter of fact, for some people, the diagnosis creates this shift in attitude. Discovering that they have PD turns their world upside down, so now they focus more intently on the positives. When you realize that life is finite, after all, you can use that knowledge as a real turning point — making you determined to live every day to the fullest. (And if your faith tells you that God doesn't test you more than you can endure, then you can start believing that higher opinion *and* start honing those survival capabilities!)

Laughter — Still the best medicine

According to the Mayo Clinic (www.mayoclinic.org) laughter boosts our intake of oxygen; stimulates our heart, lungs, and muscles (they all get involved when we laugh); and releases endorphins (those feel-good chemicals housed in your brain). Face it: When you laugh, you feel better. Your outlook improves — if only momentarily. You may even feel better physically.

Consider the angry, depressed man who had just gone through brain surgery. He told his wife he didn't want any visitors. The wife ran into several close friends at the elevator and told them, "Not today." But the friends still insisted. "We'll only stay a moment," they promised. Within moments, the woman heard the welcome sound of laughter — her husband's. While the visit went on and the friends worked their magic, that laughter couldn't be repressed.

Open up to life — Physically, mentally, and spiritually

REMEMBER

When you face a chronic and progressive illness day after day, you understandably have times when you just want to burrow under the covers and hope it all goes away. Resist that temptation!

Because we address your physical and mental well being throughout this book, this section looks at one other dimension — your spiritual needs — and how meeting those needs can enhance your life. *Spirituality* is that core inside you where your sense of well-being and desire to survive reside. Some people participate in organized rituals of religion to help them foster this core, but rituals can't be all of it; for other people, rituals and religion play no part at all.

You store your self-identity in your spiritual core. Your body may shake and twist, and your mind may play tricks with your memory and concentration, but your spirit remains unchanged.

TIP

Like PD, spirituality is different for every individual. But one way to begin focusing on your spiritual well-being is by using your senses to their full effect. Consider the following suggestions:

>> **Listen:** To a sermon, an inspirational reading, a concert, water flowing, wind in the trees, rain on the roof, your innermost hopes and dreams

>> **Look:** At the people who surround you, love you, and care for you

>> **Touch:** By taking a friend's hand; petting a dog or cat; hugging a loved one; stroking a leaf, a rock, a child's hair

>> **Smell:** Freshly cut grass, an autumn fire, cookies straight from the oven

>> **Taste:** The bitter, as well as the sweet

>> **Savor:** The unique tastes, sounds, sights, scents, and feelings that form the wonders of your life

REMEMBER

Tapping into your spiritual side takes the same focused effort as managing your physical and mental needs. And your willingness to push yourself on all three levels can pay off by facilitating a full and satisfying life in spite of PD.

IN THIS CHAPTER

» Getting on top of anxiety and depression

» Battling apathy with action

» Looking for help in all the right places

» Embracing effective lifestyle changes

» Thinking positively for you and your care partner

Chapter **13**

Combating Anxiety, Depression, and Apathy

You've gotten some bad news: It's Parkinson's disease (PD). At the moment, you don't know a lot — about the disease, about its impact on you and those you love, about so many questions. You're trying to come to terms with a diagnosis that means your life has changed and will keep changing while the years roll by. Of course, you have anxious moments — maybe some full-blown panic attacks. And news like this doesn't exactly put a smile on your face or a lot of sunshine in your outlook. When reactions like these last for a short time and then pass, that's normal human behavior.

On the other hand, feelings of anxiety, panic, depression, and apathy that persist for days, weeks, or even months aren't normal. And for people living with Parkinson's (PWP), their PD can complicate the anxiety and depression — a combination of living with a chronic, progressive illness *and* the neurochemical changes occurring in the brain.

This chapter looks at the ways PD plays a part in the onset of anxiety and depression and provides a host of proven solutions — some of them admittedly a little unorthodox — that can bring you relief.

Recognizing Anxiety — What's Normal and What's Not

Anxiety is a serious — but treatable — medical condition that can affect your quality of life and ability to function while you adapt to living with PD. And a number of circumstances (such as stress, side effects of meds, and lifestyle changes due to PD) can trigger an episode that sends you reeling.

Some situations naturally warrant anxiety and worry (the meeting with the boss, for example, or giving a major presentation or party). However, when time, accomplishment, or common sense don't relieve the panic, terror, and outright impending doom, something's wrong. Are you normally easygoing, self-confident, and optimistic? If you suddenly (and regularly!) find yourself dealing with persistent dread or disproportionate fear that impacts your ability to function throughout the day, these feelings need attention.

REMEMBER

Research studies confirm the following facts about anxiety for PWP:

>> It affects close to half of PWP.

>> It can be one of the first non-motor symptoms that make the PWP seek a doctor's care.

>> It often goes hand in hand with depression (which we talk about in the section "Depression — More Than Just Sad and Blue," later in this chapter).

Identifying the source of anxiety

Any number of circumstances can bring on anxiety, and that anxiety generally takes one of these forms:

>> **Generalized anxiety disorder (GAD):** A condition in which the person lives day in and day out with an underlying sense of worry that something will go wrong, but the worry has no real basis.

>> **Social phobias:** Persistent worry that focuses on a specific situation or circumstance related to the social environment (such as a fear of failure or of interacting with other people).

>> **Panic attack:** Anxiety that strikes unexpectedly, suddenly, and hard. Usually, a panic attack comes complete with major physical symptoms (such as a racing heartbeat, shortness of breath, and even chest pain). In fact, having a panic attack may make you think you're having a heart attack.

Circumstances contributing to anxiety may include a particularly unsettling and stressful event (such as a diagnosis of PD); existing personality traits (such as low self-esteem and poor coping skills); or the presence of an additional mental condition (such as depression, discussed in the section "Depression — More Than Just Sad and Blue," later in this chapter).

REMEMBER

One way to identify the circumstances that cause anxiety involves mindfulness of your own fight-or-flight mechanism. (*Fight-or-flight* is the most common reaction when people face situations that bring on stress, anxiety, or outright panic. In other words, they either stand and fight, or retreat or do nothing. Think of the times when you faced that choice. For example, if your boss confronted you about a missed deadline and you simply accepted their blame without responding (you do nothing), that's flight. But if you listened and then explained exactly why the delay was unavoidable, that's fight (you stand your ground and defend yourself).

So as a PWP, what sets off your fight-or-flight alarm? How persistent is it? Is your first instinct usually to take action, find answers, seek knowledge? (That's fight.) Or do you wait for others to direct you? (That, of course, is flight.) It's perfectly understandable that you'll have times when you just want to crawl under the covers and let somebody else live with PD for a while. But the more you adopt the fight mentality, the more likely you are to maintain independence and control over your life.

Measuring your level of anxiety

TIP

Although doctors use professional tools to diagnose anxiety, a short self-evaluation of your symptoms can help determine whether you should seek professional help. Mark an X in Table 13-1 to indicate the feelings or physical sensations you experience on most days and for much of the day.

WARNING

If you marked five or more of the symptoms in the table, don't take them lightly, and don't postpone getting to the appropriate professional for treatment. (See the section "Finding and Accepting Help," later in this chapter, for specifics about professional help.) In any case, talk to your doctor. You may be suffering needlessly from anxiety.

TABLE 13-1   **Feelings Associated with Anxiety**

Feeling or Physical Sensation	Happens Most Days	Lasts for Much of the Day
Anxiousness or nervousness		
Fearfulness (for yourself or others)		
Feeling out of control		
Panic or jumpiness		
Shortness of breath or pounding heart		
Dizziness or lightheadedness		
Feeling flushed or sweaty		
Inattentiveness		
Inability to take action		
Forgetfulness		
Sense of impending doom		

Depression — More Than Just Sad and Blue

According to the National Institute of Mental Health (NIMH), depression can strike anyone, but PWP may be at greater risk because both anxiety and depression could be far more than issues with your mental health. They could be non-motor indicators of PD. The following sections can help you consider your symptoms and determine whether it's time to take action.

REMEMBER

Keep in mind that some PD symptoms (such as the masked facial expression, slow movement, and lack of energy) can actually be symptoms of depression, which is a common non-motor feature of PD, and may be contributing to worsening of fatigue or PD motor features. Depression is treatable.

Recognizing the symptoms

The National Institute of Mental Health lists the following as symptoms of depression:

» Persistent sad, anxious, or empty feelings

» Feelings of hopelessness and pessimism

» Feelings of guilt, worthlessness, or helplessness

>> Loss of interest and pleasure in hobbies and activities

>> Fatigue, feeling slowed down, or decreased energy

>> Difficulty concentrating, making decisions, or remembering

>> Insomnia or oversleeping

>> Gains or losses in appetite or weight

>> Restlessness and irritability

>> Thoughts of death or suicide; suicide attempts

>> Crying, especially over little, seemingly incidental issues

Asking yourself the right questions

Although we definitely don't recommend self-diagnosis or treatment, ask yourself the ten questions in Table 13-2 if your feelings (mental and emotional) concern you on a daily basis. Mark each question as Yes or No.

TABLE 13-2 **Questions to Evaluate Depression**

The Question	Yes	No
Are you discouraged or sad?		
Are you moody or irritable?		
Are you feeling isolated or lonely?		
Have you lost interest in activities you can still do?		
Have you pulled away from interactions with friends and family?		
Is your outlook affecting your ability to work, make decisions, or make choices?		
Has your mood affected your sleep (for example, sleeping more in the day or not sleeping at night) or energy level?		
Have you experienced changes in appetite and weight?		
Have you lost interest in sex or intimacy with your partner?		
Have people you trust suggested that you seem depressed?		

If you've marked Yes for five or more of the questions in Table 13-2, you need to raise the possibility with your doctor that you may need treatment for depression.

WARNING

Finding yourself experiencing the symptoms listed here is a potentially dangerous situation:

>> Talking about wanting to die or being a burden to others

>> Feeling hopeless, trapped, more anxious or angry, or that you have no reason to live

>> Withdrawing from friends and family

>> Making a plan or researching ways to die

Get help as soon as possible by contacting the National Suicide Prevention Lifeline at https://suicidepreventionlifeline.org or 1-800-273-TALK, or the Crisis Text Line at www.crisistextline.org; text *HOME* to 741741 to reach a volunteer crisis counselor.

Dealing with Apathy and Lack of Motivation

Many PWP develop *apathy*, a condition in which a *flattening of affect* occurs, which means the mind and the spirit seem to give up on all emotions: good, bad, pleasant, or painful. Apathy is characterized by

>> Reduced interest and participation in routine activities

>> Lack of initiative; having difficulty starting or sustaining an activity to completion

>> Indifference or a lack of concern for others

WARNING

Symptoms of the PWP's apathy can trigger frustration in family, friends, and the care partner. When those around an apathetic person begin to realize that they're working harder at fighting PD than the PWP is, they tend to think that the person suffering from apathy doesn't appreciate their efforts or help. The end result can be that family and friends gradually go back to their own lives, leaving the person with apathy (and the care partner) more isolated and in need of help than before.

Apathy versus depression

REMEMBER

Apathy can be associated with several neuropsychiatric illnesses (such as Alzheimer's disease, PD, and stroke). In PD, however, apathy is more likely a direct consequence of physiological changes in the brain and lack of dopamine than a psychological reaction to disability. Although professionals can distinguish apathy from psychiatric symptoms and personality features (particularly depression and anxiety), it's not an easy task. Consider these subtle but distinguishing characteristics:

» Like people with depression, apathetic patients may be sluggish, quiet, and disengaged. They may talk slowly or not at all.

» Unlike depressed patients who may give verbal cues to their distress, apathetic PWP deny being sad, feeling guilty, or having suicidal thoughts.

TIP

Ask your primary care or PD doctor about the differences between apathy and depression, and what symptoms you (and your care partner) should watch for in either case. You can find an excellent article on the topic by Dr. Rebecca Gilbert of the American Parkinson Disease Association (APDA) at www.apdaparkinson.org/article/stress-anxiety-parkinsons-disease.

Invigorating an apathetic PWP

Recognizing apathy and differentiating it from depression in PWP is important because the medical treatment for the two conditions may be different. Patients who have apathy aren't lazy and may respond to a series of strategies that include gentle encouragement to initiate activities, as well as schedules and routines to keep them busy.

For example, consider a PWP who's always loved going to the ballpark. When that person's best friend extends an invitation to a major league game as a birthday gift, the PWP may indicate that they'd rather stay home in front of the television. But when the friend insists, they go to the park, and the PWP has a good time all day. However, the PWP immediately turns the television back on after returning home.

Finding and Accepting Help

You may have experienced depression, anxiety, or apathy before the onset of PD, or your first episode may come after the diagnosis. But the-chicken-or-the-egg question doesn't really matter. What does matter is that the symptoms are unnecessary hardships when you're dealing with PD.

Ask your doctor to recommend a consultation with a mental health professional who'll work closely with your doctor to assess your condition in the context of your PD.

TIP

Check with your insurance provider (or Medicare/Medicaid, if appropriate) to find out what services your plan covers. If your insurance provider doesn't cover mental health services (or covers only a portion), ask whether the professional you're considering has a sliding fee scale based on income.

Taking medication may help

In most cases, PWP tolerate antidepressant medications well. Your doctor will start with a low dose over several weeks to see how well you tolerate the antidepressant. Over time, if symptoms persist, your doctor may adjust the dosage to find a sweet spot where it works for you at the lowest possible dosage. But these medications can take weeks to have a real effect, and finding the right medication can require a good deal of trial and effort. As a result, many doctors recommend a combination treatment plan that may include or take the place of antidepressants. Combo possibilities include

>> Talk therapy (the services of a professional mental health counselor)

>> Changes in diet, exercise routines, and sleep habits

WARNING

Before you take any medication — whether prescription or over-the-counter (OTC) — to treat symptoms of depression or anxiety, be sure your prescribing doctor is fully aware of all your other medications. Some OTC supplements can interact in a negative or even harmful way with your other medications. Anytime you add something to your regimen, ask your pharmacist to review all your medicines and supplements. The pharmacist's job includes knowing about possible negative interactions.

Seeking a professional counselor

Your doctor may recommend a professional counselor who helps you talk through the feelings and fears that create the foundation of your depression or anxiety. In looking for the right counselor, keep in mind the different categories:

>> **Psychiatrists:** Medical doctors who have training (at least four years) beyond their medical degree. These doctors are board-certified by the American Board of Psychiatry and Neurology (ABPN) and licensed in the state where they practice. They can prescribe medications and coordinate a total care plan for any mental or emotional health issue.

- **Psychologists:** Counselors who have a master's degree (MA or MS) or a doctoral degree (PhD or PsyD) in psychology and/or counseling. Psychologists are board-certified by the American Board of Professional Psychology (ABPP) and licensed by the state where they practice.

  Psychologists are less focused on biological causes of depression and anxiety, and more focused on treating your symptoms.

- **Clinical social workers:** Counselors who are licensed or certified by the state and usually hold a master's degree in social work and/or counseling. Some social workers have advanced training in psychotherapy and may have the title of Licensed Clinical Social Worker (LCSW).

- **Other counselors:** This category includes professionals such as

  - *Psychiatric nurses or clinical nurse specialists (CNSs):* Registered nurses (RNs) who have additional training in psychiatry.

  - *Family therapists:* Hold a title or degree but focus primarily on counseling within the context of a family group.

  - *Pastoral counselors:* In addition to their religious training (in Christianity, Judaism, Buddhism, or whatever belief system they ascribe to), these clergy also have training in counseling.

Accepting the role of a counselor

Make your therapy to treat depression, anxiety, or a mental or emotional condition a collaborative process. You need to feel a real sense of trust and rapport with this person. Keep in mind that therapists push you to examine and confront sometimes unpleasant and even painful issues. They're not trying to be mean, but they are trying to get you past roadblocks that may hamper your ability to accept PD in order to live a fuller, more satisfying life.

REMEMBER

Any mental health professional has the ethical (in some cases, legal) responsibility to keep your therapy discussions confidential *unless* you threaten to cause harm to other persons or property.

Choosing the right counselor for you

In addition to checking credentials and experience, take time to really consider the connection you'll have with this therapist or counselor. Follow these steps to make sure you find a good fit:

1. **Work with your primary care physician (PCP) to rule out medical causes for your depression or anxiety symptoms.**

2. **Get at least two (and preferably three) referrals from your primary care doctor, PD doctor, or support group facilitator.**

TIP

   Consider specifics (such as the therapist's age, gender, and ethnic or religious background) that are important to you, and make those specifics known when you ask for referrals.

3. **Consider the convenience of a therapist or counselor's location.**

   You're going to see this person on a regular (perhaps weekly) basis over several months. The last thing you need is an inconvenient journey to and from the appointment.

4. **Make a plan for your first appointment.**

   Go in with the following points in mind:

   - Ask the same questions you ask your other specialists. (See Chapter 6 for these questions.)

   - Be prepared to describe the symptoms that led you to seek help.

   - Listen to the therapist's possible plan for treatment (medications, talk therapy, or both).

   - Prepare to listen for language such as "in cases like yours. . ." that suggests a generalized, rather than a customized, approach to therapy. If the therapist seems to take this one-size-fits-all approach, keep looking.

WARNING

After the first appointment, keep in mind that you need genuine trust and connection with the counselor or therapist to successfully conquer your symptoms. Give yourself time to think about the first meeting — what went well and what disturbed you — before keeping a second appointment. And if you go to that second appointment, let the therapist know what troubled you that first time around.

Sharing the emotional journey with a support group

A support group can be a real lifesaver for many people who have a chronic, progressive condition (and their care partners). Through these gatherings, you can hear about valuable coping skills and keep up with the latest myths and bona fide medical advances. Generally, each group has a facilitator who has professional experience in working with PWP and their care partners. This objective, outside facilitator is responsible for

>> Keeping the discussion moving

>> Stopping a few outspoken participants from hijacking the meeting so that quieter personalities fade into the background (and eventually leave the group)

>> Taking care of logistics: Meeting place and time, special speakers or programs, and notices of meetings

The most successful groups determine their own personality and style. The following are examples of group formats:

>> **Participants talk about PD news and personal updates.** They support one another emotionally and offer ideas for coping.

>> **A speaker such as a specialist in the field of PD or perhaps a therapist presents a specific topic for discussion.**

>> **The group has a political focus,** such as getting Congress to allocate research dollars that can put PD on the front burner for finding a cure. (See related information in Appendix B.)

>> **Some groups include multiple formats,** alternating group support with specific programs and advocacy projects.

TIP

PWP and their care partners have access to national organizations that offer support groups through their regional or state chapters. To see whether such a group is available in your area, you can check out the Parkinson's Foundation at www. parkinson.org, AIRPO (Alliance of Independent Regional Parkinson Organizations) at www.parkinson.org/get-involved/Local-resources/airpo, or the National Family Caregivers Association (NFCA), which you can find at https:// caringcommunity.org by hovering over the Resources link and clicking the Professional link from the drop-down that appears. Scroll through the resulting entries to find the NFCA.

If your area has zero groups specifically for PWP or their care partners, consider starting one. See the sidebar "Building a support group: From *me* to *we* in five easy steps," in this chapter, to get started.

Whether you join an established group or start one yourself, support groups can enrich your life beyond anything you can imagine because you

>> Connect with people who truly understand the challenges of living with PD.

>> Have the opportunity to laugh and cry together.

>> Can advocate for better treatments and a cure.

>> Can make an enormous difference for yourself and for those who love and care for you.

BUILDING A SUPPORT GROUP: FROM *ME* TO *WE* IN FIVE EASY STEPS

Follow these relatively simple steps to start a PD support group:

1. **Ask your PD doctor to tell other PD patients and their care partners that you're interested in organizing a group.**

   Provide cards that have your contact information for the doctor to give to interested PWP. These people can then contact you (not the other way around, which preserves their privacy and keeps the doctor on the right side of those infamous HIPPA laws.

2. **Gather the relevant information.**

   Ask your local hospital or home care agency whether they have anyone qualified and willing to facilitate the group.

   Find out whether your local library, bookstore, coffeehouse, or medical clinic has a room available for 10 to 12 people for two hours once a month at no charge.

3. **Consider initially combining PWP and care partners in the same group.**

   While the group grows, you may start to hold separate meetings for the PWP and care partners.

4. **When at least four people have expressed interest, call an organizational meeting and ask these people to invite other PWP or care partners.**

5. **If possible, ask an experienced support-group facilitator to lead an initial meeting.**

At the first meeting

   Have nametags and perhaps light refreshments.

   Ask attendees to briefly introduce themselves and state what they're looking for in a support group.

   Establish the working details for the group: when and where to meet; how often; for how long; dues, if any, to cover cost of refreshments or mailings; and programs or format style of the group.

   If you don't have a trained facilitator, consider professional speakers to lead the first several meetings. Then alternate the leader role within the group and assign responsibilities (meeting room, program, and participant notifications) for the next three months.

   End the meeting by confirming everyone's contact information and allowing time for people to socialize and get to know each other better.

Making Lifestyle Changes to Improve Your Point of View

Many people tie together the idea of enjoying life — feeling content — with being in control. But how much can anyone really control? The next hour, day, or year? Nope. The only control you really have lies in how you choose to react to life's circumstances and challenges.

The areas you *can* control revolve around your daily activities and outlook on life:

>> **Start with two words: exercise and diet.** (But you can check out Chapter 9 for a few more words.) It's no secret that research shows how regular exercise, a properly balanced diet, and regular sleeping habits can work wonders for your health, regardless of whether you have PD.

>> **Embrace the bright side: a sense of humor and positive attitude.** Finding humor in the mishaps and misadventures of living with PD is no different from finding humor in other life challenges (such as the impossible in-law or the service people who don't show up even with a four-hour window).

If you look, you can find humor in almost any situation. As Garrison Keillor, author and former host of the popular radio program *Prairie Home Companion*, once said, "They say such nice things about people at their funerals that it makes me sad that I'm going to miss mine by just a few days."

Making exercise a must and diet a tool

Just in case you need a refresher on some of the wonders of staying active, did you know that exercise can power-up neurotransmitters in your brain, which enhances your mood and your ability to look at life more positively? Exercise can also help relieve muscle tension in the face of stress and buck up your self-image, too. Not a bad return on an investment of only 30 to 60 minutes a day!

As for diet, start with a simple choice like lessening stimulants (such as caffeine and chocolate) that can contribute to your anxiety. Ready to kick it up a notch? Educate yourself about the mind-enhancing powers of certain food groups. (For more information on diet and nutrition, see Chapter 9.) When you combine these power foods with regular exercise, you have the right formula to make an enormous difference in your emotional state of mind and self-image.

TIP

Alternative therapies (such as relaxation and meditation) and mind-exercise programs (such as tai chi and yoga) can also be enormously effective in relieving the symptoms of anxiety and depression. See Chapter 12 for more info on these techniques.

Making sure to get your beauty sleep

A good night's sleep is one of the most important activities for the health of your brain. *Sleep deprivation* (a chronic lack of proper night sleep) can aggravate many PD symptoms, including the mood abnormalities described in this chapter (anxiety, apathy, depression), physical fatigue, and forgetfulness. Many PWPs report that medications for PD work better and last longer after a good night of sleep. Make sure to establish a proper pre-sleep routine, avoid late snacks, and don't fall asleep in front of the TV trying to catch your favorite late-night comedy — you can record it and watch later.

REMEMBER

PD can be associated with specific sleep abnormalities, such as *REM sleep behavior disorder* (acting out your dreams) or sleep apnea. Consult your doctor if you find out that you snore loudly or kick your bed partner; you may need a sleep study and specific treatment. See Chapter 9 for more information about sleep and PD.

Don't worry — be happy

No doubt you want to remind us that PD isn't exactly humorous. And the humor you find in PD is, of course, bittersweet. But don't permit the bitter to overpower the sweet. Choosing to laugh at yourself — and the frustrations and mishaps that can come with PD — offers a healthy dose of the absurd that can work better than any pill. The ability to laugh can work miracles for you and your care partner(s).

Just say the word

TIP

One PWP came up with the acronym *S.O.F.A.* (as in "Get off the sofa") to remind himself that anxiety, apathy, and depression are dangerous areas for anyone with PD. *Sadness* can lead to *Obstructions* (of physical and mental abilities) that lead to a *Fall* (the danger for any PWP), so the only cure is *Ambition* (to get moving — physically, mentally, and spiritually). This acronym may not work for you, but try one of your own — a password that empowers you and your care partner when anxiety and depression start to rear their ugly heads.

IT'S NOT ALL ABOUT YOU: WAYS TO LOOK BEYOND YOUR PD

One sure way to get past the poor-pitiful-me piece is to focus less on yourself and ramp up your attention to other people. This simple change can also remind other people to stop viewing you as someone with an incurable condition and start seeing you as the vital, loving, and giving person you've always been.

Fresh out of ideas? Not surprising. But, hey, that's why we're here. Pick any one of the following and see what happens:

- If a clerk or service person gives especially good service, tell them, and then tell their boss.

- Offer to trade seats on a bus, train, or plane to let a family or couple sit together — even if you end up with the dreaded middle seat.

- Find old pictures of family members or friends, frame them, and send them to the person with a note that recalls what the photos mean to you.

- Look beneath the surface. When a friend is in a crummy mood, know that it probably goes well beyond the surface. Acknowledge that they're having a bad day and ask whether you can do anything to help.

- Pass along a good book you've just finished or make special scrapbooks or family recipe books for the children in your family.

- If you're a gardener and need to divide your perennials, offer your neighbor some plants from your garden. (They can do the digging up!)

- Put an extra coin in an expired meter.

- Call the service people that you regularly see by name.

- Take a treat to your coworkers (even if you have to buy, rather than bake, it).

- Use the magic words, "Please" and "Thank you," and make a big deal out of someone going the extra mile for you.

Focusing on other people — caring for and about them — is possibly the simplest way to move beyond your self-pity and angst about PD. Of course, it can't cure clinical depression or anxiety, but caring for others provides a big first step in changing your destructive, negative self-talk to something far more positive and life-affirming. Bottom line? It is indeed better to give (care and concern) than to receive (pity and avoidance).

The crème de la comedy

Renowned essayist and editor Norman Cousins pioneered the idea of laughter as medical therapy. In his 1979 book *Anatomy of an Illness* (W.W. Norton & Company), Cousins describes how he watched hours of comedy classics such as the Marx brothers and *I Love Lucy*—nice work, huh? As a result of his and other researchers' finding (as in laughing until they were crying), laughter is now a respected therapy that supplements mainstream medicine.

Did you hear the one about . . .?

At your next support group meeting, suggest the group indulge in some laugh therapy for 15 to 20 minutes by sharing funny incidents. After all, who else can understand the ridiculousness of trying to chop veggies for a salad or explaining to your grandchild how partnering in a three-legged race might not be the best idea? Who else but PWP can laugh out loud and not seem cruel when you describe yourself hurrying to catch an elevator?

Tapping into the power of positive thinking

Your attitude can make the difference between taking control of this disease and allowing PD to control you. How much better to hear people marvel at your incredibly upbeat and positive attitude toward PD than to hear them talk in tones of pity and sympathy! When you choose to react with a sense of humor and a positive life outlook, research suggests three possible benefits:

>> **You greatly reduce your physical and emotional stress** and greatly enhance your relationships with other people.

>> **Your outlook will be contagious.** By setting the tone (as we suggest in Chapter 5), you can help your care partners (professional and personal) accept the diagnosis and move forward with you.

>> **You have an aura of self-confidence** that also inspires people around you (who may be tempted to nurture or baby you) to step back and let you take the lead. They're more likely to make decisions *with* you rather than *for* you.

So how can you change a glass that's half empty into a glass that's half full? More to the point, can you even change it, given your PD diagnosis?

TIP

Optimists tend to believe that good things do happen and bad things are just temporary challenges. Fortunately, you can take steps to enhance your optimistic side. Check out these tips for becoming more optimistic:

>> **Find the joy** — in work, in relationships, in everyday stuff such as preparing a meal, cleaning, repairing something, getting dressed, and meeting the day head-on.

>> **Surround yourself with hopefulness** — people who are positive, upbeat, and optimistic.

>> **Commit random acts of kindness.** We didn't come up with this idea, but we like the sound of it! Look beyond yourself to the needs of others (see the sidebar, "It's not all about you: Ways to look beyond your PD," in this chapter).

>> **Accept and work through situations you can control;** let go of those you can't. (Does the word *serenity* come to mind?)

>> **Be aware of your reactions.** Banish negative self-talk ("I can't" or "I never"), and if family members or friends irritate you, look for underlying traits that you admire (or even love) in those people.

>> **Take note of your triumphs.** At the end of every day, write or tell yourself three good things (okay, they can be really little) that happened that day.

A Word for the PD Care Partner

Given the nature of depression, anxiety, and apathy, you — not the PWP — need to stay vigilant about recognizing symptoms and getting help to break the cycle. These are a few actions you can take:

>> **Pay attention.** Look at the PWP's body language. Listen to what they say (or don't say). Sure, that *mask* (lack of facial expression) or stooped posture may be a result of PD, but is something else at work here? If the person you love seems persistently uninvolved and disinterested in the normal routine that you two used to enjoy, those clues need your attention.

>> **Don't be afraid to ask questions.** Your PWP may have a logical but curable reason for appearing to be depressed, apathetic, or anxious. Through gentle questioning, maybe you can get them to admit their concern so that the two of you can talk about it (and address it with their doctor). On the other hand, if their answer to all of your questions is something like, "There's nothing wrong," they may have more troubling them than they can manage but don't know how to talk about it. In that case, you can

   • Offer information from PD websites (see Appendix B) and books like this one that clearly demonstrates how PWP commonly face such feelings and that professionals can help them deal with those feelings.

- Suggest that they talk to their PD doctor about their emotions and ask whether that doctor has any suggestions for treating these unusual feelings.

>> **Talk to the experts.** If the PWP refuses to address your concern that they may be depressed or suffering from anxiety or apathy, contact the PD doctor yourself and ask for help. Or ask the care partners in your support group whether they've dealt with these issues. If they have, ask for some suggestions on how you can follow through.

Don't forget to take care of you

Being the primary care partner for a PWP will — over time — become a natural piece of your life. Before you realize it, the role is more than a daily routine; it's part of your identity. "That's Joan Sutton. Her husband has Parkinson's," some-one may say, implying that your husband's condition somehow identifies you, as well. But Joan is much more than her husband's PD.

REMEMBER

The processes of partnering in care and caregiving require constant adjustment. Understandably, you'll have days (and weeks) of exhaustion, frustration, and depression. But interspersed, you'll have moments of such high drama, joy, and sharing that you find the will and energy to fight on. You make an enormous difference for the PWP. The support and care that you provide is vital, important work.

WARNING

The danger comes when you try to do it all (or at least, more than you should), and you burn out. The signs of burnout aren't that different from depression (see the section "Depression — More Than Just Sad and Blue," earlier in this chapter). Decide now to watch out for these signs and give yourself permission to take a break, hand off some of the responsibility to others, and most of all, have a life of your own.

Positive steps you can take

We recommend the following ways to help you hang in there:

>> **Identify and nurture your personal support system.** You need people to be there just for you — to listen to and comfort *you*. You're dealing with a host of feelings, including grief and bereavement. If you feel so isolated that you can't think of anyone to talk to, you need to consider seeking some counsel-ing. Ask your primary care doctor to recommend a counselor, or perhaps your clergyperson can help.

>> **Join a support group.** We can't stress this enough: The underlying cause of depression in care partners is a sense of isolation. The people you meet in a support group don't replace your best friends, but they do give you a place to vent and share PD war stories.

>> **Give yourself a break** — an actual physical break — every day, if possible. Use your support network to come in and take over for an hour or two. Take this time for yourself. Go for a walk, watch a movie, grab some coffee with a friend. Don't use your personal time for tasks such as paying the bills or calling the insurance company.

>> **Keep your priorities straight.** Your health is vital to the PWP, so exercise, eat a balanced diet, and maintain your own social interactions and activities.

>> **Don't forget to sleep.** Night sleep is essential to restore mental and physical energies that you must have to cope with the challenges of caring for your PWP. According to the Sleep Foundation (www.sleepfoundation.org), the symptoms of sleep deprivation include mood changes (stress, anxiety, and irritability), slow thinking, and lack of energy — all symptoms that you as a care partner can't afford.

Chapter **14**

Clinical Trials and Your Role in the Search for a Cure

I t's one thing to say that a new drug or treatment works for a monkey or mouse, but it's quite another to take that next leap and declare the product safe and effective for people. Research scientists make that leap by conducting *clinical trials* (experiments) that use human volunteers.

"Okay, interesting," you say. But not exactly a priority for you at the moment. But maybe it should be. Why? Because you can make a difference — for yourself and for those who follow you down this path of Parkinson's disease (PD) — by getting involved.

In this chapter, you can find out how you can help in the search for better PD treatment and maybe even a cure.

What Is a Clinical Trial and Why Should You Care?

Clinical trials (also called *clinical research studies*) answer certain questions related to a specific health condition and test the effectiveness of a newly discovered medication or treatment. Such trials are also an important hurdle to clear before the U.S. Food and Drug Administration (FDA, or the government approval agency in your country) can approve any new therapy for the treatment, management, or cure of a disease and make it available to the market. Only through the process of such trials can therapeutic advancement happen. New products are usually first tested on animals or developed in laboratory experiments, but eventually these studies require human participation. That's where you and other people living with Parkinson's disease (PWP) come in.

Recently, major PD organizations have formed an alliance to build awareness of clinical trials among PWP. In addition to making more persons with PD (and their physicians) aware of clinical trials for treatments — and even a cure — these organizations offer some good reasons for participation:

>> **Shortening time to market.** If more PWP volunteer to participate in a trial, the testing and marketing periods (on average 12 to 15 years) can be cut in half, a whopping 6 to 7 years shorter.

>> **Decreasing overall cost.** If researchers can shorten the testing and marketing periods, then they can not only make new therapies available sooner, but they can also offer them at a lower cost. (For you curious souls, the average cost to bring a single new medicine to market is over $900 million. See the sidebar "Why prescription drugs cost so much," in this chapter, for more about these costs.)

REMEMBER

The statistics tell their own story. According to a 2020 report from Harvard University, Parkinson's is the second most common brain disease in the world, affecting a stunning 10 million people worldwide. And if that statistic isn't enough, a recent study funded by the Bill & Melinda Gates Foundation revealed that, among neurological disorders, PD is the fastest growing. These statistics alone are cause for stepping up and participating in research that can hopefully provide insight into the causes and course of the disease, find advanced treatment options, and make those options available sooner.

WHY PRESCRIPTION DRUGS COST SO MUCH

Unless you've been living on another planet for the last 30 years or so, you already know that prescription medications don't come cheap. Of course, pharmaceutical companies probably aren't in the market for the good of humanity — at least, not entirely. These companies are businesses, and by definition, they want to make a profit. ("But do they need to make such a *large* profit?" you ask. The answer depends on who you ask. All we're going to say is that, in America, capitalism remains king.)

Seriously though, the journey to discover and develop new therapies for treating disease is long, costly, and fraught with uncertainties. Nearly half of all new medicines and therapies developed worldwide come from laboratories and clinical studies in the United States. The system may be cumbersome, but it works.

Think of it this way: Every purchase has a value beyond its dollars-and-cents cost. Ask yourself what the value of a new therapy for PD means to you and your family. Ask yourself the value of finding a cure. Like the old commercial for the credit-card company: a prescription that relieves symptoms — so-many dollars; a new medical device that enhances movement — even-more dollars; a cure for PD — priceless. Keep in mind that your health and safety through the course of that journey is also priceless.

Examining the Clinical Trial Process

Clinical trial researchers must adhere to the strict standards of the Food and Drug Administration (FDA), the U.S. government bureau that monitors trials and approves research to move on to the next stage. (Clinical trials have multiple stages.) After a trial progresses through its stages, the developing group or company presents its results to the FDA. Once the FDA signs off, the new treatment (or medicine or medical device) becomes available to the general public. (This whole process involves a lot more red tape, but you get the gist.)

The following sections explain in a nutshell how a clinical trial usually unfolds. Like most topics in the world of medicine and science, the subject of clinical trials comes with its own unique vocabulary, so we clearly define each term when we introduce it.

Setting up a clinical trial

To get a clinical trial underway, a team of research scientists must determine the general category of clinical trial that matches their study's requirements. Their options include

>> **Observational trials:** Researchers study a specific health issue (such as aging or stress) in a large group of people in their home, work, or community setting.

>> **Interventional trials:** Scientists test experimental treatments and drugs or new ways of using existing therapies by applying those experimental approaches to groups of patients under controlled conditions.

Note: This chapter discusses only interventional trials, but you may participate in either type of trial for PD.

After determining the type of trial that they need to run, the research team documents the trial's associated research and intended *protocol* (like a roadmap) and applies for funding and for approval from an Institutional Review Board (IRB) to conduct the clinical trial. Please note that

>> Funding can come from various parties, including pharmaceutical or device companies, government agencies such as the National Institute of Health (NIH) or the Department of Defense (DoD), and private foundations such as the Michael J. Fox Foundation.

>> The IRB is a group of physicians, statisticians, researchers, community advocates, and others that meets independently of the research group. The IRB ensures that the trial protocol is ethical, and that integrity of the data and rights of study participants are protected.

After the study is approved, another group of clinical scientists is appointed to the Data and Safety Monitoring Board (DSMB). This DSMB follows, step-by-step, the implementation of the study procedures, makes sure that the study proceeds as planned, and addresses unexpected problems or side effects.

Following the protocol

After the IRB approves the trial, the team follows the study's protocol, which outlines the process, establishes timelines for completion of each step, and describes the profile of participants. The research team evaluates the safety and effectiveness of the trial drug or treatment, but the protocol also specifies safeguards for monitoring the overall health of participants throughout the trial.

Researchers conduct studies in the phases described in Table 14-1.

TABLE 14-1   **Typical Clinical Trial Phases**

Phase #	Participants	Purpose
1	Small group (20 to 80) of healthy volunteers	To assess potential side effects and risks of specific therapy
2	Larger group of volunteers (100 or more) who have the targeted condition	To evaluate the effectiveness and side effects of the therapy
3	At least 500 (or more, depending on the disease) volunteers — often from multiple countries — who have the targeted condition	To compare the new therapy with therapies currently available

REMEMBER

Although trials may go through several stages and take years to complete, they're still the fastest, safest way to discover and test any new treatment, medicine, or medical device before the general public can access these innovations.

Qualifying and grouping participants

In every trial, the research team establishes certain qualifiers for selecting participants. These *exclusion/inclusion guidelines* for the study appear in the trial's description. Criteria can cover gender, age, even weight or geographical location. For example, the study may include people over the age of 60 but exclude anyone under that age. Or, if the drug's side effects include potential liver problems, then the study excludes individuals who are already dealing with liver problems.

After the team selects participants (that could be you!), those participants sign a document of informed consent (which we discuss in more detail in the section "Considering the Benefits and Risks Before Signing On," later in this chapter). Then the researchers assign each participant to a *treatment group* (in which everyone receives the same form of treatment). The study may include one group in which all members receive the experimental drug, one in which everyone gets an existing drug that's the current preferred treatment, and one in which all members get a placebo.

A *placebo* is a substance that has no active ingredients, therefore no way of medically effecting change either for better or worse — so your symptoms remain unchanged. (You may have heard people talk about the *placebo effect,* meaning the observed effects that arise from the patient's expectations, rather than from the treatment itself.)

Trial participants usually go into one of two treatment groups: participants who receive a real treatment or drug, and participants who receive a treatment that only *looks like* the real deal but doesn't have any of the active ingredients (the placebo).

Going for real results

In clinical trials, researchers want to remove the placebo factor (discussed in the preceding section) from the equation. However, as many as 30 percent of patients who receive a placebo in a trial report improvement. This result seems to be especially true in PD because just the possibility of getting a better medicine can create the expectation of a reward and liberate *dopamine* (the chemical in your brain that controls movement). This placebo effect is one reason that researchers find trials for PD treatments so difficult and why those trials can take so long.

Double-blind studies are the preferred design for testing new therapies today because they assure objectivity throughout the study. In double-blind studies, participants don't know which treatment group they're in, and the researcher doesn't know which group is getting the test therapy. In *single-blind* studies, only the participant or the researcher (but not both) knows which group is receiving the placebo and which is taking the actual drug. In *open label* studies, both the doctor and the study subject know what drug the subject receives. Usually, open label studies do not employ placebo groups.

Considering the Benefits and Risks Before Signing On

By taking part in a clinical trial, you're taking the proactive role that we encourage throughout this book. And in doing so, you also

>> **Gain access to new therapies** before they become available to the general public.

>> **Get the expert attention** of scientists and healthcare professionals.

>> **Learn** more about your disease or health condition.

>> **Contribute to finding the cure** for a disease that you wouldn't wish on your worst enemy.

These benefits are fairly impressive — but, of course, they come with risks, and those risks can be major (although major risks are rare). You still need to know about the negatives of participating in clinical trials before you sign up. Possible risks include

>> **Unforeseen side effects.** Side effects can happen, for example if the new drug interacts with medication you are already taking for other conditions.

>> **Ineffective treatment.** The experimental treatment simply may not work for you.

>> **More doctor visits.** You may make more trips to the doctor's office than you would have normally.

>> **Unexpected costs.** The trial may have costs associated with travel to and from the trial site or additional tests not covered by insurance, for example.

Before you decide to participate in a trial (assuming you meet the needs of the study and have been invited to participate), the research organization asks you to sign a *document of informed consent*. This document is your agreement that you've received and reviewed the key information about the clinical trial (its purpose, how long it will last, what's expected of you, and the names and contact information for the research team). Your signature on this document also indicates that you're aware of the risks, potential side effects, and potential benefits of the treatment.

TIP

Take your time considering your participation in the clinical trial. Talk over the document of informed consent with your family, your doctor, and even your attorney to get a full picture of what you're agreeing to. The informed consent is *not* a contract or legally binding document for you or the company/institution conducting the trial. You have the right to withdraw from the trial at any time that you choose. But keep in mind that participation of people like you brings the world closer to a cure — faster. *Note:* If the document has way too much fine print, ask for a large print version — literally and figuratively.

WARNING

Although the informed consent is intended to protect the patient, you're still responsible for understanding all that you can about the trial before agreeing to participate. You must ask the important questions, such as what happens (to your body and brain) during the trial; and, more importantly, what the risks are and how the team handles any adverse reaction. Answers to these questions are especially important if you're participating in a study for surgical treatment of PD.

Volunteering for a Clinical Trial

To volunteer for participation in a clinical trial, you first have to know where to look. Clinical trials start all the time all over the country. You just need to find a trial that's convenient for you, that's actively enrolling participants, and that you and your doctor believe may help your individual situation.

Finding clinical trials for PD

The most efficient way to shop for clinical trials is via the Internet. Two excellent websites are the Parkinson Study Group (http://parkinson-study-group.org/clinical-trial-updates) and the U.S. National Library of Medicine's Clinical-Trials.gov (www.clinicaltrials.gov). Both sites give you important base information about locations of trials, exclusion/inclusion criteria for participants (discussed in the section "Qualifying and grouping participants," earlier in this chapter), and other facts that can help you rule out certain studies right away. If, in the off chance that you don't have access to a computer, ask a friend who has one to help you, or go to your local library and ask the librarian to assist you in browsing these sites.

Offering to participate

Volunteering to participate in a trial isn't as simple as volunteering at your local library or school. Each study or trial works under a strict set of guidelines and standards, and participants must meet certain specific criteria. These restrictions assure that researchers test new therapies under the most appropriate conditions to prove or disprove the study team's theories.

TIP

Don't get discouraged or take it personally if the study team denies your application. Keep trying to participate because the future of new treatments (and perhaps, one day, a cure) needs you.

Follow these steps to become a part of a clinical trial:

1. **Find a trial through your PD doctor or local PD chapter of a national organization or search the resources listed in the preceding section.**

2. **Read the description of the study and record the number that begins with NCT (the official assigned trial number) and all contact details.**

3. **Call or e-mail the contact.**

   In your communication, include any initial questions you have and request more detailed information about the study or trial.

4. **Discuss your interest in volunteering for this trial with your PD doctor and your family.**

   If possible, talk with people who've participated in past clinical trials.

5. **If you don't qualify for a certain trial (or the trial has the full quota of participants), ask the coordinator to stay in touch.**

   The trial may need more participants while it moves forward, or the contact person may become aware of other trials that better match your profile.

6. **Keep a record of your calls, e-mails, and conversations, noting dates and responses.**

Make follow-up calls if you haven't heard back from the coordinator in a timely manner — within two to three weeks.

REMEMBER

Trial coordinators are juggling many calls and details, so be patient about a reasonable response time. On the other hand, be persistent and ask when you can expect a response.

WARNING

Never volunteer for a trial just because you think you may get *free* medicines — you may end up in the placebo group. And always question any trial that offers you significant monetary reward if you join. Payments for expenses and medical care are one thing; pay-outs to get you in the door are something else entirely and should raise a huge red flag. Similarly, if your doctor seems overly anxious to *sell* you the idea of participating, you need to question your doctor about whether they're receiving an incentive from the trial sponsor to recruit patients. Even so, that may not preclude you from taking part. Just do your due diligence (homework) by researching everything you can learn about this specific trial and the company or organization behind it.

Asking Important Questions Before Committing

An invitation to participate or an approval of your eligibility for a study doesn't obligate you to sign up. Before you make that decision, gather as much information as possible. Address your questions directly to the research team, even though you can probably find many of the answers in the informed consent document (flip back to the section "Considering the Benefits and Risks Before Signing On," earlier in this chapter, for more on this document). We suggest you ask the questions in person, not over the phone or via e-mail, so that you can judge for yourself exactly how on-board the research team is with the information in the informed consent.

REMEMBER

Most people can't imagine not meeting their child's sitter in person or not having face-to-face interaction with the contractor renovating their home. Participating in a clinical trial can be far more important than either of those examples.

Grilling the research team

For your meeting with the research team, come prepared with your questions in writing. Bring someone along to act as scribe so that you can focus on listening to what the team actually says and assessing their unspoken responses. Better yet, bring along a tape recorder or your cellphone, and record the meeting so that you can play it back later while you make your decision.

In a face-to-face meeting, you want to ask

>> **What's the purpose of the study?** According to the National Institutes of Health (NIH), researchers can conduct studies for one or a combination of reasons that test or determine

- Experimental drugs or approaches to therapy

- Means to prevent disease

- New ways of diagnosing or detecting a disease

- Methods for improving patient comfort and quality of life during chronic illness

>> **Who's sponsoring the study?** As mentioned in the section "Setting up a clinical trial," earlier in the chapter, sponsorship for a clinical trial can come from a variety of sources, including pharmaceutical or medical device companies, private foundations, universities and medical centers, biotech companies, and even the government. When you know the *sponsor* (read that as *funding source*), you can better determine whether it's a reputable and reliable source with the funds necessary to see the research through, in spite of any glitches along the way.

>> **Who's conducting the study?** The members of the research team should be well qualified to manage the study and safeguard the health and well-being of participants during the study. Because the study team has been approved by the IRB (see the section "Examining the Clinical Trial Process," earlier in this chapter), you may want to ask this question simply to better identify the role of each member.

>> **Why does the research team believe the therapy or research question can help in the treatment or management of PD?** The answer should cover information about previous studies. Perhaps they've already tested animals; maybe researchers in another country have tested (or even used) the therapy.

>> **In what ways does this therapy differ from the current treatment regimen for PD?** The answer can help you gauge whether the difference between your current therapies and the new drug or treatment is substantial enough to warrant your participation in the test.

>> **What tests and treatments will you receive during the course of the study?** With this answer, you can start to get specific information about their expectations of you.

>> **Where will they administer those tests and treatments?** The convenience of the study site is important because you need to go there during the course of the trial. An important follow-up question is, "How often will I need to come to the site?"

>> **During the study, who will be in charge of my PD care and my general healthcare?** The answer should make it crystal clear that someone is going to take charge of your general care during the trial.

>> **Will I need to be hospitalized at any time during the trial?** If the answer is yes, be sure to ask about the length of stay, where you'll be hospitalized, and who'll pay the bill.

>> **What are the risks — the potential side effects — of the treatment or study?** One of the primary reasons for the trial is to determine the risks and side effects. Still, the team has some idea of what they anticipate, and you should know these facts before you agree to participate.

>> **How will participation in the trial affect my current treatment?** You need to discuss participation with your PD doctor to decide how the trial might interrupt, change, or stop altogether the current medication regimen for managing your PD symptoms.

>> **How long will the trial last?** Trials can last for a matter of weeks, months, or even years (usually, the longer trials focus on quality-of-life issues or long-term monitoring of unexpected side effects). The research team needs to tell you clearly about the intended length of this study, but only you can decide whether you consider that length of time reasonable.

>> **What does it cost, and who pays?** You can reasonably expect the organization conducting the study to cover expenses directly related to the study during the course of that study. In addition, you may receive a stipend for some indirect costs, such as mileage to and from the study site. Don't expect the study to cover the costs of managing your general health. In other words, a study for a new PD therapy probably won't include payment for that dental crown you need.

>> **Under what circumstances would researchers stop the trial or study?** Researchers may stop trials for any number of reasons. The earlier section "Setting up a clinical trial," discusses the role of the DSMB in monitoring data integrity and patient safety. In the most serious circumstances, the government can step in to stop a trial because side effects and risks become too common and serious. In other cases, a company may halt a trial because the

FDA has approved a competing drug that's now coming to market. Follow-up questions related to a premature end to a trial include

- *How will participants be notified if a trial is stopped?*

- *What follow-up can participants expect?* For example, will there be regular (such as quarterly or annual) check-ups to see how you're doing, and will you and your doctor have a contact person from the trial team in the event of a change in your reaction to the medication or therapy down the road?

>> **After the trial's completion, will you still have access to the trial therapy if it works for you?** Especially if you're participating in an early phase of the trial and the new therapy seems to make a difference for you, you want to know that you can continue taking the medicine or receiving the treatment.

>> **What if you agree to participate but you change your mind after a few weeks?** You always have the right to leave a study. Ask this question to understand how your decision to leave in the middle of a study may affect the overall results.

While you collect the information and ask any follow-up questions, pay attention to details such as how researchers refer to you and other participants; you want to be the *patient, subject,* or *participant,* and never (heaven forbid!) a *number.*

Consulting your PD support team

Following the interview with the clinical trial research team (see the preceding section), check with the following people before you make your final decision about volunteering:

>> **Your doctor(s):** Discuss the potential benefits and risks of participation.

>> **Your family:** Discuss any reservations they may have.

>> **Your attorney:** Review the document of informed consent.

While you weigh your decision, remember that you're a key stakeholder in this process. Don't be a passive participant; instead, take your place at this table as an equal player. The research team may have the degrees and fancy titles, but you're the key to that treasure — finding new and more effective therapies for PD and, one day, its cure.

4

Living Well with PD

Keep your relationships happy and healthy while you take this PD journey together.

Introduce your diagnosis at work in the right way.

Adjust how you live your life (but still *live your life!*) while your Parkinson's disease progresses.

IN THIS CHAPTER

» Tweaking your relationship with your significant other

» Keeping kids — young and old, near and far — in the loop

» Maintaining ties with the grandchildren

» Accepting help from your family

» Letting friends be friends

» Keeping your sense of self

Chapter **15**

Maintaining Healthy Relationships

Your relationships with family and friends (as well as those relationships you'll create with healthcare professionals, support group members, and others along this journey) can hold the key to helping you successfully manage your Parkinson's disease (PD) symptoms over the long haul. In sharp contrast, shutting yourself off from people or permitting those who have loved and supported you drift away can only make matters worse — for you and for them.

But your relationships will change. The shifts you see in balance and roles will be healthy for and vital to maintaining a full, productive life. In this chapter, we take a more in-depth look at these key relationships. After seeing how your PD can affect each of these connections, we offer suggestions for bringing those relationships back in line so that you (and the people with whom you have these relationships) understand that your bond hasn't changed just because you have PD.

Normal is a comparative term in life. With any luck, it includes the people and activities that bring satisfaction and contentment to your days. Having PD doesn't mean that you need to start from scratch on a new definition of *normal* — the fundamentals are still there. Although you do need to get creative while you adapt your routines to PD, you don't need to abandon those people and activities that brought you happiness before your diagnosis.

Life, PD, and Your Significant Other

A relationship with your significant other is likely your most important and cherished one. This person is the individual you can trust with your deepest (and sometimes most unpleasant) feelings and thoughts; who'll be there in spite of your anger, fear, and bouts of self-pity; who'll laugh with you when your performance of some task borders on the ridiculous. This person is the one who'll act as your advocate when you have difficulty speaking for yourself, who'll remind you that you both have lives outside of PD, and who'll affirm that you're the same person you always were. This person is your primary care partner and, perhaps one day, your caregiver.

Preparing to share the journey

When one partner in a relationship gets a diagnosis of PD, that diagnosis may seem to be for both of you. Both lives will be affected every day. But how the two of you face that fact and prepare for the inevitable changes can make the difference between strengthening your bond and straining it to the breaking point. The good news is that for most couples, facing a challenge such as PD as partners actually strengthens the relationship.

But sharing the PD journey is bound to put an extra strain on both of you — at least part of the time. If this relationship is new and relatively untested by life's normal challenges, be sure each of you knows what living with PD will likely mean. And if the relationship is longstanding but was beginning to show signs of wear and tear before the diagnosis, both of you need to face that situation at the outset. Consider meeting with a therapist who can help you navigate this fresh communications challenge.

If your relationship is new and untested, or established but shaky, seek the counsel of a trusted and objective third party (ideally, a trained therapist and probably not a friend or family member who might struggle to remain objective) before your significant other leaps into full-blown care-partner mode. If your significant other can't really fit the role of care partner, for whatever reason, you need to discuss what role your partner can manage. Then, decide who else in the family or close circle of friends (perhaps an adult child, a sibling, or an extremely good friend) can step up as you build a care team rather than relying on one central care partner.

REMEMBER

Traveling the road ahead with PD will certainly present challenges for both you and your significant other. You may experience strain on your emotions, and likely also financial concerns about the costs and monetary sacrifices involved. Check out Chapter 5 for more information about preparing to meet these challenges in the early days after diagnosis.

Watching out for the obstacles ahead

After you've both had time to let the diagnosis sink in, you need to prepare to face some common pitfalls that can result when one partner has PD and the other remains healthy. Here are three of the most common:

>> **Changes in the dynamics of your partnership:** With PD in the equation, roles can shift. For example, now that you have PD, your significant other's job may become more important than ever if your health insurance comes through their employer. Understand that this new dynamic puts added stress on the non-PWP partner. Not only are they facing a new role as your care partner, but they also have to deal with the stress of performing their best at work so that their job (and that vital insurance) is secure.

At the same time, if the PWP previously held the traditional role as the head of the house and breadwinner (if the PWP brings home the larger paycheck), that change can introduce added stress. You both need your paycheck, as well as your significant other's, but how will PD affect your ability to perform and longevity at work? (See Chapter 16 for a full discussion of PD in the workplace.) Prepare for such role changes by talking them through with your significant other — using a counselor, if necessary.

>> **Co-dependency (not a good thing):** Co-dependency occurs when your care partner is more invested in managing your PD than you are. The danger here lies in your partner abandoning major pieces of their own life in order to take control of the situation, to fulfill what they perceive to be your needs and wishes. When this perception and your needs don't jive, resentment quickly follows.

Your partner may resent doing their best but not being appreciated (plus, they're surrendering pieces of their own life to offer you this unappreciated gift!). You resent fighting as hard as you can to maintain independence and autonomy, and you feel guilty for adding to your partner's anxiety and frustration by refusing — however gently — to accept their solutions.

>> **"But everyone else manages so well" syndrome:** Some spousal care partners seem to do it all — and do it with style. One care partner may work full-time, cook, clean, take on the yard work, manage the finances, provide the most complex level of personal care for the PWP, deal with the professionals, and continue to maintain an active family and social life. And the most annoying part is that it's all done with an aura of serenity and calm that's intimidating, to say the least.

REMEMBER

Beneath the most serene surface lie whirlpools of unspeakable pain, anxiety, and even anger and resentment at the havoc PD is wreaking. Just like our hypothetical super-partner, you and your partner do your best —and that's more than enough in most cases to nourish the partnership during this difficult time.

Avoiding the pitfalls

In any life-partner relationship, certain passages come with the territory: transitions, such as children growing up and going on to lives (and families) of their own; lifestyle changes, such as moving to a different town, starting a different job, retiring, and downsizing; and tough times, great times, chaotic times, and calm times. Through it all, you and your partner have formed your own unique ways of managing each passage. Now, you face life with PD. It's just one more challenge — but a big one, and one that'll affect the rest of your lives.

Here are two keys to avoiding the pitfalls in your partnership while managing the stresses and strains of living with PD:

>> **Communication and caring = coping:** You'll both have times when you struggle to adapt to the changes caused by PD. Your partner may feel stressed by all the extra responsibility. As the PWP, you may be depressed and anxious (for good reason).

Take time to talk it out, to state your needs, to listen to your partner's concerns — even if you can't immediately solve the problem. If you're seeing a counselor to manage depression and anxiety (see Chapter 13), ask that person for tips about improving communications during especially stressful times.

>> **Mutual respect — the foundation of all successful relationships:** Think about all the reasons the two of you teamed up in the first place. You loved your partner's bubbly outgoing personality — so different from your shy, quiet demeanor. Your partner loved your take-charge-in-a-crisis style. The activities that gave you individual identities also strengthened you as a couple. You aren't clones; you *complement* (complete) each other. Now one of you has PD,

and the other has been cast in this new role of care partner. Just like you've adapted in the past (when the kids came along or one of you changed jobs), you can do that again.

REMEMBER

And even if yours isn't a union of marriage, but perhaps a sibling or best-friend connection, you know what we're saying about the importance of mutual respect. The section "How Your PD Can Affect Parents and Siblings," later in the chapter talks about the sibling relationship.

TIP

Few relationships remain stagnant (at least, those that survive and thrive don't). So chances are good that the dynamics of your partnership would have changed and shifted, regardless of whether you had PD. So, don't permit yourself (or your partner) to stress out about the possible changes you'll face while the years pass. And for heaven's sake, don't allow PD to keep you from enjoying the intimacy that comes with living in a loving partnership.

Keeping the magic alive — Sex and intimacy in spite of PD

For some couples, one of the most challenging shifts can come in the area of intimacy. You and your partner can either surrender to a loss in this area, or you can get creative and find new ways to share your love.

Humans take a certain amount of pride in their physical, mental, and even emotional attractiveness. The diagnosis of a lifelong, debilitating condition can play havoc with a person's sense of self, and it can be especially devastating to their sense of sexuality. The relationship you may have enjoyed with your significant other for years — even decades — suddenly comes into question. Can I adequately satisfy the needs of this person I love? Is this person humoring me by pretending that nothing's changed? Why don't I feel like being intimate even though I love this person? Doesn't this person deserve a *whole* lover?

Okay, just stop it. Take a moment to get the facts before you leap to unfounded (and, in some cases, unnecessary) conclusions; for example, that your days of having sexual relations are over. Consider these circumstances:

» When sexual needs and desires change, the root cause usually responds to medication or other therapy such as counseling. Check first with your primary care physician to see whether the cause is treatable.

» If the change comes on the heels of the diagnosis — well, duh! You just got some tough and depressing news. Talk about a mood crasher!

>> Depression and anxiety may well be symptoms of your PD (see Chapter 13), so your sexual concerns may result from the disease itself. And what about those prescription meds for depression? Read the label. Most likely, they list sexual dysfunction as a potential side effect.

>> Certainly people with PD (PWP) may experience performance anxiety, given the facts that PD is a movement disorder and good sex often involves coordination and flexibility.

>> Unfortunately, the effects of PD can play havoc with self-image. The *mask* (inability to show facial expression) is one example. Struggling to manage basic grooming (styling your hair, getting your face just right, and putting on your favorite cologne) can also make anyone feel less than desirable.

>> Women's fluctuating hormone balance in the perimenopausal years can affect desire. Women with PD need to have their gynecologist and PD doctor work together to regulate hormone replacement and antiparkinsonian medications.

>> If you're male, you may experience episodes of erectile dysfunction — another sideshow of PD — because the brain needs to work with the body for you to maintain an erection.

So, what to do? Well, you don't want to ignore any problem that may have a solution. And sexual dysfunction — regardless of gender — is one of them. Let your doctor know because treatments are available. For example, if depression is behind your change in sexual interest, counseling may be the answer.

TIP

And for both your sakes, talk to your partner, who may be having problems, as well. For example, when faced with a loved one's diagnosis, some partners leap light years ahead to the day (that may never come) when the loved one can't function at all. As a result, your partner goes into serious protection mode and tries to avoid any activity that they think may cause you more stress (including sexual relations).

Yes, you and your partner may need to explore new ways of being intimate. Gee — experiment with new ways to kiss, to hold each other, to touch, to . . . Sounds like a good thing!

Retaining personal space for each of you

REMEMBER

Receiving a diagnosis of PD may draw the two of you even closer together, but don't make the mistake of abandoning your individual activities and contacts. As much as you love and cherish each other, you still need some personal space from time to time. The richness of relationships is often rooted in the fact that each has their own unique interests (and friends). You may share news about these activities and people with each other, but you both accept that this is *my* activity or *my* friend — and that's okay.

In these early weeks, you have a lot to take in (tests, doctor's appointments, therapy sessions, and such). But if your partner enjoyed a weekly card game or volunteer activity for years, and after the diagnosis, they haven't had the chance to do it for months now, this is a problem. And *you* need to lead by example. Take stock of those individual activities and contacts that you've let slide and get them back on your calendar. Then insist that your partner do the same.

You and your partner may also be in danger of surrendering your personal space when your PD symptoms become more troublesome. While your need for assistance and care escalates, your partner may become so entrenched in caring for you that their own physical, mental, and emotional well-being is jeopardized. Make it your job to prevent that problem from happening.

TIP

Prepare in advance for ways that each of you can protect your individual life beyond PD. Don't look at this strategy as an act of selfishness; in the long run, giving attention to separate activities and personal space can bring the two of you closer and enrich the life you share. (Check out Chapter 23 for more ways to care for your care partner.)

Helping Kids Deal with Your PD

For people with Parkinson's (PWP) who have children, the change in your relationships will depend in part on the age of your children. A person who has young onset PD (see Chapter 8) may have very young children. But if your PD was diagnosed later in life, your children may have children of their own (your grandchildren) who also need your attention (we talk about the grandkids in the section "Staying Close with Grandchildren after Your PD Diagnosis," later in this chapter).

Regardless of their age, children can become confused or alarmed when they hear that a parent has PD. Some of that initial response comes from a knowledge base (or lack of one) about PD and its progression. And some of the response can be normal self-concern about life changes now that a parent is ill. In either case, you need to reassure your children and include them while you and your care partner make decisions that may affect their lives, as well. Your kids may ask (out loud or just to themselves) questions something like the following:

> "What if they need to use my college savings fund for Mom's medical bills?"

> "I thought we'd have more time before I needed to be there for my parents."

Addressing their fears about the future

You and your significant other need to discuss early on how to deliver the news of your diagnosis to your children (see Chapter 7). After you tell them, look for obvious and not-so-obvious reactions, such as withdrawal from their normal social activities or slipping grades if your child was an honor student before the diagnosis. If you see mood changes (such as increased irritability) or personality changes (your little extrovert suddenly becomes quite the introvert), talk it out. You may consider taking your preteen and teenage children with you to your next PD doctor's appointment so that they can raise their own questions. Or consider going with your adult child for some talk therapy with a counselor.

TIP

Regardless of your children's ages, your positive outlook and sense of humor can go a long way toward reassuring them that life won't change much just because you have PD. While time goes by (years — not weeks) and the PD becomes more difficult to control, your children will adapt with you.

When your children are young

In this section, the idea of "young" children covers a broad age range. Your relationship to your children and parental responsibilities change with respect to the children's ages and the stage of your PD. Consider these age groupings and how to engage with each:

>> **Very young children (under age 10):** If young children ask questions or change their normal behavior toward you, then those concerns need your attention. Just be careful not to blow problems out of proportion. For example, your child's very simple concern, "Can I catch Parkinson's like a cold?" may have an easy answer: "No."

>> **Middle-schoolers (ages 10 to 13):** Consider giving children of this age an assignment: put them in charge of staying on top of and reporting the PD e-news from the trusted sites listed in Appendix B.

TIP

Giving your middle-school child a specific assignment, such as playing PD news correspondent, can help them feel like they're a part of the solution. You absolutely must avoid allowing children of any age to feel as if they're being kept in the dark.

>> **Teenagers (ages 14 to 19):** Have them participate in development of an action plan for managing household changes. When included from the beginning, teens are more likely to take ownership and responsibility for additional chores or tasks. Whenever you and your partner reassess the plan and discuss necessary changes, include your teen.

TIP

A great way to empower children who are struggling with a parent's illness is to encourage them to raise funds for a national organization that's searching for a cure. Maybe your child can participate in an organized run or bike ride, raising money through donations. Kids like action. Help them take an active (and proactive) role to raise awareness or money for research.

When your children are adults

Adult children may live at home, nearby, or miles away. They may be single, married, have children of their own, have promising and demanding careers, be in college or graduate school, or have a combination of these. Whatever their situation, they're living their own lives now (even if they're still in your house). You're a part of that life, but not in the same way as when they were younger.

After your diagnosis, your adult children probably feel that the roles have shifted (even if you don't); they may now consider taking care of you, rather than the other way round. Such ideas can make for some interesting relational conflicts — parenting my parent, for example. Your best tactic involves clearly demonstrating through words, actions, and — most of all — attitude that you do need their support and concern, but you're still fully capable of deciding how you want to live with PD.

If you don't ask, they won't help

Maybe your natural instinct as a parent is to protect your kids from worrying about you. If you constantly respond to your children's concern with, "We're doing fine," then don't be upset when your kids take that at face value and get on with their lives. But here's a news flash — they're probably worrying anyway *and* frustrated that you won't confide in them and let them help. Give them a chance to help by stating specific needs. (Check out Chapter 7 for more on this idea.) In the worst-case scenario, you'll be disappointed by the reaction. In the best case, your child steps up to the plate and delivers a solid hit by taking on some chore, bringing over dinner once a week, or bringing the grandkids to see you more often.

When adult children live nearby

Adult children who live nearby can be a blessing for you and your care partner — especially when your PD progresses and you can use a little more help. Consider establishing some new family traditions, such as a potluck or ordered-in dinners once every other week for you, the kids, and the grandkids. This ritual can

>> Help your children and grandchildren adapt to the impact that your symptoms may have on the usual routine they might currently take for granted.

>> Open the door to the possible need for more intense regular contact down the road.

Because PD tends to progress slowly, you'll probably read the signs that your symptoms are getting worse before others even notice. (For example, your meds may not work as well, and routine tasks become more of a struggle.) When you recognize these new limits on your abilities, consider organizing a family meeting to discuss how and when you may need to modify the ways you currently receive help from family (see Chapter 17).

The following suggestions can help you in that meeting:

>> Offer specific ways that your adult children and older grandchildren (even those who live some distance away) can pitch in.

>> Clearly demonstrate that you recognize and appreciate their busy schedules.

>> Start with small requests. For example, can your grandchild cut the lawn? Can one of your children cook up a casserole once a month for the freezer? Can one of your children (even if living in another state) help compile your taxes?

TIP

Ask yourself whether you would have willingly committed to certain responsibilities when you were your kids' (and grandkids') ages. Would you have cheerfully taken on additional tasks? Would you have put these activities ahead of other items on your schedule? If the answer to these questions is "No," then perhaps your ideas about what and how much responsibility your children can handle is overly optimistic. Far better to start out with smaller, less time-consuming tasks, such as those mentioned in the preceding bullet list, and then add more requests for assistance while time and your PD progress.

The goal: Involve your adult children almost from the beginning so that they become a part of the decisions and planning and are invested in the reality that over time your needs will escalate. Acknowledge their own busy schedules. Ask for their opinion and input. The decision about how to handle PD challenges is ultimately yours, but including your children in the discussion makes them feel like a vital and valued part of the whole process.

WARNING

If some adult children live nearby and some live farther away, don't take the assistance of nearby children for granted. In many families, visits from far-away kids and grandkids are a cause for celebration, but in-town children who provide regular hands-on help (at some personal sacrifice) also need to feel appreciated. Call your in-town daughter specifically for the purpose of thanking her after she's rearranged her schedule to do something for you. Comment on how much you appreciate something specific that each of your children (in-town and out-of-town) does for you when you're all together.

When children live far away

Adult children who live far away may suffer some guilt from not being available to help out. When they visit, you may want to plan some major project (changing the storm windows and screens, cleaning the basement, or painting the kitchen) so that they can participate in a hands-on way in the household care routine. You want them to realize that they're not your guests — they're your children. Even though they can offer only sporadic hands-on help, you can encourage them to come through for you and your care partner.

REMEMBER

Long distances between parties can shut down lines of communication. Be sure to include the adult children living far away in family meetings and conferences (even if only by e-mail, phone, or videoconference). Ask for their input and include them while you come to a decision. Make a personal commitment to keep all your adult children in the loop. They need to hear your news, including major decisions or changes, from you (or your care partner) — not from a sibling.

Staying Close with Grandchildren after Your PD Diagnosis

Children and grandchildren of all ages can provide you with good medicine just with their presence. Their curiosity and sense of adventure can be contagious in a good way. Their belief that they're indestructible and immortal can be inspiring. The way kids pack 40 hours of activity and energy into a single day can serve as an important reminder: You have this day — live it or lose it!

Seeking guidance from your grandkids' parents

The first step with your grandchildren involves consulting with their parents (one of whom is your child) before you talk with the kids about your PD. How do they want you to handle their children's questions? What have the parents told your grandchildren already, and how did they tell them? After you know those answers, show your grandchildren through your interactions that nothing has really changed. You're still Grandma or Grandpa. Keep your routine with them as normal as possible.

If you've played games or gone apple-picking with them in the past, keep that up. If those tasks aren't possible for you now, find new activities. Perhaps make a game of doing your exercises with your grandchild. Or go to the apple farm and buy the apples, bring them home, and make applesauce with your grandchildren. Most of all, reassure them with simple but honest answers to their questions, and let their parents know whether you see signs that your grandchildren are holding questions or concerns inside.

Engaging your grandkids' innate sensitivity

Children are wise beyond their years and extraordinarily tuned in to the moods and vibes of the adults in their world. They may not fully understand what's going on, but they know when you're upset, sad, depressed, or angry. And more often than not, they mistakenly think they're to blame or that your mood has something to do with them.

TIP

We're not suggesting you fake a happy-go-lucky attitude around the young ones. But don't sell them short. You're the adult here. You know when your frustration causes you to lash out or withdraw. Pay attention to your reactions and to the reactions of the child you're with, and speak up when you know you have crossed a line. "I'm sorry I snapped at you. Sometimes I just get so frustrated when I can't do the things I used to do. Do you ever feel sad like that?" Now you've opened the door to a dialogue with the child and perhaps to a conversation that can reveal some of their own angst about your PD.

How Your PD Can Affect Parents and Siblings

Okay, there's the family you have now — maybe a spouse or a life partner, perhaps children, and maybe a close-knit group of friends. And then there's the family that knew you from childhood — your parents and siblings. One or more of this group may play a role in helping you in some minor (or perhaps major) way as your PD advances. In any case, this family you grew up with needs the same consideration as the family you built on your own. They deserve to know what's going on and to have their concerns (for you and perhaps for themselves) addressed.

WARNING

When you consider the current relationship you have with your parents and siblings, remember that you have longstanding histories with these people. If you never could please your mother — or if your brother always felt that he had to live up to your example — those facts have colored the way your family interacts. Don't make the mistake of expecting the foundations of your relationships to magically change simply because you have PD.

Over the course of your life, each of you has found ways to adapt to those unique interactions. Perhaps you handle your Mom's apparent disappointment in you by simply enduring her comments and moving on. Good choice. Likewise, your brother's sense of insecurity (and inferiority) is his issue — not yours. Be sympathetic but understand that he's no more likely to step up now than he was before.

Seeking parental support or offering reassurance

What if your aging parents are still around while you're dealing with your PD? If that's the case, you may want to confide in one or both of your parents, allowing them to play the role of mentor and counselor, and seek advice for balancing the demands of PD with your other responsibilities while you face this new challenge. A good way to start this discussion is to remind your parents of difficult challenges they've faced over the course of their lives.

However, if your parents are emotionally fragile and thrown by the news of your illness, your role may become one of reassuring them rather than relying on them. But, because you really don't need more emotional responsibility at this time, consider asking a sibling to reassure Mom and Dad. This arrangement can be especially helpful if your brothers or sisters are looking for ways they can offer you support and tangible help.

REMEMBER

If you were diagnosed with young onset PD (see Chapter 8), your parents are probably still living. If your parents' health is compromised and you're providing some care for them, you and your care partner need to consider how best to incorporate your dual role as adult child with PD and caregiver for aging parents into an already busy life. If you have siblings, it's time to call a sibling meeting and decide how others might take on some of the tasks you've been managing. If you are an only child, have a frank talk with your parents about what their need for help in the future might look like and discuss options available to them if you can't provide the physical care they may require.

Adapting to a sibling as a care partner

If your sister or brother becomes your primary care partner, the two of you need ground rules about the relationship, just as if your care partner were your spouse or significant other. For example:

>> **Adapting longtime roles:** You both need to acknowledge and then set aside the familial roles you may have assumed throughout childhood. For example, if your sister always played the big-sister role and you followed her lead, that

relationship needs to change. The way you choose to handle life with PD is your decision, and she needs to be willing to follow your lead.

>> **Assessing values:** You both need to face the fact that you're adults, which means you've probably gone in different directions philosophically and may have different approaches to a variety of issues. Are you on opposite ends of the political spectrum? Is your sibling of a rule-oriented, by-the-book nature while you are a free what-will-be-will-be spirit? You need to acknowledge these differences and find a way forward through discussion (perhaps with a therapist) about what compromises might be necessary.

REMEMBER

After you face the relationship issues, you need to focus on the reasons that having your sibling act as your care partner makes sense: They bring strengths to the table that you counted on when the two of you were growing up. You've chosen your sibling for those strengths, and they've agreed because history shows that you can work together in the same way the two of you faced challenges as children.

Keeping Friends Close During Your PD Journey

No matter what your friendships are like, there's nothing like a chronic, progressive, and eventually debilitating condition for sorting out friends who'll be there from those who'll eventually drift away. And discovering who's who in this process is usually surprising. The guy you thought would be there no matter what may not handle the idea that you can't enjoy the vigorous sports activities the two of you have always shared. Even though you assure him that it may be years before that happens, he doesn't hear you. Meanwhile, a coworker you've always seen as a casual acquaintance (nice to have a beer with after work and such) steps up, intuitively understanding how to be helpful but not intrusive for you or your care partner.

The following suggestions help you make this transition with your friends as smooth as possible:

>> **Tell it like it is.** Friends may want to help but don't know how. And, like everyone else, they'll take their lead from you. If you repeatedly assure them that everything's fine and reject their efforts to understand PD and figure out how to help, then shame on you. And if you shut them out with self-pity, depression, and a nobody-can-help attitude, don't be surprised when they drift away.

IT'S ALL IN HOW YOU LOOK AT IT

At the foundation of your ability to maintain healthy relationships is your ability to maintain a healthy sense of self. With respect to PD, you certainly have an impressive roster of celebrities to emulate (Muhammad Ali and Michael J. Fox, to name two great examples). But, to understand the importance of this sense-of-self on a personal level, go to a PD support group meeting and look around.

Joan sits over there in a corner. Diagnosed two years ago, her symptoms are well controlled with medication. Yet Joan is always looking for the downside; her conversations project a dire future. She likes to report disastrous cases, like the person who fell, hit his head, and became demented almost overnight. (Take this opportunity to move on as quickly as possible!)

You notice Charlie in another part of the room. He's had PD for over a decade. His hand shakes uncontrollably at times, he has trouble swallowing, and you have to lean in close to hear him. But you discover that he still runs his own business, attends social functions with his wife, and is an active volunteer in the fight to find a cure for PD. He's telling a story about his latest doctor's visit:

"Doc asked whether I had vivid dreams . . . and whether I was in my dreams," he says. "I told him I was in my dreams, and I didn't have PD — just me moving freely with no tremor."

You ask Charlie what the doctor said about that and Charlie replies, "He said I must have one whopper of a positive outlook!"

You can be Joan, you can be Charlie, or you can be someone in between. The choice is yours. No doubt Charlie has his bad days. But how he's chosen to get through those days is worth finding out.

>> **Ask for the usual treatment.** Okay, you don't want to lose your friends, but you also don't want them treating you any differently. Tell them that. Be open to their questions. Give them the facts. Seriously consider their suggestions for treatments, doctors, and such, rather than reject them out of hand. But remind your friends that you've done a lot of research and have the backing of your professional care team as you make decisions. Let your friends know you'll have good days and bad. And then decide together how they can best support you.

>> **Seek a sympathetic ear.** Friends are terrific at playing the role of confidante for you and your care partner. And, by the way, we hope you and your care partner have one really good friend (not the same one!) that you can trust to hear you vent, whine, and feel sorry for yourself now and again.

>> **Know their strong suits.** Recognize that some people are good listeners and counselors, and others need to offer hands-on help. Surely you know these folks well enough to know the difference. So when the inevitable question of "What can I do to help?" arises, be prepared with concrete and specific ideas — in the same way that you do with your children and other family members (as we discuss throughout this chapter).

>> **Keep a balance.** Beware of accepting too much help. Some people (friends and family) may start strong, practically smothering you with their help. But the odds are good that these people will over-promise and under-deliver, eventually burning out. By the same token, the more you permit other people to do for you — especially early on — the less you push yourself to remain active and independent for as long as possible.

And Then There's You

Having Parkinson's is a life–changing situation — one that will continue to affect you for the rest of your days. But are you a PD patient, or are you still the same active, involved, in-charge person you were before you were diagnosed PD? You can choose to allow a diagnosis of PD to dominate your daily routine, even in the early stages, or you can take the proactive approach — doing what it takes to maintain as much of your preferred lifestyle as possible despite having PD. Or to put it more bluntly: Don't allow PD to define you.

You and those around you had a life before you were diagnosed, and you still have that life. You may have to accept changes, but your ability to participate in those activities that gave your life purpose and meaning are still possible. And that can-do attitude goes a long way toward keeping friends and family close and in the fight alongside you.

Consider these two questions:

>> **How many work hours do you average each week?** For most people, the answer to this first question is between 40 and 60 hours. If you're retired, you likely devote these hours to hobbies and household tasks.

>> **Between what times do those hours occur?** This second answer likely falls between 8 a.m. and 6 p.m.

So, one way to look at adapting PD is to focus on those daytime hours and how to use them in meaningful ways. At first, this focus may require you to schedule the activities (reading, biking, or coffee with a friend) for the times when you know you're at your best. In time, your daily routine can hopefully settle into a pattern that feels familiar and less programmed.

Although you certainly can't schedule your PD symptoms, you're still the same person you were before you got diagnosed. Your life's activities may need to change over time — just like they do for everyone with or without PD. But for now, it's likely most of your normal routine is still viable.

TIP

As a matter of fact, you may be able to get back to some activities you dropped while your PD symptoms went untreated. Perhaps you can partially relieve your stiffness and slowness through physical therapy and a regular exercise routine (see Chapter 9). Maybe those feelings of anxiety, persistent sadness, and depression that you thought were job-related are treatable with counseling and possibly medications (see Chapter 13). And maybe you can manage your hand tremor by working with your doctor to figure out an effective medication routine (see Chapter 10).

Chapter **16**

PD in the Workplace

dapting to life with Parkinson's disease (PD) works best when you can partner with other people. We hope you're already partnering with your healthcare team (see Chapter 6) and your primary care partner (along with your family and friends — see Chapter 15). For some, the third angle of this partnering triangle is your partnership with your employer and coworkers, a relationship that permits you to stay on the job and takes into account your employer's need to run the business effectively. In this chapter, we offer some ideas for delivering the news and building the workplace version of that team-oriented partnership.

WARNING

Don't assume that our suggestions are exactly right for your situation. Every employer-employee relationship is unique, just like your PD is different from other people's PD. You know the specific climate that surrounds your workplace, and only you can decide the best approach for telling your employer — or employees, if you happen to own the place — that you have PD.

Doing Your Homework Upfront

If there's one message we pound home in this book, it's this: Your best course of action in all facets of managing your PD is to prepare, prepare, and then prepare some more. That advice is never truer than when you're about to tell your employer that you have a chronic and progressive condition. And those words are exactly (and probably only) what your boss is likely to hear. Therefore, your job is to prepare to fight any preconceived misperceptions about what having PD means with every resource you can muster.

Before you tell your employer, you have some homework to do — and yes, we do mean you! In broad strokes (with details in the following sections), here are your assignments:

>> **Assess your abilities.** Put together an honest assessment of your position requirements and whether or not you can continue to fulfill them. Our friend, Gary (to whom we've dedicated this book), was an orthopedic surgeon. No way he could continue his work indefinitely.

>> **Verify your assessment with your doctors.** Discuss your job responsibilities with your PD doctor and get a written medical evaluation of your ability to perform those duties.

>> **Explore workplace accommodations.** Research what the company can offer to accommodate your changing needs and what it has offered other employees in the past (such as a different workstation configuration or a flexible schedule so that you can work in-house when your symptoms are well managed or work from home).

>> **Know your workplace policies and legal options.** Familiarize yourself with options that the Americans with Disabilities Act (ADA) or other government programs may offer.

Honestly assess your ability to continue in the job

Before you start spreading the news that you have PD to your boss and coworkers, decide how and if you can continue working. First, you need a clear understanding of your job requirements and performance demands. You and your PD doctor both need this information so that you can honestly assess your ability to continue in the job while your PD progresses. For example, if your job requires fine handwork and you already have a significant tremor in one hand, you can't ignore this problem.

Keep in mind that PD progresses at different rates for different people, and neither you nor your doctor can really predict its course. However, you can acquire information to help you and your doctor make the best possible assessment by

>> Reviewing the written job description from when you were hired

>> Analyzing recent performance review sessions or upcoming performance criteria in which your employer restates the expectations and requirements of the position

TIP

If you didn't receive a printed job description or your next performance review isn't in the near future, then consider asking for an informal conversation with your supervisor — especially if that's not the same person who hired you. Their expectations for your performance may not be the same as your former supervisor's were. Keep the meeting informal and conversational. If you say something like, "I wonder whether you'd give me a written, detailed description of my position," you're going to raise all sorts of red flags (especially if you've been working there for some time already).

If you have no job description and can't have a chat with your immediate supervisor, take time to think through and document the tasks required of you — physical, mental, and emotional (stress-related). Be as specific as possible.

REMEMBER

Be brutally honest now — *before* you sit down with your supervisor to deliver the news that you have PD. Before that conversation, no one else is asking these questions or listening to your answers. But if you try to fudge the answers when you know your PD's already making some tasks difficult, you're only harming yourself.

Discussing your job obligations with your doctor

At your next appointment with your PD doctor, discuss your job requirements and how to adapt your PD symptoms — those you're experiencing now and those that are most likely to occur over the next year or so — to the demands of the job (and vice versa). Take notes. If you think your employer may have safety concerns but your doctor indicates that you can continue the job, ask your doctor for a letter stating that you're capable of performing the tasks in question.

Assess the job aspects in Table 16-1 and use the right column to note your thoughts and the results of any discussion with your doctor.

TABLE 16-1

Fitting Your Job Requirements to Your PD

Job Aspect	Examples	Adaptations for PD Symptoms
Physicality	Desk job; manufacturing station; hands-on artisanship	
Time commitment	Regular schedule; overtime; at-home work	
Mobility requirements	Mostly standing or sitting; regular movement; travel	
Mental requirements	Quick decisions; complex problem-solving; coordinating team activities	
Stressors	Productivity and sales goals; deadlines; multitasking	
Emotional investment	Supporting team members; client needs; balance with home life	
Demand potential	Long hours; short deadlines	

Consider job options that may be available

Depending on the size of your company, you may have an entire list of options to help you stay on the job and perform effectively — or you may have no options at all. If you work for a larger company, your employer may be able to offer flexible hours, job-sharing, working from home one or two days a week, or a reduced workload (which, of course, may have a reduction in pay).

But even the small business owner may still have some options. For example, if you work in a restaurant that's busiest at breakfast and lunch, your employer probably doesn't have much leeway for adapting your hours. But can they assign you to work a later shift when the restaurant has fewer customers to serve?

TIP

Think outside the box for solutions to job challenges. Your employer's not the only one responsible for devising options for you. The employee who needs to be on the job by seven but struggles with getting up, dressed, and out the door in time to meet that start time may need to make adjustments: get up an hour earlier and talk to their doctor about adjusting the timing on their medication routine to accommodate this early-morning start time.

Exploring company and government policies

If you work for a larger company, you probably received an employee handbook as a part of your new hire information. As part of preparing to tell your boss about your diagnosis, dig this employee handbook out and read it. Better yet, go to the company's internal website (if it has one) and get the latest version. If your company (or the company your care partner works for) provides group insurance for employees, read those policies. Make notes so that in the meeting with your boss — and eventually the person from Human Resources (HR) — you have a firm understanding of the company's policies regarding special accommodations or coverage for short- or long-term disability.

Also, find out what Title 1 of ADA (the Americans with Disabilities Act of 1990) says about employment considerations for people with disabilities. Through the ADA, you have some protection against discrimination in the workplace that might occur because of your PD. You can visit the website at https://ada.gov/employment.htm to find links to the text of the ADA, a fact sheet, regulations, and related resources.

Deciding When to Disclose Your Diagnosis

Although PD is progressive, it isn't one of those you've-got-six-months-to-live situations. You have some time to tell your employer about your PD. On the other hand, you also want to choose the best time for your specific situation. We help you make that all-important decision in the following sections.

From your perspective

Depending on your job, your PD may not have any real impact on your ability to perform satisfactorily for years. In the meantime, make use of the initial days and weeks following your diagnosis to accept that you have PD and that it's going to be a factor in every facet of your life, including your work. (See Chapter 5 for more specific ideas on getting through those first weeks after diagnosis.)

REMEMBER

Only you can decide the appropriate time to tell your employer; aim to minimize the fallout from sharing this kind of news.

Consider these two scenarios and their possible outcomes:

>> **You rush into your boss's office within days of the diagnosis and announce that you have PD.** The danger in this scenario lies in the potential for your employer (and coworkers) to view you *and* your performance differently. In other words, well before your PD symptoms have any effect on your ability, other people may perceive a problem and attribute it to your PD. Subconsciously, your employer may label and pigeonhole you (possibly passing you over for a better position) because of their misperceptions.

>> **You withhold the news until your symptoms become more difficult to control and begin to affect your performance.** In this scenario, you may think you've been controlling your symptoms, but your news comes as no surprise to your employer or coworkers. If your colleagues have already become aware of a change in your performance, they may wonder why you took so long to come forward. Or worse, if facial *mask* (lack of facial expression) is one of your symptoms, they may have interpreted that symptom as disinterest or apathy, and then attributed the decline in your performance to that misinterpretation.

REMEMBER

If your supervisor has expressed concern about your recent job performance (via questions such as, "Is everything all right?" or "How's everything going at home?" — or even at a more formal review of your performance), they're giving you a good hint that they're concerned about you and the work they need from you. Don't procrastinate (with informing the boss about your PD) so that the situation doesn't get to this point.

TIP

If you know that safety will eventually become an issue, stay ahead of the curve by considering other positions within the company that you can handle while your PD progresses. If your company offers training for such positions, take it to maximize your options. Remember our mantra: Prepare and plan ahead.

From your employer's perspective

Keep in mind that bosses can't look at a situation in isolation. Employers must consider how your situation affects other people and, yes, ultimately, the bottom line. This fact of life may seem harsh, but the point of opening a business is to make enough money to reinvest in the company's future and keep the business going. Consider these points:

>> **Most employers want very much to maintain good employees.** If you're a person who delivers on the job and adds value to the company, your employer will probably be eager to help you stay on the job for as long as possible.

>> **If safety is relevant to job performance in your position, your employer can't put the company, you, or your coworkers at risk.** And in this case, the bottom line isn't about making a profit; it's about security for you, your coworkers, and your families.

The first person to tell at work is your immediate supervisor (and then the folks in your HR department). In rare circumstances, employers can be short-sighted when it comes to supporting employees in tough personal situations. Maybe you and your supervisor already have an adversarial relationship, so you're concerned your PD will tip the situation over the edge.

WARNING

Resist the notion of bypassing your immediate supervisor for your PD reveal. If you believe that your relationship with your supervisor is adversarial, you may be tempted to seek out someone else in the company who seems more supportive. But this plan only makes the problem worse and can actually backfire on you. Your supervisor may resent being passed over and make it more difficult for you to convince other people that you're still a valuable asset to the company. Consider asking for a meeting that includes both your supervisor *and* someone from HR.

Telling Your Boss

Okay, the moment's at hand. It's time to deliver the news of your PD to your employer. Follow these steps (or something like them — adjust as needed to your particular circumstances):

1. **Request a meeting.**

   This can be informal if you and your supervisor have a relationship that permits you to say, "Do you have 20 to 30 minutes today or tomorrow? I need to talk to you about something." If the request needs to be more formal, follow the company process for requesting and scheduling a meeting with your supervisor or manager. Allow at least 30 minutes for the meeting. It may not take that long, but it's important not to rush this.

2. **Prepare and practice your talking points.**

   You want your boss to hear these key points after you say, "I have Parkinson's."

   Keep the points short and simple. Don't try to educate your boss about the intricacies of PD right after you announce your diagnosis. For example, you may say, "I've been diagnosed with Parkinson's disease." (Allow time for a short response — hopefully a sympathetic one.) You continue, "The good news is that progression is slow, and my doctor agrees that it may be some time — even years — before symptoms really have an impact."

3. **Demonstrate that you've done your homework.**

   Your boss may hear very little after you say, "I have Parkinson's." And inevitably, they'll start thinking of its short- and long-term impact on the business. You can offer them a simple fact sheet about what PD is — and isn't. (One excellent resource is the publication available online from the Parkinson's Foundation at www.parkinson.org/sites/default/files/FactSheet_051616.pdf.)

Then, follow up the PD fact sheet with

> *Documentation from your doctor(s):* Produce a copy of any letter your neurologist, movement disorder specialist, or other doctor has provided that states your ability to continue in the job.

> *Demonstration of the effort you've already put into the situation:* You've reviewed your job description and performance expectations set out for your position; you've met with your doctor and gone over the demands of the job; as a result, your doctor has given you the documentation.

4. Maintain a positive and can-do attitude throughout the meeting, regardless of the response you get from your manager.

You know that having PD is a challenge but not a deal-breaker when it comes to your ability to contribute. In this meeting, demonstrate through your can-do attitude that PD is just one more challenge that you can conquer.

REMEMBER

All your homework and advance preparation pay off in giving you a good basis for a discussion with your boss. But keep in mind the way you deliver the information you've prepared:

> *Keep it short and simple.* You don't want to inadvertently raise red flags by saying something such as, "And as for the travel piece of my job, well, I'm pretty sure that won't be a problem as long as the travel doesn't increase."

> *Keep it positive.* You don't want to come off as threatening or adversarial at a time like this, so don't present your message as, "I have PD, and I know my rights." Instead, say something like, "I know this news raises all sorts of questions, but I'm confident that together we can find answers and solutions that will allow me to continue to contribute effectively."

5. Direct the meeting away from immediate job changes.

Understand that your manager needs some time to take this information in, so don't agree to any option or accommodation that your supervisor may offer off the top of their head at this initial meeting. Acknowledge any such offer as a possibility but one that perhaps you should both discuss after the manager has had time to digest the news — the same way you needed some time to digest your diagnosis (which we talk about in Chapter 5).

6. Address the subject of coworkers at some point in the meeting.

Tell your supervisor that, with their permission, you want to meet with the members of your immediate department and give them the news about your diagnosis along with the brief fact sheet that answers frequently asked questions about PD (which you already gave to your manager in Step 3). You also want to ask them to help squelch rumors or misinformation while the news spreads.

7. Let your manager know that you plan to contact the HR department to gather information about your benefits and options.

8. Thank your manager for their support and concern and ask whether the two of you should set a time to meet again.

9. Get back to doing the great work you've always done.

Getting the Facts from HR

Your HR department can provide answers to most questions related to your insurance options and work options if or when you can longer do your current job. In the same way that you prepared for your meeting with your manager (see the preceding section), prepare a list of questions for this meeting and be ready to write down the answers (or get printed materials that provide the information).

REMEMBER

When you meet with your HR representative, you're actually on a fact-finding mission. You're not necessarily going to act on any of the following factors right away, but you need to clearly understand your employer's policies related to

» Disability

» Early retirement

» Availability of any pension or 401(k) funds

» Government insurance programs, such as COBRA

» Health Savings Accounts (HSAs)

» Social Security Disability Insurance (SSDI)

» Medicare and Medicaid

» Any available state health insurance pools

TIP

The Americans with Disabilities Act (ADA) can be a real resource of options while your PD progresses. But be aware that the ADA doesn't apply to all employers, and it does have limitations. (See the sidebar, "The Americans with Disabilities Act — your golden parachute — maybe," in this chapter.)

THE AMERICANS WITH DISABILITIES ACT — YOUR GOLDEN PARACHUTE — MAYBE

According to the Equal Employment Opportunity Commission (EEOC), the Americans with Disabilities Act (ADA) gives civil rights protections (similar to those for race, color, sex, national origin, age, and religion) to individuals who have disabilities. The ADA prohibits discrimination in all employment practices: job application procedures, hiring and firing regulations, promotion opportunities, benefits, and compensation.

The broad protection given by the ADA sounds very promising. But keep in mind the fine points, as well — points that can affect your rights under the law. For example

- If your workplace employs fewer than 15 people, you may not be covered under this legislation.

- As a person with PD, your disability must substantially limit major life activities such as seeing, hearing, speaking, walking, breathing, performing manual tasks, learning, caring for oneself, communicating, and working.

- You must be qualified to fill the requirements of the job, and your employer maintains the right to establish performance and production standards that all employees must meet, disabled or not.

The ADA further requires your employer to consider whether you can continue to do your job with certain "reasonable accommodation." Examples of this requirement include special products (such as voice-activated computers), changes that make your existing workspace more accessible, or restructuring the job itself.

Because every disability and its effect on an employee's ability to do a specific job is slightly different, keep the following suggestions in mind:

- Your employer will rely on you to speak up and suggest possible solutions. If you don't have a suggestion, do some research and work with your employer to find one.

- Understand that the company is expected to pay for any equipment or necessary accommodation, but your employer isn't required to provide an accommodation that causes an *undue hardship* on other employees or the business. If cost is a factor (and you can afford it), you may consider offering to pay part of the cost.

- The ADA doesn't give you a free ride. Your employer can hold you to the same standards of performance and production as people without disabilities. You have a responsibility to be honest with yourself and your employer about your ability to meet those standards.

We strongly urge you to

- Become familiar with the pros and cons of the ADA for your situation.

- Not assume an adversarial or threatening attitude with your employer when it comes to applying ADA regulations to your situation.

For more information about ADA, call 800-514-0301 (voice within the USA), 800-514-0383 (TTY), or 202-514-0301 (outside the USA); or check out www.ada.gov.

Positioning the News for Coworkers

The type of job you have and the people you work closely with will influence what and how much you tell your coworkers. You have two possible scenarios given that you may be a supervisor or an equal-weight team member.

When you are the boss

Suppose that you're in a management or supervisory position and have several people who report directly to you. After you tell your boss (and have gotten their agreement that you need to break the news to your team), call a meeting of your group. Keep it informal. (In some business settings, this meeting is called a *huddle*, like a football team huddling to get the play before going into action. The huddle's a great analogy for the kind of atmosphere you want to create for delivering this news.) Consider making these tips a part of your meeting:

>> **Deliver the news plainly.** Do it with humor, if possible, but keep it direct and simple.

>> **Hand out a simple fact sheet about PD.** We talk about this kind of fact sheet in the section "Telling Your Boss," earlier in this chapter.

>> **Lay out the ground rules.** Tell your team what aspects may change but emphasize that it'll be business as usual — you're still a team.

>> **Offer some gossip guidelines.** How do you expect your team to handle any gossip or rumors that they may hear about you or PD? (Remind them that they can squelch any such nonsense by using the simple facts you provide in the fact sheet.)

>> **Request direct feedback.** Let your coworkers know that they can come directly to you with any concerns or questions. Then, you can assure them that you're most definitely still you and send them back to work.

When you're an integral team member

Suppose that you're part of a close-knit group whose ability to succeed relies on everyone pulling their weight. Your teammates react to the news with one of two attitudes: "Poor Mary. How will she manage? What can I do to help her?" or "Poor me. This is going to end up meaning more work for me." Be prepared for either reaction by

>> **Maintaining that same upbeat, can-do attitude** that you demonstrated when you told your boss (discussed in the section "Telling Your Boss," earlier in this chapter)

>> **Offering your PD fact sheet** and stating outright that, according to your doctor, you're going to be around for years to come

>> **Assuring everyone** that you're not expecting special considerations from them, and you'll continue to pull your weight on the team

REMEMBER

The manner in which you deliver the news of your PD to your manager and coworkers forms their attitude when they carry that news forward. If you're positive and upbeat, they're more likely to assure others that you have a real handle on it. And you want to project exactly that image to everyone.

Taking Steps to Protect Your Income

Working people have a variety of ways to protect themselves and their dependents if they can no longer work. Two types of protection come from income-generating plans and insurance coverage options.

REMEMBER

Although the following sections provide general definitions for a variety of options, we aren't recommending any one of these programs. If you need to leave your job and rely on other sources for your income and insurance coverage, consult with a qualified financial planner or counselor (see Chapter 20).

Checking out income-generating plans

You can find sources of income-generating plans through employers and the government:

>> **Employer disability plans:** Such plans can be short- or long-term, and eligibility requirements differ from one employer to another. In general, these plans allow employees to purchase short- and long-term disability insurance

as a part of their overall company-sponsored benefit package. If you need to leave work because of a disability, the plan pays you a percentage of your salary while you're disabled. Some plans pay that full percentage, even if you're also eligible for and receiving benefits from Social Security; other plans may prorate their payments based on what you receive from the government. *Note:* For specific information about disability benefits, talk to your HR department.

>> **Social Security Disability plans:** This segment of Social Security is different from the more common retirement benefit payout. Two programs are available: Social Security Disability Insurance (SSDI) and Supplemental Security Income (SSI). Both programs have stringent eligibility requirements:

- *SSDI:* For people who have an established work history; the amount you receive is determined by your work history and specific earnings.

- *SSI:* Based on financial need, serving people who have little work history and very limited financial assets.

For more information on becoming eligible for either program, call 800-772-1213 or go to www.ssa.gov.

Looking into insurance coverage options

Insurance coverage options can come through employers, from private companies, or from the government:

>> **The Consolidated Omnibus Budget Reconciliation Act (COBRA):** This option permits employees who lose their employer-sponsored benefits to pay out-of-pocket for the same health insurance coverage they received while working. Coverage can be quite expensive and the normal period you can pay for coverage is 18 months after you leave. unless you're determined to be disabled, in which case you can extend coverage to a total of 36 months. (For more information, talk to your HR department.)

>> **Long-term care (LTC) insurance:** LTC insurance plans provide coverage for care necessary to help a person with the basic activities of daily living, such as bathing and dressing. You can usually choose from benefits for a range of settings — the home, an assisted-living facility, or a nursing home.

REMEMBER

A growing trend among employers is to offer an LTC insurance option as a part of the employee benefit package. If your company provides this option and you haven't taken advantage of it, check into it again. (For more information on LTC insurance, talk to your HR department or call your state government's insurance department.)

>> **Medicare:** People under the age of 65 can qualify for Medicare (the federal health insurance and drug coverage plan). For current information on qualifying if you aren't yet 65, call 800-633-4227 or go to www.cms.gov. (For a more complete explanation of the Medicare program, see Chapter 21.)

>> **SHIP Programs and Medicaid:** Every state has some form of a State Health Insurance Assistance Program (SHIP) to help its citizens find the best insurance options, regardless of the person's financial or health situation. The website www.shiphelp.org/about-medicare/regional-ship-location gives links to SHIPs by state. In addition, every state offers Medicaid, the federally funded and state-managed program that provides health services based on financial need. (For more information on Medicaid in your state, go to www.medicaid.gov.)

IN THIS CHAPTER

» Easing into new routines and daily rhythms

» Keeping the family up to date and in focus

» Befriending your friends and going public

» Making room for R&R

» Moving forward with your care partner

Chapter **17**

Adjusting Your Routine While Your PD Progresses

I n the first months after the onset of your Parkinson's disease (PD) symptoms, you may be surprised how few accommodations your symptoms require. In fact, if your doctor recommends regular exercise and a balanced diet, and you follow their advice, you may be feeling better than you have in some time. Your symptoms may actually be more of an annoyance than any real concern. You may even have avoided going to see the doctor for that reason — the symptoms weren't really interfering with your routine.

As time goes by, however, your symptoms become troublesome enough to affect your life and routine — perhaps significantly. But this advancement of symptoms doesn't mean you can't live a full and active life. In this chapter, we offer tips for managing your symptoms — even while they worsen — *without* letting PD be the driving force in your life.

You're the same person you were before the diagnosis. You hold the same importance to your family and friends, and you retain many of the talents and skills you developed through your life. You may need to adapt — doing activities a different way, at a slower pace, or even with the help of others — but nothing about your essential identity has changed.

Exploring Ways to Make Daily Activities Easier

You can take a number of positive and proactive steps to keep your daily routine from overwhelming you. In the following sections, we look at some key ways that you can stay in control — as long as you're willing to adapt and not dig in your heels with a my-way-or-the-highway attitude.

Your occupational therapist (OT) can offer ideas and explain proven techniques for adapting your routine to accommodate your symptoms. Appendix B also recommends a number of resources and devices available to make life easier.

Don't allow other people's expectations or your own internal demands to direct your activity. The added stress of trying to compete or live up to last year's successes (big and little) can have an adverse effect on your overall health. Stress and performance anxiety can actually inflame your symptoms and undermine your daily efforts — at least momentarily.

Timing your activities

The main difference in your life now is timing — it can be everything. Understanding when you can and can't do something may provide the key to continuing many (or most) activities that you've always enjoyed. We're not talking about timing your meds (which you and your doctor need to work out together) or performing activities during your on times (we discuss on and off times in Chapter 10). We're talking about accepting and understanding that everything is a matter of time. You take longer to get ready to go places and longer to get from here to there. You take longer to do a task (such as dressing or brushing your teeth) that you used to knock off in a matter of minutes.

Even if you take four or five times longer, you're still independent. Continuing to perform these basic activities with little (if any) help for as long as possible can foster your ongoing sense of autonomy and being the one in control of how you will live with PD.

Make sure that those around you — family, friends, employers, co-workers — understand your need for extra time. Work out an appropriate time schedule for tasks that you perform personally or on the job. Be realistic. If you used to take 15 minutes to do something, let your cohorts know that you may now need an hour.

Reserving your energy

Accept that you have limited energy and that you must conserve it and use it wisely. This attitude can help protect your right to live independently and fully for as long as possible. Some days, you just might feel downright pooped, unable to complete the list of activities you have planned. So what? Are you saying that you never fell short of completing an ambitious list before the onset of your PD symptoms? Yeah, right. Everyone overestimates their potential for accomplishment from time to time. You're just wise enough to say, "Okay, I'll tackle that tomorrow — or the next day."

Approach each day with an I-don't-have-to-do-everything-but-will-do-as-much-as-I-(and my PD)-can attitude. The following are a few more tips to help you manage your energy bank:

>> **Prioritize tasks.** Take the time to think through the demands on your schedule each day. Determine what you need to tackle right away and what you can put aside for later.

>> **Schedule important tasks.** Choose a time when you're at peak performance.

>> **Implement energy-boosting suggestions.** Discuss with your doctor the advantages of regular exercise and diet changes for improving your levels of energy; then make those changes.

Taking tips from other PWP

Your ability to manage basic tasks may vary greatly from hour to hour and depend on where you are in your medication dosing cycle. But the ingenuity of the nearly one million people with Parkinson's (PWP) in the United States and a history of nearly 200 years can provide you with more than a few tricks to make your life with PD easier. The following sections share ways that other PWP maintain independence in spite of their symptoms.

Other people respond more positively to people who take an interest in the way they look. And looking your best empowers and keeps you in control of your own destiny. So make the effort — put your best face and foot forward every day. Some days, you may think, "What's the point of getting dressed? I'm not going anywhere and no one's going to see me." Yes, you are going places — even if it's just around the house. And your family (and any friends who happen to stop by) are hardly nobodies.

Strategizing

REMEMBER

Your determination to be as independent as possible — no matter how long a basic task takes — begins with curiosity and imagination. Take advantage of these general tips to make each day run a little more smoothly:

>> **Take baby steps.** Try to approach each situation as a separate challenge and break each task into individual steps. Focus on one step at a time. Try to start with the simplest one; after you conquer that, move on.

>> **Plan your meds and activities.** Keep in mind that timing is everything. Coordinate the timing of basic tasks with your medication routine to avoid off symptoms (we talk about off symptoms in Chapter 10) that can make each step even more frustrating. In addition, consider planning your exercise sessions, physical therapy, doctor's appointments, and so on to coincide with the time of day when you're feeling the best.

>> **Share the load.** If you have a partner, let them know that you find the difficulties you face as frustrating as they do, but you have to continue to try because doing so is one way you fight back — mentally and emotionally as well as physically. Discuss ways that your partner can help without taking away your opportunity to do as much as you can. For example, your partner can put toothpaste on your toothbrush and leave it out for you. Or while you shower or bathe, your partner can remain nearby in case you need help; they can also lay out your clothing for the day.

Grooming

Personal grooming is probably so much a part of your day that you barely think about all the individual tasks. Brushing your teeth, washing your face, shaving (whatever body parts you shave), applying makeup, and combing your hair are routines you've performed for decades.

But now your symptoms make these simple tasks next to impossible and even exhausting. Are you at the point where you need to ask for help? Not necessarily. Give these proven techniques a try:

>> **Sit down instead of standing.** You not only conserve energy, but also lower the risk of losing your balance and falling.

>> **Prop your elbows on the counter.** Steady your hand and support your shoulders while you shave or apply makeup.

>> **Use electronic appliances.** An electric razor, toothbrush, and so forth do a lot of the work for you.

>> **Try a simpler hairstyle.** Go with a style that's easier to manage and dries quickly without a hair dryer. In a pinch, try one of the dry-shampoo products available at drugstores or beauty supply shops.

>> **Treat yourself to regular pampering.** Everyone deserves a little TLC:

- *Getting styled:* Treat yourself to a regular appointment for a shampoo and styling at a discount hair salon or a local beauty school. (Getting your hair done is great therapy for relieving stress!)

- *Doing your nails:* Suggest that friends and family get you a certificate for a professional manicure or pedicure when they ask for birthday or holiday gift ideas. Or check with a local beauty school for a less-expensive session with a student.

Dressing

Before your PD symptoms started getting in the way, you probably never thought about the many balance and flex movements that are necessary just to put clothes on.

TIP

Before you begin breaking down this task into manageable steps, take the time to go through your closet and assess your wardrobe. Are the clothes easy to put on and take off? Table 17-1 gives some ideas for managing your attire.

Think through the steps of dressing — from choosing what to wear to putting on each item — and allow plenty of time. These tips make the tasks easier:

>> **Prepare the night before.** Choose your clothing and lay out all the pieces (from underwear to accessories).

>> **Sit on a sturdy armchair.** Don't use a rocker or the edge of the bed; and use the armchair's arms for support while you dress.

>> **Have a small footstool close at hand.** This stool can provide support when you put on socks and shoes.

>> **Lie down on the bed.** If lying down makes it easier for you to put on certain items such as pants or socks, go for it.

TABLE 17-1   Clothing Management for PWP

Clothing Item	What to Look For	What to Avoid
Jeans or slacks	Easy closures, such as elastic or drawstring waists	Buttons and zippers
Shirts or blouses	Magnetic snaps or Velcro; you can replace buttons on your favorite shirt with either	Buttons (especially small ones); consider sewing buttoned openings closed if you can pull on a top that's loose or stretchy
Sweatpants or workout pants	Relaxed fit	Elastic at the ankles
Shoes	Elastic shoelaces or Velcro closings	Lace-ups, heavy-weight shoes (no wingtips), and high heels
House shoes	Non-slip socks (like the ones hospitals have)	Bedroom slippers
Socks and hosiery	Knee highs or shorter	Pantyhose
Fabrics	Stretchy, non-clingy	Fabrics that cling — such as flannel, velour, and corduroy

Bathing and showering

Bathtubs and showers can be falls waiting to happen, so you first want to make them as safe as possible. Your OT can help assess the need for safety bars, tub mats, shower chairs or stools, non-skid rugs, and such. (Read more about OTs in Chapter 6.) Better yet, ask your OT for a scheduled walk-through of your home to identify safety concerns and how to fix them.

Next, you need to determine whether your normal bathing routine still applies. For example, when you consider the extra effort a shower or bath takes with PD, is your former daily routine realistic or even necessary? *Note:* One symptom in the mid-to-later stages of PD is excessive perspiration. If you have this symptom, you do need at least a daily sponge bath.

WARNING

Because of the danger of falling, never attempt a shower or bath when you're home alone. Although you may want the privacy of managing this routine on your own, make sure you have your care partner or someone in the family close enough that you can call for assistance if you need it. (Besides, what's so bad about having someone else wash your back?)

Whatever schedule you and your care partner decide on, these additional tips can make bath time less stressful:

>> **Prepare.** Cut down on trips that can drain precious energy by gathering everything you need (soap, towels, shampoo, robe, and such) in one place. Perhaps a plastic container in the bathroom can keep it all together.

>> **Make it pleasant.** Check that the bathroom is free of drafts and that you like the water temperature. You want to make your bath time a pleasant, relaxing experience, not a time when water that's too hot or too cold surprises you, potentially leading to a dangerous loss of balance or a fall.

>> **Remember your OT techniques.** Undress and, using the techniques you practiced with your OT, get into the tub or shower. If your PD doctor hasn't prescribed occupational therapy and you're beginning to struggle with movements such as getting in and out of the tub, ask for an OT referral. The OT can come to your home to work with you. In the meantime, be safe. Let your partner assist you in and out of the tub or shower, or plan to take sponge baths.

>> **Take your time.** The sensation of washing yourself should be a pleasurable one. Pour your bodywash into a container with a pump for easier use. If you still insist on using bar soap, consider using a bath mitt, which is a glove-like washcloth that's available at most drugstores and a good alternative to a loofah. And speaking of soap, go easy on the bath oils. They can make the shower or tub floor slippery (even with a rubber safety mat). Better to rub on bath oil as part of the drying process after your bath.

>> **Dry yourself thoroughly when you finish.** Again, take your time. Apply any lotion or cream to dry or chafed skin, and then put on your robe. In fact, a thick terrycloth robe is a super way to dry yourself if you lack the flexibility needed to towel dry.

WARNING

Don't attempt to get even partially dressed in the bathroom; the danger of falling while you attempt to dress in such close quarters is huge. Put on your robe and go back to your bedroom to dress, following the guidelines in the preceding section.

Personal hygiene

One symptom PWP can develop while their PD progresses is urinary incontinence (see Chapter 18 for a discussion on the impact incontinence may have on your PD). This problem not only presents a health concern but also a real hygiene issue due to the potential for odor. Of course, first discuss these problems with your doctor. Also consider these tips:

>> **Use disposable products.** Disposable products include sanitary pads available in varying degrees of thickness. Many of these products are far more discreet than wearing an adult diaper.

THINKING OUTSIDE THE BOX

Dr. Gary Guten — yes, the guy we dedicated this book to — had battled PD over a decade when it occurred to him that playing the piano could be a way to maintain flexibility and coordination in his fingers and hands. Over the years, Gary — an orthopedic surgeon, marathon runner, and expert in the field of sports medicine — had found several innovative ways to meet the various challenges of his PD's advancing symptoms. Taking up the piano was one way.

Gary and his teacher developed various techniques — such as placing 2-pound weights on Gary's wrists to help steady his hands and creating a system for remembering notes and reading music. After several weeks of lessons and practice, Gary joined 20 other students (average age of 13) to present his first recital. As Gary said, "At my age and at this stage of my PD, what else could I do to earn the applause of 75 people?"

Remember the words of the famous writer Gilbert Keith Chesterton: "If a thing is worth doing, it is worth doing badly." Like Gary, you and your healthcare team can get creative about what works for you in the fight to maintain your balance, mental alertness, and independence.

>> **Give yourself easy access.** Make certain that the pathway to and from the bathroom is well-lighted and free of obstacles. Or ask your doctor to prescribe a portable commode that you can place near your bed to avoid trips to the bathroom at night.

>> **Make a bathroom clean-up kit.** Keep moist towelettes, disposable pads, and other products within easy reach in your bathroom so that you can clean yourself as needed.

>> **Make a portable clean-up kit.** Keep a few pre-moistened disposable wipes and an extra set of clean underwear and clothing in a plastic bag in your car, in a bag, or in a backpack for whenever you go out, just in case.

Maintaining the Family Dynamic

Collaborative management is a relatively new term in managing the symptoms of a chronic condition such as PD. In medical circles, the term applies primarily to the healthcare team (see Chapter 6) that helps you plan for and manage your PD symptoms. But you can also use the term to describe families that need to include a chronic and progressive condition into their daily routines. The elements of collaborative management within a family unit may include

>> **Defining the issues to be managed:** Medical, mental, and physical health, as well as the emotional impact of PD on the PWP and the family. For example, if the PWP's been the family's chief financial manager, the PWP can train another family member in the details of managing the finances, paying the bills, investing and saving, and so on.

>> **Targeting each issue:** Establish realistic goals, achievable objectives, and a satisfactory plan of action for the PWP and the family. Goals can be simple and short-term, such as planning a family trip. If the PWP has always handled the planning, preparations, and details, then other members of the family need to step up and define ways they can take on some of those tasks.

>> **Supporting and encouraging the PWP's autonomy and independence:** Medical interventions, lifestyle changes, and emotional support systems can allow the PWP and their family to maintain as normal a routine as possible. Often, a family member responds to the PD diagnosis by jumping in and trying to do everything for the PWP. Because that person wants to deal with this challenge through action, find ways that they can contribute. For example, maybe they can prepare a salad or side dish for dinner while the PWP — an accomplished cook — makes the rest of the meal just as they did before PD.

>> **Monitoring the status of the PWP's role within the family unit:** Also keep an eye on the family's ability to adapt to the presence of PD. Ongoing and open communication — such as regular weekly or bi-weekly family meetings (see discussion of initial family meetings in Chapter 7) — can accomplish this goal and provide a safe haven for members to voice concerns. The agenda starts with an update from the PWP. Then other family members engage in a round of *concerns and joys,* in which each person can talk about possible needs or red flags and then mention something that's working well or brings special delight.

REMEMBER

As much as you might feel that the challenge of living with PD (or living with a family member who has PD) is all about you, in fact, it affects every family member. Whenever you have these family gatherings, make sure that you listen to everyone's honest concerns (and sometimes outright frustrations), whether you're the PWP or a loving family member. Acknowledge the concern, focus on the specific issue rather than the emotional overtones, and open the discussion to everyone to seek the best solution together.

Socializing with Friends

Every circle of friends has the person or persons who drive the social calendars of getting together, going places, calling, e-mailing, and the like. Each circle also has people who wait to be called, e-mailed, and the rest. Before your diagnosis, which role did you play? Were you the extrovert or the introvert? The social butterfly or the hermit? If you're an introvert by nature, maybe the friends you counted on to call and set up get-togethers seem to have turned into a bunch of loners. If you were the social cheerleader of the group, maybe you've dropped that ball now that you have PD — not wanting to impose yourself and your symptoms on your friends.

TIP

Get over it! If your friends are real, they're waiting for you to show them the way. If the usual extroverts seem to be hanging back, call them and clear the air. Chances are they've been hanging back while trying to figure out what you want. If you were the social leader, get back in the game. Call the old gang together and have an open discussion about your PD, how you're handling it, and most of all, how you hope *they'll* handle it. Then get back to doing whatever you did together before your diagnosis.

Whatever activity you decide on, don't make your PD the focus of (or reason for) getting together. You want to bring the relationships back to some semblance of normalcy. After your friends see you in action and enjoying the activities you've always enjoyed (maybe with a bit more effort and a little less speed), they can relax — and the friendships can move forward.

Going Out and About in the Community

You may as well get used to it: You'll have times when total strangers stare at you with pity (or worse, disgust), children point and snicker, and people even cross to the other side of the street to avoid passing you on the sidewalk. Some people might misread your balance symptoms as intoxication. Others may read your facial mask and lack of expression as a sign of mental illness or not being very bright. (This reaction is fairly obvious because the person speaks ver-r-r-y slowly and LOUDLY, as if instructing a small child or a non-English speaker.)

You can choose to take this ignorance and lack of good manners personally, or you can choose to understand that this stranger is the one with the problem — and then get on with your day. In either case, what do you care about the opinions of strangers? Are you going to permit people like that to stop you from living normally? Aha! We didn't think so.

Attending public events

Try to schedule your medication timing and dosing to your greatest advantage during the planned outing. Talk to your doctor about your plans and let them suggest any modifications to your normal dosing routine. (Chapter 10 dives into the medications for PD.) If you plan to go to a play, movie, concert, ballgame, or restaurant, some simple preparations may help:

>> Call ahead to get answers about accessibility (ramps, not stairs; seat on the aisle if you prefer an easy exit; room for a wheelchair if you need one; and so on).

>> Get plenty of rest before the event.

>> Allow plenty of time to get ready.

>> Arrive early so that you can get seated and settled without rushing.

REMEMBER

Make social outings as enjoyable for your care partner as they are for you. Don't use this time to try to prove your independence. For example, if helping you get ready (such as putting on your shoes for you) allows more time for your care partner to get ready, accept the help — *appreciate* the help. If using a wheelchair makes life easier and the occasion less stressful for your care partner, use a wheelchair. Think of this acceptance not as a surrender of your autonomy but as a gracious way of caring for your care partner.

Traveling

Taking a trip requires careful planning to make the trip a pleasurable experience, rather than a hassle. Like everything else, when you consider taking a trip, break it down into more manageable chunks:

>> **Choose where you want to go.** At this point in your PD journey, figure out what's realistic (a theater tour of NYC?) and what's not (scaling Mt. Everest?):

- Talk to a travel agent about special tours available for folks traveling with a disability.

- The website for the National Center on Health, Physical Activity and Disability (NCHPAD; www.nchpad.org) provides information on a variety of topics for people who have disabilities. Go to the site and enter the keyword *travel* in the Search box for firsthand information about travel.

>> **Figure out the transportation.** Plane, bus, car, train? Or maybe all of the above? If you go by car, you and your travel companions are probably well aware of your limitations and needs. If you're taking a plane, train, or bus,

contact the company well in advance to discuss provisions they offer to special-needs travelers.

REMEMBER

» **Be very specific about your needs.** For example, you may need your seat to be close to the bathroom. On the other hand, you may find navigating the entire length of a jumbo jet while you board just so that you can be close to the economy-class facility more trouble than it's worth. Ask whether you can have a seat closer to the front and permission to use the closer facility in business or first class. *Note:* If you'll be using a wheelchair — not a bad idea to conserve energy while you get from place to place within airports and train stations — the carrier needs advance notice.

» **Select your overnight accommodations carefully.** You may love an old, historic bed and breakfast, but can you navigate the stairs (which in old buildings can be steep, winding, and narrow)? If you're fine with a traditional hotel and it publicizes accessibility for people with special needs, don't take them at their word. Call and ask specific questions. For example

- Does the bathroom have grab bars and a walk-in shower (not a shower in a tub)?

- Are the doorways wide enough to accommodate a wheelchair or walker?

» **After you arrive at your destination, plan to get out and about.** Most tourist attractions in major cities around the world are well-prepared to accommodate visitors who have special needs. But often the trick is to locate those entrances, facilities, and other special services:

- *Call ahead.* Gather complete information about what services the attraction offers. Then, on the day of your visit, call again and let the staff on duty know that you're on your way. (You may want to call the day before to give advance notice.)

TIP

- *Contact member services.* If you or your traveling companion holds a membership in the museum or site that you want to visit, call the member services department and let them know that you're planning a visit. They may offer you and your party more than the standard accommodations for special-needs visitors.

» **Be prepared — just in case.** Emergencies happen even on vacation, so take the following suggestions seriously:

- Keep your medications on hand, don't put them in your checked baggage.

- Take along an extra supply (two to three days' worth) of your medications, as well as their prescriptions in case you have to replace medications.

- Carry a list of your medications (including over-the-counter products) and the emergency information listed in Chapter 6.

- Ask your PD doctor to recommend a colleague in the place you're visiting (or if you're taking a trip in the U.S., check online at https://doctor.webmd.com/find-a-doctor/specialty/neurology for a complete listing of certified neurologists by state).

Volunteering — The double blessing

Giving back to your community and making a real difference in the lives of other people pays double dividends. Not only are you contributing to the betterment of society — locally, nationally, or globally — but you're permitting yourself to turn your attention away from your own problems.

Whether you were an active volunteer before your PD or never had the time because of work and family responsibilities, PD shouldn't stop you from volunteering. When you give of your time and energy in spite of your own challenges, you inspire other folks and give them hope. If you can manage your PD while also mentoring a troubled teen, managing the volunteer program for the blood drive, or coordinating a fundraiser for your church, then you move other people to action. And that's something.

And speaking of getting involved, don't overlook this golden opportunity to really make a difference for yourself and other PWP. See Chapter 24 for ways you can build awareness of and increase knowledge about PD locally or even nationally. The national PD community is active, organized, and inspiring — not to mention a great deal of fun.

Taking a Breather — Respite for the Weary

You might find living with a chronic, progressive condition (or living with someone who has such a condition) stressful and even overwhelming while the months and years go by. Watch out for these warning signs:

- **Communication problems:** Increased frustration, irritability, short tempers
- **Physical symptoms:** Stomach upset, shortness of breath, headache
- **Unhealthy lifestyle behaviors:** Overeating or not eating enough, increased smoking or alcohol use, sleeping too much or too little
- **Emotional symptoms:** Depression, anxiety, feelings of deep anger or sadness

Take action before you lose control of these symptoms. Plan regular respite for yourself and your care partner — separately and together — as part of your daily routine. (Even the lowest-paid laborer is supposed to get a break at least a couple of times a shift!) In addition, you and your care partner need to consider the following:

REMEMBER

>> **Independence:** Your diagnosis doesn't require the two of you to be joined at the hip. You had separate activities before (and probably enjoyed telling your partner about the experiences). That arrangement shouldn't change simply because one of you has PD.

>> **Relaxation:** You both need to identify (in some cases, remember) the ways you individually relaxed and found respite before PD. Perhaps your partner spent an afternoon with the grandchildren. Maybe you had a regular card game. Maybe each of you gave time to a favorite charity.

>> **Trips:** Try to plan vacation-type respites together. The travel industry tries to accommodate the special needs of travelers like you.

TIP

If long-distance traveling becomes more stressful than fun, then perhaps you can go on vacation in your own community. Ever notice how much you enjoy the special sites and events of your community when you have out-of-town company? Treat yourself — move to a hotel or accessible bed-and-breakfast for a few days; eat meals out at restaurants that you've been meaning to try; visit a tourist attraction, such as a concert, play, or sporting event; and buy souvenirs for your friends or the grandkids. Just remember to pace yourself and get the rest you need to enjoy the around-your-town trip.

>> **Activity:** While your PD progresses, you may find that you don't have the freedom to physically get away. Respite for you may come in the form of alternative and complementary therapies, such as meditation or yoga, which we discuss in Chapter 12. And you may be surprised to discover the ways in which regular exercise can also provide you with respite therapy (see Chapter 9).

A Word for the PD Care Partner

You can find watching your loved one struggle to perform simple tasks frustrating and even emotionally painful. You may instinctively want to do whatever you can to make the task easier. That compassion certainly isn't bad, but you really need to fight the follow-through.

Managing the symptoms of PD means the PWP must fight to maintain as much movement, flexibility, and independence as possible for as long as possible. If you permit yourself or your loved one to give up on an activity that they can still do, you're actually (in a small but significant way) inadvertently accelerating the process that leads to your loved one needing real hands-on care.

Instead, discuss ways that you can help without taking away your partner's ability to manage on their own. For example, show your complete confidence in their ability. If your PWP usually drives the two of you to dinner, assume that they will be behind the wheel (as usual) whenever the two of you go out. On the other hand, if the PWP suggests you drive, don't make a big deal. Just agree. At the local coffeehouse, if the PWP's tremor makes you shudder every time they try to transport a cup of coffee from the counter to the table, ask if you can carry it instead. If they refuse, accept that.

Respite is vital for you and the PWP while you face the progression of current symptoms and the onset of new ones (see Chapter 18). Take advantage of available support so that you can care for yourself without guilt. You have every right to this self-care. Those supports may include

>> Family and friends who assume the role of primary care partner for brief periods while you take a break

>> In-home or respite care or adult daycare programs (see Chapter 20) when care partnering becomes caregiving

5

Coping with Advanced PD

IN THIS PART . . .

Plan for when your Parkinson's disease symptoms (eventually) progress.

Consider how the progression of your PD will affect your care partner.

Map out your future, both financially and legally.

Investigate living options for when your current home is no longer viable.

Chapter **18**

Facing the Progression of PD Symptoms

Sooner or later, you have to accept that a progressive disease such as Parkinson's disease (PD) just refuses to remain in the background of your life. In this chapter, we tackle the symptoms that may be brand new for you — perhaps even unexpected. Or maybe you've been dealing with some of them already. Our suggestion? The best defense is a good offense. Decide to fight back:

» Discuss openly any changes in your condition with your PD doctor.

» Explore options for additions to your current treatment or therapy.

» Prepare for lifestyle changes that may become necessary (such as relying on a cane or walker, or changing your living space arrangements).

In this chapter, we look at PD symptoms that usually occur later in the progression of the disease, and we also suggest some realistic ways to combat these symptoms.

Noticing Changes Caused by Your Meds

You may face some challenges after you've been on meds that control your PD symptoms for a while. Not everyone will experience *motor fluctuations* (wearing off of the effects of medication or the equally bothersome onset of dyskinesia). But for those who do experience these fluctuations, their timing during the progression of PD is different for everyone. Some PWP develop motor fluctuations earlier than others. Although one cause (for wearing off or dyskinesia) is related to increased medication, it's important to understand that the progression of your PD is also at play here.

When medications wear off

REMEMBER

The first medication-related challenge is *wearing off*, which occurs when your medication can't control symptoms over several hours. Suppose that you currently take your dosage of carbidopa/levodopa every six hours and don't notice a real difference in motor symptom control throughout the day. Over time, as the disease progresses, you may find that you start to experience the emergence of *off symptoms* (such as worsening tremor, slowness, and stiffness) prior to the timing of your next dose.

>> **At first:** Symptoms simply return earlier than usual, initially on a predictable basis (for example, you notice the symptoms return half an hour or an hour sooner than they used to).

>> **After a while:** An unfortunate evolution (the *on-off syndrome* discussed in Chapter 10) occurs where you can't predict the length of symptom control from one dose to the next. Some people with PD (PWP) get to know the pattern and may elect to simply live with the off times rather than increase medication.

TIP

Keep note of this wearing-off situation. It's a balancing act — one you need to discuss with your PD doctor — so that your doctor can adjust your medication regimen to meet your changing needs. For example, they may recommend adding a dosage so that you are taking your carbidopa/levodopa every four (instead of six) hours.

Counteracting uncontrollable movements

A challenge brought on by increasing meds plus the progression of your PD is *dyskinesia*, that twisting, writhing movement (see Chapter 10). Dyskinesia is the result of a complex interaction in the brain between the disease progression and the chronic administration of dopamine medication. As a result, dyskinesia

>> Usually appears after you've been on the meds for some time (somewhere between two and ten years)

>> Affects PWP in varying degrees that range from mild to severe, depending on their disease progression and their dose of levodopa (a common medication for PD, see Chapter 10).

Your PD doctor may be able to lessen or control your dyskinesias through a change in your medication or the dosing routine. If the situation becomes intolerable, your doctor may suggest another solution such as deep brain stimulation (DBS) surgery. (See Chapter 11.)

Keeping a diary and keeping your doctor informed

TIP

To help your doctor control your symptoms, keep a diary of the symptoms, including the time of medication intake and the time you feel the symptoms begin to return.

Doctors treat on-off problems in a variety (or combination) of ways:

>> Prescribe medication doses closer together

>> Add a second medication

>> Increase the dose to reduce wearing-off

>> Reduce the dose to control dyskinesia

REMEMBER

Whenever you notice a different reaction to your antiparkinsonian medications, talk to your PD doctor before making any changes in your dosing routine on your own.

When Communication Becomes Difficult

PWP can find the phenomena of speech changes in PD — *hypophonia* (softness of speech, or lower volume) and *palilalia* (repetition of words or syllables) — to be especially disheartening. These problems in communicating can make you feel downright depressed and frustrated. The following sections break down two major problems: difficulties with vocal and written communication.

The challenge to vocal expression

You can recognize changes in your normal communication by paying attention to the dynamics of a conversation. Consider the following scenarios:

>> You start to notice people (not just your significant other) leaning in or straining to hear and understand what you're saying. They do a lot of nodding and smiling but don't appear to comprehend your ideas.

>> People often ask you to repeat what you just said or to speak up.

>> People seem to be talking over you or finishing statements for you.

>> You can't have a normal conversation because you're asked to repeat yourself, or worse, you're ignored.

TIP

Do these situations seem all too familiar? Try to minimize these frustrations by asking your family and friends to do the following:

>> Be patient and look directly at you when the two of you are talking.

>> Try to conduct conversations away from background noises such as televisions, car radios, or other competing conversations.

>> Keep in mind that your *mask* (lack of facial expression) doesn't reflect your level of interest in the conversation. (See Chapter 3 for an explanation of this symptom.)

You can help yourself, too, by taking care of your voice:

>> Take a deep breath and project, without straining or shouting.

>> Allow time to rest your voice.

>> Slow down if your words come out too fast.

>> In any case, use your voice (talking, reading aloud, and singing). Use it or lose it!

While symptoms progress, you may want to seek help outside of yourself and your care partner. We help you explore your options in the following sections.

Speech pathologists

Speech pathologists (specially trained speech therapists) have the training and tools to improve symptoms or delay their worsening by using therapy in conjunction with your medication regimen. Your therapist can assess your needs, design a program of exercises to help strengthen your voice, and offer tips for making communication a more productive and pleasant experience.

If you have no speech professional in your area, consider ordering one or more of the following tools:

>> *Speech and Swallowing: A Body Guide to Parkinson's Disease*: A free book from the Parkinson's Foundation that includes exercises to help you strengthen vocal and facial muscles. (You can find it available online for download at www.parkinson.org/pd-library/books/speech-swallowing.)

>> **BIG and LOUD therapies:** The LSVT Global LOUD therapy (which you can find at www.lsvtglobal.com) has documented that PWP who follow this program (administered by a certified therapist) show improvements in loudness and intonation of their speech. Other secondary improvements include clarity of speech, changes in swallowing, and improved facial expressions.

Special devices

Several devices (such as message boards or more complex voice-activated software for your computer) can also help by amplifying your voice or making communicating easier. *Note:* These devices can be expensive, and you may find them awkward to use or carry around. Your speech professional can advise you on these tools, or you can contact the American Speech-Language-Hearing Association (ASHA) at www.asha.org or 800-638-8255.

You can get amplifiers that you wear to facilitate communication. Also, to improve communication via telephone, look for apps such as Loud and Clear (https://loudandclear.io) or ask your phone company about any special equipment they may offer at very low prices (or at no cost for customers who qualify).

Handwriting: Telling the story of your on-off cycles

Micrographia is characterized by writing that starts out normal-sized but becomes increasingly smaller and more cramped. This symptom may appear early in the progression of your PD, later in the progression, or not at all. When medications manage your symptoms well, handwriting may appear normal. But when medications wear off and you get closer to the next dose, you may see your fine motor skills compromised. When this happens, your writing may start strong and normal, but it quickly trails off into small, cramped letters and words.

TIP

Consider these tips to help you compensate for the writing challenges:

>> **Write a sentence at your next** PD doctor**'s appointment,** and then repeat that exercise at each check-up to see how much (or whether) your micrographia is progressing.

>> **Talk to your occupational therapist (OT)** about tips to help you manage this symptom.

>> **Use an electric typewriter or computer** for your written communications.

>> **Use lined paper that's sold with school supplies** to help your pen stay in line.

Swallowing: Don't Take It for Granted

In some PWP, *dysphagia* — swallowing difficulties — becomes a problem while PD progresses. Don't just write off the symptoms to an unrelated condition; have them evaluated by a doctor, speech therapist, or speech pathologist. Don't ignore the onset of swallowing difficulties. Watch for these symptoms:

>> Difficulty in eating and the need for a beverage to wash food down

>> Episodes of food going down the wrong way or food seeming to get stuck in the throat

>> Coughing or throat-clearing during or immediately after consuming food

>> Unexplained weight loss

>> Refusing food or drink because of the difficulty in swallowing, which has made eating an unpleasant experience

>> Fever due to aspiration in the lung

>> An increase in saliva or thickened mucous-like saliva

>> Drooling — a little or a lot

TIP

Lack of regular swallowing can cause problems with excess saliva and drooling. Two tips to prevent drooling and control saliva include the following:

>> **Keep your head up and your mouth closed** when you're not talking or eating.

>> **Take frequent sips of water** throughout the day, not only to remind yourself to swallow and stay hydrated, but also to water down that thicker saliva.

Your doctor or speech professional may perform an X-ray procedure that uses barium to assess the swallowing muscles in action. Your doctor may ask you to eat a sample of various foods and beverages so that they can evaluate how different foods and drinks affect your ability to swallow. And they may test you at various times in your dosing cycle to determine how your medications may affect your swallowing.

After the evaluation, your doctor can recommend ways to ease your swallowing difficulties and make eating and drinking easier. Possible suggestions include

>> **Timing your meals** during the on cycle of your PD medications

>> **Cutting food into small bites**, chewing thoroughly, and taking a sip of water before the next bite (yup, the old dieter's trick)

>> **Blending fruits and veggies** to create a drink — the popular *smoothie* that you may be able to swallow more easily than actual foods

WARNING

These may sound like simple solutions, but don't attempt to self-diagnose a swallowing problem. You could have a condition completely unrelated to your PD. Definitely check with your doctor if you start having swallowing problems.

Your Vision: A Bump in the Road

Another significant problem that can crop up while your PD progresses involves the potential for changes in your vision — blurred vision, difficulty focusing (and reading), dry eyes, and such.

Dealing with normal eye changes

REMEMBER

The aging process frequently includes some eye conditions that have easy solutions. For example, your doctor may prescribe a special eye drop or suggest an over-the-counter (OTC) product for dry eyes. Also, if you start experiencing blurred vision, you might just need a change in your lens prescription.

On the other hand, your dry eyes may result from the decreased number of times you blink due to your PD. Fortunately, the irritation and discomfort respond to the same artificial-tears products that your doctor recommends for similar problems related to aging.

Treating other eye conditions

Other vision problems that can affect PWP include spasm of the eyelid, excessive blinking (*blepharospasm*), and double vision. Interestingly, the popular cosmetic injection *Botox* (the brand name for a botulinum toxin) can treat the problem of excessive blinking. When you develop slowed and uncoordinated movements of your eyes, double vision can result; you can control it by using special lenses (prism lenses). Wearing a patch over one eye can help while you wait to see the eye doctor.

WARNING

Like with any health issue, don't attempt to self-diagnose or treat. See your eye doctor, describe your symptoms, and let the expert prescribe a solution.

Freezing and Rigidity: When Your Head Says Go, but Your Body Says No

Advanced PD often affects your ability to walk safely. Unconscious, easy maneuvers of yesterday that you took for granted now present you with major hurdles, just waiting to trip you up. This section discusses three of the most common problems: freezing, festination, and rigidity. Also, it includes suggestions to minimize the greatest concern — your risk of falling.

Freezing in your tracks

You're walking along fine and then — bam! — like the cartoon character who steps in glue, you're stuck! *Freezing* is the sudden inability to step forward, and it typically happens in three situations:

>> **While you step out:** *Start hesitation* classically occurs when you attempt to take the first step forward. You feel like your feet are glued to the floor, and you may also feel like you're walking in place. Although your feet are stuck, the rest of your body may lurch forward, placing you at great risk for falling.

>> **In mid-stride:** Even after you get started, freezing often happens with changes in thresholds, such as walking through a doorway or moving from hard surface to carpeting. You can also freeze when you need to take a step while you perform another action, such as turning the doorknob.

>> **When stopping or turning:** Freezing and hesitation can really complicate the act of turning around or changing direction — another circumstance that's ripe for a fall.

Freezing is mostly helped with *cueing* (visual hints such as bright yellow tape on the floor) that cue PWP to make a big step, or step over, in order to break the abnormal messaging telling your body to freeze. Another maneuver to help break the message is marching in place. You can work with your physical therapist on these techniques.

Assistive devices are also important to prevent falls and some walkers, for example, the U-Step rolling walker, have laser features that help by providing visual cues via a laser beam. You can find a growing number of products designed specifically to address the problem of freezing, such as some of the walking aids listed in Appendix B. In addition, exercise DVDs, online programs (check out You-Tube), and booklets offer programs specifically for PWP. Check out Appendix B, as well as Chapter 9.

When you get hasty with festination

Another typical walking problem in advanced PD is *festination* (from the Latin word *festinato*, meaning *haste*), where you take several short, almost running steps in an effort to regain your balance. This usually occurs when you break out of an episode of freezing.

You can use several tricks to maintain the rhythm of your walking:

>> March in place or hum a marching tune.

>> Take a step to the side before attempting to move forward. (This change in direction seems to interrupt the freezing sensation and allows you to continue your forward movement.)

>> Step over an imaginary line on the ground.

>> Visualize your foot moving through space three feet forward.

Rigidity: When your whole body locks up

Rigidity (stiffness in the muscles and limbs), which we discuss in Chapter 3, may first become evident in a reduced arm swing when you walk or when you display the *mask*, the loss of animated facial expression (see "When Communication Becomes Difficult," earlier in this chapter). While PD progresses or if medication needs to be adjusted to meet the progression of your symptoms, the severity of rigidity can escalate. Rigidity can also result in muscular pain. In normal movement, activating one muscle (the *agonist)* is offset by relaxing the muscle that performs the opposing action (the *antagonist)*. In rigidity, the opposing muscle fails to relax.

Your doctor can determine the degree of rigidity by gently moving the arm, leg, torso, or shoulder while you're standing or sitting in a relaxed position. One classic type of rigidity is known as *cogwheel,* where an arm or a leg can move only in short, jerky, or ratchet-like movements. Cogwheel rigidity is usually associated with *resting tremor* (a tremor that appears only in times of inactivity). Another common type of rigidity is *lead pipe,* when the muscles feel heavy and weak, and using them causes fatigue.

TIP

A program of regular exercise and stretching (see Chapter 9) can give you the most effective weapon to fight increasing stiffness and rigidity. Many communities offer special exercise programs through the local YMCA or hospital for people who have conditions that cause muscle stiffness, weakness, and rigidity. Talk to your physical therapist (PT) or support group about the availability of such a program in your area (or about getting a program started).

PD and Falling: A Tricky Balancing Act

The greatest risk while PD advances is the danger of falling. By some estimates, two-thirds of all PWP experience falls in the mid-to-later stages. And falls rank as the number one cause of hospitalization for PWP because of fractures or head injuries, as well as the role of falls as the precipitant factor in worsening of symptoms.

REMEMBER

Your PD symptoms contribute enormously to your possibility of falling. Think about the following scenarios:

>> Your shuffling gait practically begs for the opportunity to trip over a rug or uneven pavement.

>> Your general stiffness and slowness affect reaction time, so you can't stop yourself from falling by grabbing onto something.

>> Your tendency to overcompensate for impaired balance by swaying backward when you turn or stand compromises your balance.

As a PWP, four situations can increase the likelihood that you'll fall. The following sections cover those situations and the steps you can take to reduce your risk of falling.

Recognizing side effects from those meds

Most medications that you can take to manage PD symptoms have side effects, including "may cause dizziness." Medications for other health conditions (such as high blood pressure) can add to the problem. If you experience any change in maintaining your balance (stumbling, dizziness, lightheadedness, overcompensating to stay upright, and so forth), report these changes to your doctor immediately.

WARNING

Be sure to stay hydrated to help avoid risk of light-headedness, which can be a side effect of your PD meds. Monitor your BP as well and if you experience new symptoms of dizziness or imbalance after a recent change in meds, the med change may be contributing to the problem. Don't try to guess what's happening — call the doctor.

Anything you can do to prevent a fall is worth the effort. The following suggestions may help:

>> **Ask for an assessment of your current status by a PT and OT.** (See Chapter 6 for info on these specialists.) Ideally, the therapist(s) can compare this assessment to one that you had shortly after your diagnosis so that they can evaluate the amount of change.

>> **Implement suggested ways to prevent falls.** The therapist can evaluate your movements and risks for falling, and then advise you on making anti-fall changes in your home environment. (See Chapter 21 for tips on conducting this home survey yourself.)

>> **Seek productive changes to medication and environment.** Ask your doctor whether your meds come in a dissolving tablet (you take them without water) so that you can take a dose before you get up. At some point, you may want to ask your doctor to prescribe a hospital bed that you can raise and lower for greater assistance.

Cutting back on activity (Don't!)

WARNING

Falls (and possible injuries that require hospitalization) can lead some people to reduce their normal activity level. If your fear of falling limits your activity, you may be doing more harm than you think because staying active — physically and mentally — goes hand in hand with staving off PD symptoms (and thus preventing more falls). Talk to your doctor about the possibility of a PT or OT assessment and therapy that helps you adapt and get active again.

Adjusting for impaired balance

Your PD's progression can include impaired balance (because of your increasing muscle stiffness, rigidity, a stooped posture, and/or more frequent episodes of freezing). See the section "Freezing and Rigidity: When Your Head Says Go, but Your Body Says No," earlier in this chapter. Never is your team of professional care partners more important than now.

REMEMBER

Training and adaptive devices (including the proper cane or walker) can help you move safely and independently. Please don't just assume that Uncle Dan's old cane is right for you. Ask your therapist to properly fit a device to you.

Heeding the advice of your care team (Do!)

Your doctor, PT, and OT can assess your needs and make recommendations to help you maintain your balance. In the meantime, this short list of suggestions can help you prevent a fall:

>> **Use that cane or walker** that your doctor or PT ordered and customized for your needs.

>> **Avoid footwear that has rubber soles,** which may stick to the floor. Ask your PT to suggest the best footwear for you.

>> **Use a trick to maintain a rhythm** while you walk. Check out the section "Freezing in your tracks," earlier in this chapter, for some suggestions).

>> **Focus on walking,** rather than distractions. For example, don't try to talk on a portable phone and walk around at the same time.

>> **Take time to turn (TTT).** If you walk a few extra steps to make a wide turn, you can get where you're going; unlike if you pivot suddenly and lose your balance.

Overcoming Sleep Disturbances

Doctors consider anything that causes a disruption of normal sleep on an ongoing basis and prevents you from getting the rest you need a *sleep disturbance*. Disturbances may have a number of causes: genetic factors, environment (such as shift work), age, medications, and diet. Sleep disturbances are also non-motor features of PD. PWP often suffer from insomnia, excessive daytime fatigue, OSA (obstructive sleep apnea) and of course, REM behavior disorder (dream enactment).

Common causes of sleep disturbance

PWP are particularly prone to develop sleep disturbances for a wide variety of symptom-related reasons:

>> **Difficulty turning in bed** or medication-induced dyskinesias may disturb the level of muscle relaxation necessary to sleep.

>> **Urinary urgency and frequency** may force you to visit the bathroom several times during the night.

>> **Medication to treat your PD symptoms,** if taken too close to bedtime, may cause vivid dreams or agitation that awakens you.

>> **Anxiety and depression,** which frequently affect PWP (see Chapter 13), can make falling asleep difficult (anxiety) and can cause you to wake early or sleep too much (depression).

In addition, PWP may experience a number of specific sleep disturbances. The most important one is *rapid eye movement (REM) sleep behavior disorder,* a condition that makes you act out your dreams, unknowingly talk out loud, move your limbs, and sometimes even hit your bed partner! All of these actions can create a state of chronic sleep deprivation that leads to fatigue, excessive daytime sleepiness, and visual hallucinations.

Improving sleep habits

TIP

Keep in mind that you can improve many sleep disturbances simply by developing better sleep habits. The American Academy of Neurology offers the following tips:

>> Sleep only when drowsy and only in the bedroom.

>> Keep lights and noise low when trying to sleep, but keep a night light on to prevent falls if you need to get up in the night.

>> Limit your intake of tobacco products, caffeine (chocolate, coffee, non-herbal tea, and such), and alcohol.

>> Don't eat a heavy meal or participate in strenuous exercise for four to six hours before bedtime.

>> Make use of relaxation and stress-relief techniques (see Chapter 12).

Of course, like any new or troublesome symptom, discuss a sleep disturbance with your PD doctor especially if you are experiencing excessive daytime fatigue and/or frequent sleep interruptions at night. The problem could be a side effect of your medications, or it might a signal of a more serious condition, such as *sleep apnea syndrome* (breathing stops and starts repeatedly during sleep), which requires specialized management.

Those Embarrassing Constipation and Urinary Issues

The good news: Although a nuisance for PWP, you can often treat and manage urinary and bowel issues, even while your PD progresses.

REMEMBER

As we note in Chapter 17, never automatically dismiss urinary or bowel problems as unrelated to your PD. If you begin to have problems with incontinence or constipation while your PD progresses (or you've had issues in the past, but they seem to be worsening), tell your doctor. Although both conditions are common side effects of many medications (even common OTC meds), simply stopping or changing meds may not relieve symptoms.

Tackling an errant bladder

In some cases, PWP may suffer from an overactive bladder and feel an urgency to get to the bathroom as soon as possible, especially at night. Other PWP may experience an inability to fully empty the bladder, so they need to go again within a short time. PD often includes malfunction of the bladder. If you're experiencing such symptoms, tell your doctor. In males, you may have an enlarged prostate gland; in women, you could have an infection (called a *urinary tract infection*, or *UTI*). In either case, your doctor may recommend that you see a urologist to rule out other causes.

When even BMs slow down

The slowed movement that's a core part of PD can make constipation a relatively common problem for PWP. Because of other issues that can crop up with the progression of PD (such as swallowing difficulties that lead to a poorer diet, not drinking enough liquids, and infrequent exercise due to impaired movement and balance control), constipation can become a recurrent problem for many PWP.

Let your doctor know of any changes in your normal bowel or urinary habits. In the meantime, you know the routine (your mother probably drummed it into you when you were a kid):

- » **Drink plenty of water.** Yes, even if you need to go (#1) all the time.

- » **Eat your roughage.** Also known as fiber (fruits, veggies, and whole grains). See the USDA's MyPlate website (www.myplate.gov) for more information on healthy eating.

- » **Get daily exercise.** No, reaching for the remote doesn't count!

Dealing with the Big D — Dementia

Dementia (a change in your thinking or memory that impacts your ability to function independently) may be one of the most frightening and unsettling words in the English language. Just to be very clear, dementia can

- » **Impair a person's intellectual function** to the degree that it affects normal and routine activities (such as decision making, keeping track of monthly bills, and such) and relationships with other people.

- » **Possibly cause changes in behavior and personality.** A person who has dementia may experience delusions or hallucinations. The key word here is *possibly*. Not everyone with cognitive impairment or dementia will develop hallucinations or delusions. But other changes may occur — a person who was always calm and controlled becomes angry and agitated, for example.

- » **Affect at least two normal functions of the brain.** These functions include memory, reasoning, perception, and judgment. (Memory loss by itself is not dementia.)

Note: Dementia — senile or otherwise — isn't a normal part of aging.

You probably have this question uppermost in your mind: Is dementia part of PD's progression? Here's the answer: It can be, but it might not necessarily be for you. For those who develop dementia, the timing of when it occurs varies, but for most, the longer you have had PD (think 10-20 years) or the older you were when first diagnosed, the more likely you will develop dementia or cognitive impairment.

REMEMBER

Everyone experiences the progression of PD in a unique way. So find out what you can about dementia and consider how you and your care partner may handle its possible onset. Then, get back to living your life.

PD is not Alzheimer's disease

Today, Alzheimer's disease (AD) is one of the most commonly recognized conditions associated with dementia. A person who has AD faces a progressive loss of intellectual and mental function. If a person has AD, they have a *primary* dementia, which means the dementia doesn't result from any other disease or condition.

In contrast, for people who have conditions that affect movement or other functions (such as PD), dementia is a *secondary* dementia. According to the Johns Hopkins Medicine website (www.hopkinsmedicine.org/health/conditions-and-diseases/parkinsons-disease/parkinsons-disease-and-dementia) dementia occurs when nerve cells degenerate, leading to chemical changes in the brain. For more in-depth information about dementia related to PD, see Chapter 8.

REMEMBER

The point is this: The onset of dementia in a PWP isn't a foregone conclusion, and dementia isn't the same as AD. You need to report any sign of cognitive malfunction to your doctor because your sudden hallucinations, or excessive sleepiness and dull mind, may have a perfectly logical (and treatable) explanation.

Reviewing those cognitive symptoms

Although Chapter 3 has a full discussion of cognitive symptoms, a quick review can help you collate those early symptoms with this chapter's context of PD progression.

TIP

If you have some cognitive symptoms, don't think that you're definitely headed for full-blown dementia. Don't panic, but do talk to your doctor if you're experiencing any of the following:

>> **Anxiety or depression:** Part and parcel of PD. Focus on the fact that they're treatable. If you ignore or refuse to acknowledge these symptoms, shame on you. (If you haven't read Chapter 13, do it soon.)

>> **Executive dysfunction:** Can include troubles with keeping track of your monthly bills, following directions, making routine decisions, and such. Fortunately, you can strengthen and exercise your mind and possibly keep this problem at bay. (See the following section for tips to keep your body and mind healthy.)

>> **Hallucinations:** A potential side effect of your medications, *hallucinations* are when you see objects that really aren't there — perhaps a child or animal passing quickly by your door. Or you may simply feel the presence of a person without actually seeing that person. Hallucinations can be *visual* (sight), but

they can also be related to other senses: *auditory* (hearing), *tactile* (touch), or *olfactory* (smell). They can occur in the presence or absence of medication and also in the presence or absence of cognitive impairment.

But while your PD advances, you may also develop a cognitive disorder that leads to these usually harmless hallucinations. Like with anything that seems out of the norm, you (or your care partner) need to let your doctor know. They might prescribe simple medication changes or add other medications to block hallucinations.

To Drive or Not to Drive

Changes from the progression of your PD can potentially seriously impair your ability to safely operate motorized vehicles, and for a PWP, losing the ability to drive can equate with a loss of independence and autonomy. In addition to vision problems, you may see these symptoms while your PD progresses:

>> Your meds wearing off at inopportune times so your ability to properly operate the vehicle is compromised.

>> Possible worsening of your rigidity that impairs the coordination you need to operate a motor vehicle

>> Slowed reaction timing — hazardous for any driver

TIP

How to continue to drive in spite of your PD? How to know when you can just no longer drive? Follow these suggestions to assure your safety (not to mention the safety of other people) before you get behind the wheel:

>> **Be smart about when you drive.** Consider limiting (or eliminating) driving after dark. A lot of people struggle with night driving while they age, not just PWP.

>> **Don't drive if another driver's available to take the wheel.** Consider taking public transportation when you can.

>> **Don't drive after consuming even the smallest amount of alcohol.** You really can't predict the effects of combining a drink with your meds.

>> **Visit a Driver Rehabilitation Specialist or an OT with expertise in this area.** If you (or your partner) question your ability to drive, play it safe by asking your occupational therapist (OT) to refer you for this visit. Let the specialists assess your ability and, if possible, recommend changes (such as not driving at night or for long distances) that can allow you to keep driving.

> » **Have your doctor note in your chart that you're capable of driving — day or night.** For legal reasons, if your PD doesn't affect your driving ability, this written verification can help protect you if an accident occurs and you're not at fault.

Especially for men, driving is a mark of independence — that macho thing. Get over it. If the end of your driving days isolates and depresses you because you refuse to consider alternatives, that's on you. You have choices, including asking a friend or family member (who just happens to be looking for a concrete way to help) for a lift.

When Medical Treatments Are Limited

Identifying the various symptoms that may worsen or appear while your PD advances can give you confidence for the next step: addressing those changes. What options do you have when medical treatments can't provide the answer? You have a number of resources — all within your grasp — for fighting back if you have to face the onset of new symptoms or the progression of your present symptoms. The following guidelines can help you stay the course:

» Continue to eat a healthy diet rich in antioxidants (see Chapter 9).

» Continue your daily exercise program (also discussed in Chapter 9).

» Continue to exercise that mind! Mental activities such as playing games, working crossword puzzles, and so on (no, TV doesn't count) can help to keep your mind agile.

» If possible, consider taking a class or starting a new hobby.

» At the very least, remain socially active and engaged in the world and the community around you.

REMEMBER

Yes, you may be approaching the point where you rely on other people more. But you don't have to surrender all decisions and control. Your lifestyle and life choices can play an enormous role in your ability to postpone your PD's progression. Keep fighting! Keep moving! Keep living!

A Word for the PD Care Partner

While your partner's PD progresses, you may face some tough challenges, such as having to persuade your partner to give up driving or acknowledge that their recurring signs of cognitive impairment can impact their safety. You may see such challenges as even more difficult because you've both been living with PD for a number of years. Obvious symptoms that let you know the PD is getting worse can add strain to the relationship. The following tips may help you hold it together while you and your PWP enter this new phase of living with PD:

>> **Acknowledge changes when they come** and seek the advice of the PD doctor, especially if you notice any unusual progression of symptoms (such as sleep disturbances or onset of visual hallucinations) or recurring behavior (excessive eye-blinking or increased urinary urgency).

>> **Continue to prepare for potential lifestyle changes** that may become necessary (such as a change in living accommodations) and check out the availability of options in your community.

>> **Let someone else be the villain** when it comes to taking away driving privileges. If you're concerned, let the PWP's doctor know. The doctor can order a driving evaluation and make recommendations based on that.

>> **Contact a representative in your state motor vehicle department** if the doctor doesn't respond to your concerns about your partner's driving. Ask the representative to require a road test as a step in renewing the license.

>> **Talk to people in your support system.** Reach out to your support group contacts or facilitator, your clergyperson, or the counselor you found when you and your PWP set up the healthcare team (see Chapter 6). If you begin to feel overwhelmed with responsibilities (financial, physical, emotional), ask for some concrete tips for coping.

>> **Realize that you're in danger of burning out.** To keep on keeping on, address your need for regular short-term breaks and an occasional long-term respite. Plan for these breaks; they're as vital to living with PD as your partner's timely medications.

If you and your partner have prepared for this day, you've already discussed some difficult decisions. Your partner now needs to accept and appreciate that you're simply carrying out those decisions that you both made months or years ago. If your partner can't seem to understand (or appreciate) that fact, remind yourself that your PWP is still in control. But you need to remember: Having made the choices together, you're now simply carrying out those wishes. (For more advice on coping with progressing care, read Chapter 19.)

Chapter **19**

When Care Partners Become Caregivers

Y ou probably have many years left to live, in spite of your Parkinson's disease (PD). The future is hopeful as every day brings us all closer to a cure. But while your PD progresses, the day may come — possibly following a fall and maybe a fracture, or the worsening of another medical condition (diabetes, for example) that requires hospitalization — when you need more hands-on, direct care.

We hope you have a care partner while you make your PD journey to this point. But having a care partner comes with both good and bad news. The good news is that this person represents the most likely candidate to become your primary care-giver, and they're probably very familiar with you and the path your PD has taken. The bad news is that you're pretty used to being in charge in that care-partner relationship. Handing off that control takes some adjustment.

While your need for care increases, you almost certainly have different tiers of care around you. Your *primary caregiver* is the person who takes the lead, manages your care day to day, and acts as your spokesperson if you can't speak for yourself. But you also need *secondary caregivers,* people (usually other family members and friends) who take on a specific role, such as handling your finances or doing the grocery shopping.

In this chapter, we consider that transition from care partnering to receiving care because of your symptoms' progression (see Chapter 18 for more on how your symptoms will likely progress). This chapter covers specific changes in your caregiver's new role and how your relationship with that person may adjust. We also offer alternative arrangements that you may need over time, give you a heads-up about the biggest challenges of this transition, and suggest ways to foster your secondary caregivers. Finally, we offer straight talk and important suggestions for your care partner.

Understanding Your Primary Caregiver's Role

By definition, *caregivers* provide some type of hands-on assistance to other people. That assistance may be in the area of handling finances, managing legal affairs, providing emotional support, attending to routine chores, administering personal care, or any combination of these categories. According to the Family Caregiver Alliance, as many as 65 million family caregivers in the United States provide care for a family member or friend who's an adult (age 20 and over). Most caregivers (75 percent) are women, and about half of all caregivers are employed elsewhere full-time.

Your caregiver takes primary responsibility in providing more intensive home and personal care assistance. You trust this person to abide by your wishes — those plans that you made clear in better times — and to speak for you if you can't speak for yourself.

REMEMBER

Your caregiver isn't the person with PD (PWP). Life will go on for this person after the time for giving care has passed. Your caregiver deserves to attend to that life while still attending to your needs. This person may have been right there with you, acting as your care partner to this point; if so, your relationship must adjust to a new balance of roles. Your care partner, who's becoming your caregiver, well knows the emotional and psychological impact that these challenging times have on both of you.

Giving care versus partnering in care

You and your care partner's roles are changing now. More and more, care-partner-turned-caregiver must take charge of decisions and actions that affect your welfare and safety. Decisions that used to focus on your needs must now increasingly focus on your caregiver's needs, abilities, and emotional strength in order to deliver what you require when you need it without sacrificing their normal routine.

Never will you face more temptation to give in to the anger and resentment that this widening chasm can create. Never will your care-partner-turned-caregiver deserve your love, appreciation, and emotional support more.

And yet an important element of partnering remains. If you and your partner have prepared for this day, discussed the difficult decisions that you knew you might face, and explored options to address your increasing needs, then keep in mind that your partner is simply carrying out the decisions you both made months or even years ago.

Is your care partner a novice or a natural caregiver?

Some people are natural nurturers. Others aren't. Some come to the role of caregiver with years of experience already under their belts. Other folks who are new to the role may find themselves entering a strange world that they're not prepared to tackle. But most caregivers have one fact in common: One day, a care partner's loved one is managing fairly well, and then the role shifts seemingly overnight. The care partner suddenly must become caregiver and intervene. More often than not, this ongoing level of care becomes not only necessary, but essential.

TIP

Keep in mind that not everyone is up to the job. Even though a person may seem like the most obvious candidate — your spouse, significant other, or adult child — they may not be physically and emotionally prepared to take on increasingly complex caregiving duties. You and your care partner must keep an open mind and consider creative ways to decide how best to manage your care while your PD progresses.

It's called the 36-hour day for a reason

For over 30 years now, the gold standard guide for caregivers of people with Alzheimer's disease is a book called *The 36-Hour Day* by Nancy L. Mace, MA and Peter V. Rabins, MD, MPH (Johns Hopkins University Press). The concept of giving a loved one care that escalates over time makes the book title into a truism for caregivers in all sorts of circumstances.

No one can give an accurate estimate for just how long you'll need care. It can be anywhere from a year to decades. But if your caregiver devotes 20 to 40 hours a week (as statistics indicate) to giving care, in addition to juggling other roles (such as parent or employee), then the exaggerated idea of a 36-hour day fits.

In addition to selecting the best caregiver for the job, it's essential that you and your care partner get real about how much time your care will require and where that time will come from. Two lives are at stake here — yours and your caregiver's. At this stage (just like in the earlier stages), each of you has the right to maintain some semblance of a lifestyle that fills your physical, mental, emotional, and spiritual needs. (Chapter 15 can help you set up the ground rules for your relationships, and Chapter 17 suggests ways to bring clarity to your roles.)

Considering How Your Relationships May Change

If you prepared for this day (which we talk about doing in Chapters 5 and 6), you and your significant other (or adult child, or other care partner) have discussed the what-will-happen-when questions. And you thought about how to address the increasing necessity to rely on other people. You may think that the most likely candidates for caregiver are pretty obvious, but each situation comes with a history that can affect this shift in roles.

When you rely on your spouse or significant other: A balancing act

"Grow old along with me! The best is yet to be," as the quote from Robert Browning goes.

In a marriage or union between two people, each person settles into a role. Maybe one pays the bills and manages the day-to-day budget, and the other handles their long-term financial and healthcare security. One is the gardener; the other is the cook. One is the social butterfly; the other prefers staying home with a good book. Through the years, they develop ways of compromising, moving out of their comfort zones, and reinventing themselves individually while they find their way as a couple.

So, what happens if everything shifts? Suppose that the former cook has advanced PD and can no longer safely prepare the meals. The gardener must now take on the responsibility of meal preparations. When going out becomes more difficult for the PWP, the social butterfly adapts by staying home to be with them. The PWP feels guilty that the PD impacts their lives so much, and the partner reassures the PWP but can't deny a sense of mourning about how their lives have changed. While the caregiving becomes more intense, perhaps the partner abandons more and more of those activities that gave them identity.

REMEMBER

When one partner becomes the caregiver, both partners need to maintain balance while their duties and responsibilities shift. The most effective way that you and your care partner can accomplish this shift is by accepting the help of other people — even outsiders whom you pay to perform some specific care task. This help can free the PWP's partner to pursue (in moderation) their life, and if they accept this help as your contribution to the relationship, it can relieve guilt for wanting a life beyond your PD.

When your adult child steps up: You're still the parent

Some people call the relationship that comes from an adult child caring for a parent *parenting our parents*. Wrong! Roles may shift when you turn to your child for advice on finances or assistance with daily chores, but the relationship between you and your child has a history. There's no reversal here. (See Chapter 15 for more discussion on this relationship.)

If your adult child becomes your primary caregiver, your history influences the relationship that you forge. Although the ways you've communicated (or not) through the years may have mellowed, the base of your relationship doesn't change just because you now need help. And this reality may be good, or it may cause some rough moments.

TIP

The key to making any caregiving relationship a success involves mutual respect. As an adult, your child deserves the same trust and respect that you would extend to any person of maturity and experience. At the same time, that child needs to accept that — regardless of your frailties and even childlike dependencies — you're still a grown-up with a history of managing your own life (and their life when they were young).

When your sibling comes to your aid: Rivalries remain

Family history plays a part with siblings, too. Your position within the family order (eldest, middle, youngest) continues to impact the relationship. The feeling that "Mom always liked you best" doesn't go away, although someone may only mention it in jest these days. Old jealousies, wounds, and slights that you never addressed after you became adults can still fester. Labels from when you were small can linger. "Mary was the smart one." "Jim was the family comedian."

If a sibling seems the most likely candidate to become your caregiver and spokesperson, mend those fences way before you need them to take that role. Also, set ground rules about the way you live your life and interact with other people. If your sibling can't respect your ways and expects you to adapt to theirs, you may have a stressful caregiver relationship from day one. And, trust us, the last thing you need in your life is more stress. Hopefully, you and your sibling had this discussion early in your PD journey and realized that — although they might make an excellent care partner — you might need to look elsewhere when a caregiver is needed.

When your friends offer to help: Are they in it for the long haul?

If you're single and have no family member close enough (geographically or emotionally) to consider as your caregiver, you may turn to a long-time friend for help and support. Although this pattern can and does work for many people, be careful. A lifelong friendship can be destroyed if both sides aren't absolutely upfront about giving and receiving care.

TIP

Identify the specific ways that you anticipate requiring help and make sure you indicate that any help offered is not a life sentence for the helper. Start with one task — perhaps you need your friend to provide transportation to and from doctor appointments, or to make a daily call or visit to check on you. Friends are usually quite willing (even anxious) to step up, but they crave direction. And if they must eventually back off, they want to know you'll understand and that you can find another source for help.

Exploring Alternative Arrangements

If you live alone, you may have to look outside your immediate home for the care partner who can and will take on caregiving while your PD progresses. In fact, you may want to split the job up and enlist more than one caregiver.

Long-distance care with emergency backup

In today's world, family members often scatter across a wide area. The most obvious caregiver may be someone living miles away. Short of you or this person making a major move, what choices do you have?

One caregiver in Wisconsin managed care for her parents in Virginia over an eight-year period without anyone having to move. When long-distance caregivers take care of loved ones, both of you have to go into the challenge with knowledge and preparation. As the PWP, take these two steps:

1. **Prepare: Find out ahead of time what programs and services your community has for support and care. Then share that information with your potential long-distance caregiver.**

2. **Identify local emergency caregivers (friends, neighbors, or paid caregivers) who can step in for a short time until the long-distance caregiver can arrive.**

Emergency caregivers are people who can step in when something unforeseen arises. They have a temporary, but important, role. Your emergency caregiver may be a neighbor who can step in until your long-distance caregiver can arrive or a friend who's agreed to assume this key role. For example, your clergyperson might marshal the forces of the congregation to step in until more permanent help arrives.

TIP

Whoever you identify for this emergency backup role, you — and especially your long-distance caregiver — need to establish a plan for emergency action, sooner rather than later. If you fall and your primary caregiver is miles away, who can come to your aid?

A caregiving community instead of an individual

In rare cases, no single person can step in and assume the role of primary caregiver. When that happens, don't despair. You have options for preparing for the day when you need more direct care. Start by watching the YouTube video (presented by the Parkinson's Foundation) called "PD Solo: Living Alone While Living with Parkinson's Disease." You can find this video online at www.youtube.com/watch?v=F0N66n9Q73U. If you don't have access to that online resource, consider these arrangements:

>> **Remain in your home and get the help you need.** If you're still pretty mobile and on top of your monthly bills, but you need daily check-ins and help

with shopping, you can remain in your home if you get a little help. You can set up some aspects of this arrangement more easily than others. For example,

- Sign up for delivery services. Many pharmacies and grocery stores offer a delivery service for medications and food.

- Address safety issues by installing a phone service and wearing a medical alert monitor. If you don't contact the service by a specified time each day (or even twice a day), then the service contacts someone to come and check on you. Or if you fall and need help, you can activate the monitoring device (some systems can actually detect your fall and send help!).

>> **Change your living arrangements, sooner rather than later.** Some facets of personal care are more complex than grocery shopping or general safety. Perhaps you struggle to manage routine tasks (such as showering, shaving, or shampooing). Maybe you can't keep a handle on your financial matters or begin to experience diminished mental capacity. You still have options, such as

- *Community services:* Many communities offer meal delivery services and in-home assistants who visit regularly to help with personal care and monitor medications.

- *Retirement or other care communities:* Consider moving into an assisted-living facility or *multi-level community* (where care progresses from independent living to nursing care). For a full discussion of care and housing options, and how to manage the costs, see Chapter 21.

Making the Transition

When the transition from partnering to caregiving (and care accepting) begins in earnest, you may find your relationship changing in unexpected ways. Consider these new challenges:

>> **For the PWP:** Moving from independence to the necessity for assistance, and from blind stubbornness to acceptance

>> **For the PWP's care partner:** Shifting from partner to caregiver, a seemingly full-time job

>> **For both of you:** Consciously recognizing the emotional roller coaster you've boarded — right when your physical and emotional defenses may be waning

TIP

The best coping tactic for the PWP involves acknowledging the difficult feelings (see Chapter 22) that come with increasing challenges and dealing with those feelings head on. Talk to your mental health therapist for help dealing with the transition if you need it.

Agreeing to accept help

Many people have fiercely independent natures, and perhaps never more so than when illness or other circumstances beyond their control threaten that autonomy. Just make sure that you recognize accepting help from others — regardless of how independent and self-sufficient you've always tried to be — as simply one more tool that you and your primary care partner can use. Allowing others (friends, extended family, the community) to provide assistance gives you much-needed support in preserving your energy to live life as fully as possible for as long as possible.

One of the concepts we try to instill throughout this book is that fighting PD is a team effort. If it takes a village to raise a child, it takes a contingent of healthcare professionals, family, and friends to maintain a rich life when you have PD. You may be the quarterback, but you need every one of those other players to help you run those plays and live on your own terms.

REMEMBER

Don't feel shame for accepting the help of other people. As a matter of fact, you're often helping them. You empower them by needing them. And you enrich their lives by giving them a way to tangibly demonstrate their love and respect for you.

You know how much you hate this PD being all about you — the glances, the murmured comments when people think you're out of earshot. You have just one way to change that: Take control and accept the help you require. If you're still not convinced that the time has come to seek additional help, think again. Maybe you're reading this chapter because you already suspect that you and your care partner can no longer manage totally on your own.

WARNING

Refusing to acknowledge that you need help (and then making the necessary changes to accept help) can result in serious setbacks for both the PWP and the care-partner-turning-caregiver. These possible setbacks include

>> A toll on your relationship

>> Costs associated with emergencies (brought on by your refusal to accept help) that affect your financial well-being

>> Isolation that comes from managing your PD to the exclusion of everything and everyone else

>> Ignored warning signs — such as confusion, anger, depression, and guilt — that result when managing alone becomes too much for you

>> Damaged health — physical, mental, and emotional, all caused by stress — for you and your care partner

Whether you enlist the help of other people or make a more permanent change (such as moving to a different residence where you have access to the support and care that you need), don't be stubborn about this. Don't toy with your life and the life of your beloved, devoted care partner. Snap out of it!

Remembering that your PD isn't your caregiver's fault

An old song (first recorded by the Mills Brothers) says, "You always hurt the one you love." And it happens fairly innocently. Your care partner knows that you aren't always at your best, and they don't expect you to be. With this person, you can let go of the brave façade, the "I'm doing great" demeanor.

WARNING

But avoid going too far with burying those not-so-positive feelings and hurtful behavior. The dark side of this denial comes out when you start taking out your anger and frustration on your care partner. This emotion may come in the form of a short temper, snappish comments, or lack of any appreciation for your caregiver's sacrifices. It may also come in more subtle ways, such as shutting the person out through silence or isolating the person from their own life through your neediness.

Your care partner has surrendered a piece of their life to continue this journey with you. You can help determine just how great a sacrifice they have to make.

Dealing with burnout

If you or your care partner weren't dealing with this less-than-ideal situation, if both of you were living lives without the influence of PD, wouldn't you make room for regular breaks from your routines? Consider how most jobs include breaks, holidays, vacation time, and personal days. You and your care partner deserve at least that same consideration.

TIP

Take charge by establishing a routine for daily, weekly, and long-term breaks and by accepting the help and support that's within your reach.

Review your current situation

Burnout is common in the workplace, and even more so among caregivers. However, rarely do you hear about burnout in the PWP or in people who have other chronic, progressive conditions that require constant adjustment and adaptation. Ask yourself and your care partner the questions in Table 19-1, and write Yes or No, depending on your answers.

TABLE 19-1   **Questions That Can Reveal Burnout**

Question	PWP's Answer	Care Partner's Answer
Do either of you find facing the daily challenges of your PD increasingly difficult?		
Is the care partner showing signs of health changes — sleeplessness, under or overeating, headaches, or vague complaints of aches and pains?		
Do either of you react to good news or complaints with irritation, cynicism, or sarcasm? (In other words, do you have a compromised ability to show interest in or concern for others?)		
Do the two of you often feel irritable and impatient with each other?		
Do you see signs that either of you are becoming increasingly isolated, sad, lonely, or resentful of others?		

If you or your care partner answered yes to at least two of the five questions in Table 19-1, think *burnout*.

Now, ask these big questions and give brutally honest answers:

» Do you or your care partner reject suggestions and offers of help because you believe that other people just don't get it? (They haven't had to live with this disease, so they can't possibly understand.)

» Do you honestly believe that only your care partner and you can make your care routine work?

If you answered yes to one or both of these two questions, you need a break and possibly some counseling — and you need it now.

Ask for additional help

Ideally, when you decide to look for additional help, sit down with your care partner and follow these steps to identify and strategize ways to get the help you need:

1. **Identify the personal support networks for you and your care partner.**

   List the one or two people whom each of you would call if you just needed to vent. Then, add the names of three or four people whom you'd call for specific help or the occasional favor.

   Note: The PWP and care partner networks don't necessarily contain the same people.

2. **Consider the abilities and availabilities of each member of your support networks.**

   Of these people, have you or your care partner turned down help from one or more of them? If so, are you ready to swallow your pride and ask if they might still be available to help in some specific way? For example, could they pick up a prescription or stay with you for an hour while your caregiver takes a break?

3. **Strategize for enlisting specific help.**

   Based on the results of Step 2, identify specific ways each person in your support network is offering to help. Then talk through how that might happen: will this be a regular one-time-per-week assistance or errand, or something more spontaneous? The important thing is to plan with that other person. Never assume that they are available or will continue to help, and *always* show them appreciation.

TIP

If a person whose offer of help you formerly rejected accepts your overture and asks what you need, be prepared with specifics. For example, "Can you just stop by for a visit while my care partner goes to the store? It's getting harder for me to go along — and, frankly, the break does us both good."

Consider counseling to get your head and spirit straight

Depending on how far you've distanced yourselves from other people, you may need professional counseling to help you find ways to reconnect. But you have other choices that carry built-in benefits of community and social interaction. Check out these three possibilities:

>> **Support groups:** Okay, you may have resisted this option up until now, but get over it — if not for yourself, then for your care partner. Properly facilitated support groups can provide you with a real source of new ideas, local

information and updates, and even inspiration for managing your PD more effectively.

You may need to visit more than one group to find a good match, and smaller communities may not have a group specifically for PD. To find support groups in your area, go to the Parkinson's Foundation website (www.parkinson.org). For more general information, go to the website of the Caregiver Action Network (www.caregiveraction.org).

>> **Community:** Every community has counseling resources for low or even no cost. For example

- *Religious communities* have one or two clergypersons well known for providing comfort and counsel. The clergyperson doesn't need to be yours (or even of your faith).

- *Hospitals, your local library, and civic groups* may offer community programs that host experienced speakers who address topics of loss, aging, living with chronic illness, and so forth.

- *Funeral homes* often offer grief counseling by a professional who's trained in helping people work through a loss. Certainly, you and your care partner have suffered loss while your PD has progressed.

>> **Professional:** At some point you or your care partner may benefit from the guidance of a professional counselor. You have no reason to feel shame about taking this step — it is another resource that keeps you independent and in control. Your physician, hospital, or home-care social worker, as well as the local Office on Aging can provide good resources for referrals.

Plan for the healing power of R&R

Good news: You can avoid much of the damage caused by burnout if you build regular respite into your routine — early on. Plan daily and weekly breaks, as well as the occasional (but just as regular) longer hiatus:

>> **Daily short-term respite:** At least two timeouts — separately or together. Perhaps your care partner takes a walk while you watch a sports event on television; or you call a friend while your partner takes a long, hot bath; or the two of you order takeout from a favorite restaurant and watch a favorite movie together. Whatever the respite, plan it, schedule it, and don't cancel it (okay, short postponements are acceptable).

>> **Weekly breaks:** May include trips to the beauty salon or manicurist, card night, choir practice, a movie, or a club meeting. These breaks last a couple of hours. And support group meetings don't count because *respite* means getting away from *everything* to do with PD. Plan the breaks, write them on the calendar in ink, and make them non-negotiable — unless the house is on fire.

>> **The longer hiatus:** Usually lasts several hours to several days. Only you and your care partner can best identify the rest and relaxation you need. Maybe you take a trip to the city for shopping, dining out, and seeing a play. Or you could choose a place more off the grid giving you time to unwind with a book, take a walk in the woods, lie in a hammock by a lake, and so on. Such breaks take careful planning, but you can certainly do them. And you get an enormous pay-off, for you as individuals and for your relationship.

REMEMBER

If your care partner receives vacation, holiday, and personal time away from work, that time off doesn't count as *respite* if they spend it maintaining a household and a family, and dealing with your PD. Labeling time as *vacation time* doesn't mean it counts as respite; you have to use that time in a way that gives you a chance to take a break and get away from the daily focus being on managing care for your PD.

Recruiting Secondary Caregivers

Okay, your chronic PD has progressed. Little tasks that you used to do with little trouble now leave you nearly exhausted — and frankly, you don't always see them as worth the effort. You may find spending the day in your PJs easier than the hassle of getting dressed. Brushing or styling your hair is a joke, and shaving or trying to apply make-up? Forget it!

These days, you carefully time your appointments or activities to your PD's on-off cycles. You don't have the concentration that you used to, and you're beginning to worry that you may be forgetting to follow through on important details (such as paying the electricity bill).

On top of all these changes and worries, you're seriously concerned about your partner — the worry lines around their eyes and mouth, their constant exhaustion, and the lack of attention they pay to personal needs, activities, and grooming. Your partner needs some help — and so do you.

Calling another meeting

We hope you and your family met soon after your diagnosis to talk about the ways PD would likely impact your lives (see Chapter 7). Now, while the symptoms worsen and new symptoms seem inevitable, you need to gather the troops once again. This time, you go in with a different agenda.

In some cases, your adult children may jump the gun and bring everyone together. This family meeting may take on the trappings of an intervention if your family believes that you and your care partner are stubbornly refusing to ask for and accept help. You can prevent others taking over if you acknowledge early on that you need additional help and plan this meeting on your terms.

Extending the invitation

According to the book *Daring Greatly* by Brene Brown (Avery), "Sometimes the bravest and most important thing you can do is just show up." And that definitely applies when you have a family meeting to discuss help and support — you need the family to actually show up. Although we don't suggest subterfuge for getting family members on board, you need to do what you can to gather the family in one place at one time. If that seems next to impossible, then choose a family holiday when you plan to be together — Thanksgiving or either your or your care partner's birthday.

Consider these suggestions to help organize this meeting:

>> Make it clear to family members that the day will include a discussion of the future for you and your care partner.

>> If the gathering involves young children, make plans to occupy them for two to three hours. Ideally, arrange for them to be at another site so that they don't interrupt the meeting.

>> If a family member refuses to attend the meeting, assure the other family members that you plan to speak with this person privately about a commitment to your care.

If a person who doesn't attend the meeting clearly doesn't want to take part in the discussions at that meeting, then drop it with them for now. Perhaps down the road (maybe when someone else is burning out), this person can step up.

Preparing the agenda

The meeting to recruit secondary care givers (helpers) can cover arrangements for immediate needs, as well as planning for future needs. Perhaps the immediate needs include help in doing regular chores (such as mowing), tackling seasonal tasks (such as cleaning gutters), providing transportation, and so on. Future needs might include personal care tasks such as bathing. For this meeting, you have three goals:

>> **Disseminating the facts:** You and your roster of potential caregivers need to face the music. Your PD has advanced, and your spouse, significant other, adult child, or other rock whom you've been leaning on can't do it all.

>> **Defining the care you need:** You now need more hands-on and supportive care for you and your primary care partner. Specify the tasks that you need someone to do and how often. For example, perhaps you need help showering twice a week or for someone to stay with you while your caregiver does the weekly grocery shopping.

>> **Focusing the care efforts:** Everyone needs to understand the situation and figure out how to make some definitive contribution. Attendees must focus on what they can do (perhaps driving you to a doctor's appointment), not what they can't (being available to dispense your daily medication).

REMEMBER

In some situations, family either can't help or doesn't want to help. In that case, you can follow a similar guide for a meeting with friends and neighbors who have expressed a desire to help. Just keep in mind that your friends and neighbors aren't family — they have their own families and responsibilities. You should not expect your needs to take priority.

You probably don't need help with everything — at least, not immediately. Table 19-2 offers some ideas about areas where you may need help now and in the future. When you need that help, fill in the table with which care helpers you can engage to provide that help.

TIP

When you prepare these lists, don't surrender a task (such as grocery shopping) if it gives you or your primary care partner a break from confinement to the house. If you see that task as a positive event (providing the opportunity for socialization, for example), participating in that event may offer greater value than someone's assistance in doing it for you. Perhaps someone can visit with you at home while your partner shops (and enjoys the shopping). Then that secondary caregiver can assist in bringing in the groceries and putting them away.

Turning over the meeting

Surprise! We suggest that you open the meeting, lay out the agenda (see the preceding section), engage the attendees (see the next section) — and then leave. Why should you leave a meeting all about discussing you and your life? Simple. Family members may find it difficult to admit limitations and aversions to giving care; they find voicing these concerns to your face even more difficult.

TABLE 19-2   **Engaging Care Help**

Care Area	Related Tasks	Who Can Help
Hygiene	Bathing, oral hygiene, dressing, personal grooming (hair, nails, and so on), other personal hygiene	
Medications	Organizing and storing, dispensing, refilling prescription and over-the-counter medications	
Transportation	For medical appointments, community or social events, shopping	
Exercise and Recreation	Assistance in flexibility and strengthening exercises, yoga or tai chi, hobbies, and leisure activities	
Basic Nursing Tasks	Walking (from room to room), transferring (from bed to chair, for example), caring for medical equipment (such as a catheter)	
Emergency Care	Basic first aid; wound care; getting the help needed if you fall, faint, choke, or experience an adverse reaction to medications	
Household Chores	Exterior home maintenance (mowing, painting, clearing gutters, interior home maintenance (cleaning, changing the furnace filter), errands (grocery shopping, trips to the post office), meal preparation	
Financial Tasks	Bill paying (utilities, medical, and household bills), taxes (preparing, filing), money management (investments, pensions)	

When you leave, let your primary care partner take over the facilitation of the meeting; or, better yet, you may want to ask a third party (such as your support group leader or clergyperson) to conduct the meeting. Create an environment where those in attendance feel free to express concerns and limits without worry about hurting your feelings.

TIP

Especially in families that have a history of discord, you can make the meeting much more amicable by asking an objective third party to direct it. Possible candidates include a trusted clergyperson, a counselor (perhaps your mental health therapist), or the facilitator of your support group. If you enlist the help of a third party, both you and your primary care partner leave the meeting after the opening.

Getting everyone talking and committing

Open the meeting by stating that you fully intend to manage as much as you can for as long as you can. But you do need their assistance (not control) and patience because tasks may take you longer than before and require more effort.

Distribute printed copies of the agenda that includes your list of tasks (see the section "Preparing the agenda," earlier in this chapter, for ideas). Then excuse yourself (as we suggest in the preceding section). Your care partner or a third party then facilitates the meeting. Before the meeting, talk with your facilitator about how to make the meeting a productive one. If you or your care partner plan to conduct the meeting, follow these steps:

1. **Give everyone time to consider the list of possible tasks and their willingness to commit to becoming an active participant in providing the help you need.**

   Allowing 10 to 15 minutes should give everyone the time they need.

   Note: Although we suggest a time for consideration, don't try to limit any part of this meeting to a specific schedule. Make this meeting an open discussion, not one constrained by time.

2. **Ask everyone to mark tasks that they might consider taking on alone or in partnership with others.**

   Explain that people don't have to take on every task that they mark. You want to use the results of this process to assign specific tasks, establish back-up help for a task, and identify gaps that may need outside help. Ask that they focus on what they *can* offer rather than why they cannot.

3. **Open the floor to questions, discussion, and additional suggestions for the list.**

4. **Go through the items one by one and identify coverage (or lack thereof).**

5. **Tally the cost of outside help for the apparent gaps.**

6. **Ask family members to indicate (in writing for your or the facilitator's eyes only) what amounts they can and will contribute monetarily to that total for outside help each month.**

7. **After the meeting ends, express your appreciation for the progress made, and let everyone know that you'll hold a follow-up meeting.**

After you and your care partner go over the information from this meeting and make a tentative schedule, it's time for that follow-up meeting, in which you can get actual commitments for hands-on help and financial contributions (which we talk about in the following section).

Teenaged children, grandchildren, extended family members, close friends, and other people may welcome the opportunity to help you and your care partner in concrete ways. Don't leave them out of the discussion, although you may want to approach them separately. If you do propose to include others in your care plan, talk to them shortly after the meeting with your family's adults — perhaps that same afternoon.

Accepting aid with appreciation and gratitude

After you have the commitment of family members (or close friends), as discussed in the preceding section, you and your primary care partner have an important task: You need to accept their willingness to help by making specific assignments.

You can't possibly divide the contributions equally or fairly. Everyone needs to face that fact from the outset. A family member who lives nearby faces a very different physical and emotional toll than a member who lives at some distance. Similarly, one family member may be uncomfortable with the idea that they might be expected to help with such personal tasks as taking a shower or going to the bathroom.

You and your primary care partner must not pass judgment, but you do need to try to find ways in which each personality can contribute. If someone can't manage the hands-on care, assign them to tasks that are less personal, such as home maintenance, shopping, finances, taxes, and so on.

Some individuals are just naturally more nurturing. One of your adult children or siblings may mark practically everything on the list. Resist the urge to take them up on that offer. Don't let these secondary caregivers burn out when you need them most. (See the section "Dealing with burnout" earlier in the chapter.)

You and your care partner probably have a realistic idea of the time and effort each task takes (especially the ones involving personal, hands-on care). You also understand the emotional toll of dealing with PD better than these relative newbies. Keep all these concerns in mind when you consider who may provide assistance for each task.

Whatever the contribution, as long as the provider gives it with love and the best of intentions, accept it and say, "Thank you."

A Word for the PD Care Partner

Even though you didn't ask for this role as a PD care partner, you need to find a way to attend to the growing list of help tasks the PWP requires, in addition to other facets of your own life. Many of those facets may be (probably are) vital to the situation. For example, your work may be the prime source of income these days. It also may provide the insurance that both you and the PWP need.

You also need to keep your health in mind. You can hardly manage the escalating tasks of a caregiver if your own health is compromised. So, good eating habits, daily physical exercise, and adequate rest are more than good ideas — they make a huge difference in your overall ability to tackle this new challenge.

Get real about the time that giving care will take

The Family Caregiver Alliance (www.caregiver.org) estimates that the average caregiver spends 18 to 20 hours each week giving care. One-fifth of family care-givers provide 40 or more hours of care per week. Even if you don't work outside the home or work only part-time, you have other facets of your life that need your attention. You have *you*, who needs and deserves your attention.

REMEMBER

You don't have PD — your partner does. And you won't have PD after your part-ner moves beyond your ability to provide full-time, hands-on attention. You'll have a life — and we hope it's still filled with the people and activities that have sustained you since before PD became a part of it.

Consider the roles you play now: spouse or significant other, adult child, parent, sibling, employee (or employer), homemaker, civic or community leader (in your town, religious community, or such), volunteer. Add to these official roles a list of the activities you enjoy, such as reading, biking, traveling, gardening, and so on. Finally, add any additional hobbies you enjoy (and don't necessarily share with the PWP), such as needlework, photography, sports, playing cards, and such.

When you write it all down, you probably see a life that's pretty full. Add one more item: Besides the PWP, do you have other family members (such as an aging par-ent or in-law) who may need your care and support in the next few years?

So, how can you fit caregiving for your PWP into that busy life? Put another way, what do you have to put aside or give up altogether to be an effective caregiver over possibly several years?

Get creative about finding the time

Time management experts advise you to look at time as blocks. Start with your five weekdays — that's five 24-hour blocks. Block out the non-negotiables: work (say 8 hours per day times x days a week) and sleep (at least 7 hours a night). Work and sleep account for up to 15 hours, leaving 9 hours available.

Now, you need to figure out the time you take to get ready for work, travel to and from work, do shopping and errands, take care of laundry and other housework, and prepare (and eat) meals. Whew! Chances are you just knocked off another two to three hours a day, and you still have to find time for checking up on other family members, catching up with friends, making time for choir practice or a workout — and, oh yes, providing the extra care the PWP needs. Where does the time go? Better question: Where does the time come from?

America, as a society, has gotten very good at multitasking, and that practice may save you time in a few places. For example, can you make phone calls while preparing a meal or doing the laundry? Can you work part of your week from home so that you can do the actual job in the evening and open up the day for something like a doctor's appointment, grocery shopping, and that workout?

TIP

How about taking advantage of available community services, such as adult day care and in-home services (see Chapter 21)? Can they provide the PWP some of the care you currently give (such as a hot meal or hair care) in order to free up time for you?

You can find the options out there. You and the PWP just have to look for and accept the help — and accept the fact that others may not do things your way or as well as you do them. But if these options can give you back the time you've surrendered to mundane tasks so that you can once again enjoy a quiet evening of television or visiting with friends, then certainly consider them.

Be prepared to delegate

When giving care, you face the temptation to simply do it yourself. Maybe it seems faster and easier than trying to explain what you need. And maybe you get energy from the praise and admiration you receive when you handle everything on your own.

The world has its super-moms and super-dads. Are you becoming super-caregiver, trapped into believing (and convincing other people) that you and the PWP are managing fine when you really aren't? Are you sending signals that let these people think they can go about their lives without feeling overly concerned? *Whoa!*

In the early and mid-stages of PD, you and the PWP managed for some time without relying on others. Then, you realize one day that the PD — its physical demands, and its mental and emotional demands — are falling squarely on your shoulders.

You need to get others involved (see the section "Recruiting Secondary Caregivers," earlier in this chapter, for the details):

>> If you haven't already, open the door (and your mind) to accept the help of other people.

>> If you haven't held a family meeting, do it now.

>> If you had the meeting, call the family together and let them know that the need for help and support has reached another level.

>> Review what else friends and family can do to help and what they can add to their present financial contributions.

WARNING

When you work with others to figure out who can take on more care responsibilities, don't make the mistake of ignoring the PWP. Ask yourself whether you (or others) are

>> Assuming that the PWP can't perform tasks or make decisions that they in fact still can

>> Making sure that the PWP still participates in the discussion and decision-making

>> Keeping in mind that, for your loved one who has PD, this increased need for assistance marks another loss in the battle to maintain autonomy and independence

REMEMBER

This PD journey isn't about you. Presumably, you have years ahead of you, but your PWP faces a progressive decline. And you still have choices that the PWP no longer has. On the other hand, no one expects you to martyr yourself for the cause of giving care. That's where respite comes in — for you and your loved one. If you haven't read it yet, be sure you check out the section "Dealing with burnout," earlier in this chapter, for specifics on healthy respites.

BILL OF RIGHTS FOR THE PD CARE PARTNER

As the care partner for someone with PD, you perform an incredibly valuable and loving service. Anyone willing to put their life on hold in order to make the life of another better deserves the respect and appreciation of everyone involved. Just in case you have days when you feel like no one is showing that respect (and you will have such days), make a copy of the following Bill of Rights for care partners, carry it with you, and take it out now and then to read through.

I have the right to

- Take proper care of myself because doing so makes me a better care partner for the person with Parkinson's (PWP)

- Seek the help and support of others and have the PWP accept that we need such support

- Maintain certain facets of my life beyond the PWP, just like I would have if that person didn't have PD

- Occasionally (and humanely) express anger, sadness, and other difficult feelings

- Reject any attempt by others (including the PWP) to manipulate me (either consciously or unconsciously) by using guilt

- Receive respect, appreciation, and acceptance for the support and care that I provide, knowing that I'm giving it my best possible effort

- Take pride in my efforts and recognize the courage and sacrifice required to provide that support and care

- Protect my individuality and my right to make a life for myself beyond the support and care of the PWP

- Expect and demand that, even as new strides are made toward the treatment and cure of PD, similar strides be made toward aiding and caring for those of us who partner in care

IN THIS CHAPTER

» Organizing: A place for everything

» Checking the pulse of your financial
health

» Maneuvering through the
insurance maze

» Making your choices known — and
legal

Chapter 20

Putting Your Financial and Legal House in Order

Managing long-term illnesses such as Parkinson's disease (PD) has more than a physical, mental, and spiritual price tag. The financial cost is also significant. And closely related to financial considerations are the legal issues that need your attention throughout the journey.

Like with the rest of this book, in this chapter, we preach planning and preparation. Chances are good that before receiving the PD diagnosis, you had made financial plans for your future, so you already have a lot in place. If not, you need to attend to these matters sooner rather than later because PD can progressively affect your capacity for decision-making. The information in this chapter gets you through the financial and legal red tape of protecting your assets and the futures of loved ones.

Gathering Important Information

The first step in managing your financial and legal affairs is to gather all the information and documents in one place. Some people are already terrifically organized; they can put their hands on key documents from three years ago in a flash. But other people don't do as well with organizing. Some folks think nothing of showing up at the tax preparer's office toting shoeboxes stuffed with receipts, cancelled checks, and handwritten notes; they dump it all on the poor preparer's desk and then assume that the preparer can make sense of it.

Whichever group you fall into, set aside some time, get a notebook and pen (or work from your computer, if you prefer), and prepare to get organized with your financial, medical, and legal documents. Doing so is an important piece of preserving your security.

Inventorying legal and financial documents

You need a clear and accurate inventory of key identity information, such as your Social Security number, insurance numbers, bank account numbers, and so on. Also, if you've appointed a power of attorney for legal or health matters, that document (and copies of it) must be readily available. Your health history is also a vital piece of this inventory. In fact, everything that may be needed — when you're unable to provide it or give its location — needs to be a part of this inventory.

TIP

Here's a big picture look at the inventory process: Create a document in your computer files or make a list in a notebook with the information noted in the following steps. Then carefully store this information where it's secure from theft or fire (such as in a home safe) and be sure your care partner and others you trust can readily access it.

Your steps for compiling and documenting all the information you need to have available may happen in a different order, but you still need to make sure that you have each of the following steps covered. Follow these steps (or a version of them that works for you):

1. **Gather and document information for any online personal or business accounts.**

   For each of the following accounts, include user ID, personal identification number (PIN), and password clue (or actual password); contact name and phone number for technical support; and online addresses, as appropriate:

   - E-mail and voicemail accounts

   - Social media accounts

   - Personal and business websites

- Online banking, shopping, and monthly bill accounts

  You can also include credit cards that you manage online, electronic transfer accounts (ETA), or bills paid automatically and managed online.

2. **Gather and document the location of your personal identity documents and family information.**

   These documents include

   - Medical history and records
   - Family history, including their relevant medical history
   - Your dependents' names, birth dates, and contact details
   - Birth certificate and adoption documents, if applicable
   - Naturalization papers
   - Marriage license(s) and divorce decree(s)
   - School records
   - Employment history
   - Social Security card (including the number)
   - Driver's license (including number and expiration date)
   - Passport (including number and expiration date)
   - Military discharge information (including branch of service and service ID number)
   - List of memberships such as civic or professional organizations or the local art museum (including name of organization, contact information, and membership number)

3. **Gather and document the location of all financial and tax-related information (both personal and business-related, if applicable).**

   In addition to providing information about document locations, include the names of the companies or institutions involved; contact names and phone numbers; account or file identity number(s); and name(s) on the accounts for the following:

   - Income tax filings
   - Property tax obligations; liens (existing or paid) against property
   - Credit cards (if not covered in the online account information)
   - Savings certificates and bonds; stock certificates
   - Safe deposit box (including information about location of the key and a list of its contents)

- Personal or installment loans or mortgages

- Business accounts and loans

- Social Security or disability income

- Pension and retirement accounts

4. **List physical possessions and their locations.**

These items can include

- *Home inventory:* Fixtures, furnishings, appliances, equipment, and so on

- *Personal valuables:* Jewelry, artwork, antiques, books, clothes, mementos, and so on

- *Business inventory:* Fixtures, furniture, stock, and so on

- *Contents of storage units:* What they contain, as well as the units' rental agreements (including location of unit, name and phone number of company, unit number, and location of key or combination)

- *Home and business safe(s):* Including key or combination

TIP

In addition to making a list of your physical possessions, consider taking photos of them. Store the list and photos in an online file and keep a hard copy in your safe deposit box. For especially valuable items, get appraisals and keep the appraisals with a photo of the item in your safe deposit box.

5. **Gather and document the location of insurance policies and related information.**

For each of the following entries, include the name of the company or institution; contact name and phone number; policy and any group number; and name(s) on the policy:

- Health insurance and Medicare

- Vehicle insurance (including registration number and location of the title)

- Other insurance (life, disability, long-term care, homeowner's, renter's, business, liability, valuables, and so on)

6. **Gather and document the location of (original) legal records and papers.**

These records and papers include

- *Your will and living will:* Including name and phone number of attorney and other people who have copies

- *Durable power of attorney (finance and healthcare):* Including name and phone number of the person(s) appointed, the attorney, and other people who have copies

7. **Compile and document the location of items related to end-of-life activities.**

   These documents and files will help your loved ones make sure your wishes are carried out:

   - *Religious papers:* Including the name of a preferred place of worship, a clergy person and phone number, and important religious records.

   - *Organ donor wishes:* Give a copy to your physicians for your medical records.

   - *End of life and funeral instructions:* Including funeral home and cemetery names, contact names and numbers, and the location of original documents — especially if you pre-pay

   - *Name of your favorite charity:* For donations in lieu of flowers

REMEMBER

When you list the contents of your safe deposit box, be sure that you include the following items in it:

>> Copies (possibly photos) of your home, as well as physical personal and business inventories

>> Appraisals and photos of especially valuable items

>> Original documents and files

>> Original Social Security card

>> Your passport

>> A copy of your driver's license

>> A copy of your health insurance and Medicare cards

>> A copy of other insurance (life, disability, long-term care, homeowner's, renter's, business, liability, valuables, and so on)

Getting the info into the right hands

Gathering and documenting all the information about your life is quite a task (the preceding section can help guide you through it). But you aren't finished yet. In addition to completing the inventory, you need to tie up these other loose strings:

>> Make your care partner and other trusted family or friends aware of this inventory (electronic, hard copy, or both) and how to access it.

>> Place all of the documents and files in a safe deposit box (keeping a copy of everything at home) or in a fireproof file container at home.

>> Let someone other than you and your care partner know where you store the documents and files.

As an alternative, file a copy of key documents with your physician, attorney, or financial advisor, as appropriate.

>> Give copies of your medical information (your Social Security number, insurance cards, list of medications, and so on) to your care partner and one other trusted family member or friend.

>> Make your checking and savings accounts accessible (if you're incapacitated) by putting your care partner's name on the accounts.

>> Make your safe deposit box accessible by putting your care partner's name on the account (especially if you're going to store key documents there, such as your will or living will, or the originals of your power of attorney documents).

>> Give your doctor(s) copies of any advanced directives, such as Do Not Resuscitate (DNR) orders.

REMEMBER

Also, have a copy of your advanced directives available to hand to the admissions representative any time you check in to the hospital or the emergency room.

>> Give your doctor(s) written permission to discuss your health with your care partner.

Assessing Your Financial Health

Your ability to orchestrate your healthcare and solid financial future for you and your family is tied to your ability to understand the complexities of healthcare in America today. In many cases, the decisions that insurance companies and government programs make are based on generalizations, not your specific situation.

So, getting a handle on your specific economic well-being is a wise move. The information you put together in the following sections can provide a better idea of your financial health at this stage of your life, and this understanding can help you and your care partner make the best decisions to protect your futures.

Tracking income and out-go

In addition to an inventory, you need a clear idea of your resources versus your expenses. In your notebook or on your computer, set up a table with columns for *Resources* and *Expenses*. The information you enter under each column is pretty self-explanatory. You can use Table 20-1 as a guide to create your own records of resources and expenses. Of course, the categories, examples, and amounts will be specific to your situation.

TABLE 20-1   **Resources and Expenses**

Category	Example Items	Amount Per Item
Resources		
Cash on hand	Checking and savings accounts, actual cash in your hands	
Annual income	Salary, Social Security, trusts, royalties, dividends, property rental	
Pay-outs due you	Pensions, investments	
Property value	Home, car(s), antiques, jewelry, land	
Expenses		
Standard household expenses	Food, utilities, rent or mortgage, insurance payments, property taxes, payments on loans	
Medical expenses	Doctor visits, medications, medical equipment, therapy sessions	
Occasional but regular expenses	Clothing, household items, service for the car	

Projecting costs over the long term

You have a progressive condition, meaning that it will change over time. Predicting how that will translate into dollars and cents is difficult, to say the least. But you do know that costs increase while your income decreases. What to do?

Yep, you need to make another list. So get out your trusty notebook or open a file on your computer and enter your best estimates for the following additional expenses that you can anticipate while your PD progresses. Estimate the cost per month for each of these items:

>> Lost wages

>> Lost benefits

>> House changes or remodeling

>> Transportation expenses

>> Medical expenses

- Medications

- In-home assistance (aides)

- Medical equipment (walker, wheelchair, hospital bed)

- Therapy not covered by insurance (physical, occupational, speech)

- Medical bills not covered by insurance

>> Respite costs (for you and your care partner)

- Day care

- Vacation care

- Weekly in-home relief

- Counseling

Using assets to cover medical expenses

A home or other real estate can be a financial asset to cover the escalating costs of medical care. If you're still making payments on your home, you may be able to get a second or a refinanced mortgage. If you own your home outright, a reverse mortgage may be an option.

With a reverse mortgage, you receive monthly payments from a lender (usually the bank) while you continue to own and live in the property. The amount of cash you receive is based on your equity in the home, your age, current interest rates, the value of the property, and its location. You can receive payments in one of three ways:

>> **Term plan:** Fixed monthly payments over a specific time period

>> **Tenure plan:** Fixed monthly payments for as long as you continue to live in the house

>> **Line-of-credit plan:** Cash advance withdrawals from a fixed total sum

Eligibility requirements for a reverse mortgage don't include income limits but

>> You must be at least age 62.

>> You must own the home outright.

>> The home must be your principal residence based on voter registration information.

Do reverse mortgages have a downside? Yep. Here are two of the significant downers:

>> Up-front fees can be steep for insuring and administering the reverse mortgage.

>> If you choose to use part of your cash advances from the reverse mortgage to pay those fees, those sums plus interest are added to the bottom line of those fees.

How do you repay the loan? After the borrower moves out of the home or dies, the home can be sold to repay the loan, or family members can retain the home and repay the loan in other ways.

REMEMBER

The good news? The total of the reverse mortgage loan can never be greater than the value of the home at the time the loan is repaid, even if the loan balance is greater than the home's value at that time.

WARNING

Deciding to take a second or reverse mortgage isn't as simple as it may appear. Before you take such a step, engage the services of a professional (such as your financial planner, your attorney, the bank's reverse loan officer, or all three).

For more information, check out the U.S. Department of Housing and Urban Development (HUD) website at www.hud.gov, type the search terms *reverse mortgage* in the search box, and click the search icon.

Know the Intricacies of Health Insurance

With the seemingly gazillion insurance products on the market, figuring out which product best meets your needs can be a full-time job. For people diagnosed with young onset PD (YOPD) or people with PD (PWP) who are still working and receiving employee benefits, check out the information about insurance in Chapter 8 and Chapter 16.

TIP

Before choosing an insurance policy of any type, ask your insurance agent for the company's standing with A.M. Best, a company that rates insurance companies. You want to see a rating of at least A+, preferably A++. A high rating assures you that this company is financially stable and likely to be around when you actually need the benefits.

Also check whether the company has raised premiums on existing policies. When an insurance company's management has to make this move, one or two reasons are behind the raise:

>> They didn't do their homework before setting the premium.

>> They're planning to raise rates on a regular basis; unfortunately, just when a person needs the benefits, they have to drop the policy because they can't afford the high premiums any longer.

For most people 60 years and over, the insurance game is a little more straightforward, especially once you qualify for Medicare. The important point is to understand the term "accepts assignment" (see more information below). If you're a veteran, you may qualify for veterans' benefits that include insurance. Or your state may offer a special state health insurance plan to cover people who are not yet old enough for Medicare, but who have no coverage through their work.

Whatever your options, your goal is pretty clear: You want to work with your insurance advisor to protect you and your family against the ravages of long-term illness on your financial security.

Qualifying for federally funded programs

Here's some good news: You can find federally funded healthcare programs (insurance) through the Affordable Care Act website at www.healthcare.gov. Medicare and its sister program, Medicaid, are the two most prominent. But as the following sections illustrate, all federally funded programs aren't created equal, and although they're certainly a big help, they're simply not going to pay all your healthcare costs.

Be sure your doctors accept Medicare assignment — not every doctor does.

Medicare

Medicare is a federally funded and administered national health insurance program available to any American citizen who's age 65 and older or who's eligible for Social Security Disability benefits. Enrollment is automatic regardless of health, income, or political persuasion.

But all is not rosy. The original Medicare program was designed in 1965, when the goal was to provide financial help for seniors due to the rising costs of *acute* (immediate) care. In other words, the program was intended to help pay for care following a catastrophic event such as a heart attack, a fall that results in a hip fracture, and so on. Unfortunately, the program can be confusing in terms of what it covers and what it doesn't cover.

The Medicare program works on a system of *assignment,* which means the government assigns the number of days you can be hospitalized and the payment levels for each service. So, if your final hospitalization bill reads $75,247.63 and Medicare has assigned only $50,000 to the procedure, a $25,247.63 shortfall exists. Whoa! What happens then? (See the following section for more info on this equation.)

TIP

For more information on Medicare coverage, you can call 800-MEDICARE (800-633-4227) and request that they send you publication #CMS-10050-28 — or go to www.medicare.gov and search for *#CMS-10050-28* — to get the annual update on Medicare programs and coverage.

Medigap: Medicare supplemental insurance

Medigap is the slang expression for Medicare supplemental insurance policies. You need one of these policies if you're receiving Medicare benefits because — drum roll, please — a gap (sometimes a cavern) exists between the cost of medical care and Medicare's payments. A gap also exists between the services Medicare covers and the services you need.

TIP

As a minimum, you need a Medigap policy to cover the 20 percent remainder of charges that Medicare covers at 80 percent. But beyond that, look for a policy that covers what Medicare doesn't cover at all:

>> Hospitalization expenses for a year or more past the Medicare allowance

>> Coverage for most excess charges not covered by Medicare (such as doctor bills beyond allowable fees)

>> Coverage for care received outside the United States or Canada

Fortunately, several policies are available, and these companies must accept anyone who's eligible for Medicare. The concept of pre-existing condition is not part of their vocabulary, and you have no wait period. For more information on selecting a policy, call 800-MEDICARE (800-633-4227) and ask for CMS publication, *Choosing a Medigap Policy.* You can also go to the Medicare website (www.medicare.gov) and search for *choosing a medigap policy* to find more information.

Medicaid

Medicaid is another federal healthcare program — with a twist. Although the funding comes from the federal government, each state runs its own programs. And the rules can vary wildly. However, all programs base eligibility on income, and that amount is very close to the federally determined poverty level. Income is the only factor in Medicaid; age doesn't affect eligibility.

When you're at a certain level of income (and remain there), Medicaid covers care costs for the rest of your life. What's the catch? Most states get to decide where, when, and from whom you receive that care.

For more information about your state's requirements for Medicaid eligibility, contact your state's office that focuses on aging (for example, Indiana has a Department on Aging and Elder Services).

Looking into long-term care insurance

We hope you've already looked into a long-term care (LTC) policy well before being diagnosed with PD (either because you're reaching the age where people consider such issues or because your employer offers a plan). Ask your insurance agent to help you research the most viable plans for you — and your care partner.

TIP

Although many people can benefit from LTC coverage, two instances where LTC insurance isn't essential are

>> When your income is low (or you're willing to spend down to lower your assets, as noted in the preceding section)

>> When you likely qualify for Medicaid

At the other end of the spectrum, perhaps you're in the Fortune 400 crowd of multimillionaires, in which case, your assets are such that you can afford to cover the costs of your care without seriously impacting your lifestyle. Just remember: Some estimates place annual costs of managing healthcare with a chronic progressive condition between $65,000 and $100,000. Did you catch that? That's the per-year cost. If your assets need to stretch to cover 10, 15, or 20 years, you do the math.

Using private health insurance, disability benefits, HIPAA, and COBRA

For many people, health insurance is a benefit offered by their employer, but too many people fail to examine the actual benefits of their coverage until they need it. Don't make that mistake.

Take a look at your current coverage and identify where it may be leaving you exposed. For example, does it include coverage for medications? If not, is there a rider or supplemental policy you can add to help cover those costs? Review the following discussion of health insurance basics; then, you (or your partner, if they have the policy) may want to sit down with someone in Human Resources and review the gaps in coverage. Here's the breakdown of health insurance options:

- **Private health insurance** comes in two forms:
  - *Individual policies* that you purchase on your own give you choices and coverage that last until age 65. These policies can't be cancelled, and premiums can't increase on the basis of your health condition.

    Coverage can be expensive, and at the outset, you can be turned down or denied coverage for treatment for PD or other pre-existing conditions.
  - *Group policies* are funded at least in part through your employer. You may have little or no choice on features, but the coverage is usually available with no penalties for pre-existing conditions when you start a job.

- **Long- and short-term disability coverage** is available through many employers or as an individual product. The ground rules are essentially the same as for health coverage:
  - For individual policies, you need to be in good health when you apply.
  - The group policy may require a period of employment (typically 6 to 12 months) and a waiting period of several months, during which the employee has not sought treatment for the condition before being eligible for disability benefits.

    Benefits are based on a percentage of base salary, but that salary is still taxable. No adjustments are available for inflation or cost-of-living increases. For more information on disability benefits, see Chapter 16.

- **Health Insurance Portability and Accountability Act (HIPAA)** is a government program designed to protect working people.

  In a nutshell, HIPAA requires states to make all health insurance portable. So if you leave one job for another, or leave to start your own business, you can't be denied coverage regardless of health, as long as you're under age 65. Each state decides which carrier provides this portable product, but you can't be denied coverage. For a fact sheet on HIPAA, visit www.dol.gov, search for the document "Fact Sheet: The Health Insurance Portability and Accountability Act."

- **Consolidated Omnibus Budget Reconciliation Act (COBRA)** has another federal government alphabet soup acronym. This program protects and benefits the employee, giving you the option to continue your employer's group insurance for up to 18 months at your expense after leaving your job. For a fact sheet about COBRA, visit www.dol.gov and search for the term *COBRA*. Links to several related documents appear, including "Fact Sheet: Celebrating 25 Years of COBRA."

  This option guarantees that your coverage isn't interrupted. You pay the group rate (including what your employer was contributing on your behalf).

Relying on other resources to pay for care

While the government continues to wrestle with the issue of affordable health insurance, Congress and many states continue to enact legislation that partially addresses the problem.

For example, a growing number of states have established health insurance co-ops or pools for people who are denied coverage (usually due to a pre-existing condition). *Note:* Such programs usually have a residency requirement, and the cost of coverage runs higher than similar coverage if you were completely healthy. To find out whether your state offers such a program, contact your state's insurance department (for example, in New York, you contact the Department of Financial Services).

In 2004, Congress created Health Savings Accounts (HSAs) for people who purchase a government-approved, high-deductible health plan (HDHP). The buyer pre-funds a substantial percentage of the deductible each year in a tax-deductible savings account similar to an IRA. Funds deposited in the account can be used to

>> Pay the deductible

>> Cover the costs of medical and dental services not covered under your policy, including alternative medical treatment

Any part of the deposit not used in a given year carries forward. While your PD progresses, you're likely to meet or exceed the deductible in any given year, but this plan may be an option for your care partner.

To find additional information about programs and disability coverage, check out Chapter 16 or go online to www.ssa.gov.

REMEMBER

Check that medical bill *before* you pay up. Managing your medical costs is one way that you can maintain control while your PD progresses. Requesting an itemized statement and questioning services you didn't receive or were overcharged for delivers the message loud and clear: You may have PD, but you're still in charge. (By the way, the billing office isn't allowed to charge you for making a copy of the bill, even if it runs into a couple hundred pages.)

TIP

Making Your Wishes Sacrosanct

One key to good long-term planning is to put certain documents in place well before you or your care partner needs to access them. These documents include

- >> A will, of course

- >> Trusts in your children's names if you have children to protect

- >> A durable power of attorney for finances and healthcare if your state has provisions for them

- >> Your end-of-life wishes

- >> Advance directives (make sure you've shared those wishes in writing with your doctor[s] and your family)

Powers of attorney: durable and otherwise

Appointing someone to act on your behalf is the purpose of a simple *power of attorney* (POA). The standard document allows you to assign someone the right to manage financial and personal matters for you. The catch is that this person's appointment lasts only as long as you remain capable of making those decisions yourself.

For the time when you can't make your wishes known, you still need a spokesperson whom you can trust to move forward in the way you want. At this point, the *durable* POA comes into play. Two types exist:

- >> **Durable power of attorney:** You appoint someone to speak on your behalf for financial and other non-healthcare matters when you no longer can.

- >> **Durable power of attorney for healthcare:** You appoint someone to make medical and healthcare decisions for you when you're unable to make them yourself.

REMEMBER

Not all states recognize the same documents. Check with your attorney or your state's office that focuses on aging to understand your state's laws on these issues. If these documents are available, don't put off officially naming your non-healthcare and healthcare representatives. Whether you're living with PD or you're perfectly health, stuff happens; none of us can guarantee that we won't end up unconscious in an emergency room, unable to make our wishes known.

Advance directives and living wills

The trend in medical care today has moved away from the paternalistic model where the doctor makes decisions for the patient. Today, the patient has the autonomy to state medical and end-of-life choices, and to expect that those choices will be honored. But what happens when you can't speak up for yourself?

Give advance consent to all your doctors, as well as your lawyer, to talk with your care partner, as needed. The rules and forms for doing this vary from one state to another, so ask your lawyer to make sure this consent is a part of your legal portfolio.

Advance directives and living wills are tools for stating your desires regarding decisions that the doctors and your family are facing when you're unable to participate in the decision. This concept has dual benefits:

>> You take the pressure off your doctors and family members for making emotional and tough decisions when they're under enormous stress.

>> You can make your exact choices clear in a legally binding document.

For example, the choice of terminal sedation is legal in most states. *Terminal sedation* isn't considered assisted suicide or euthanasia because the goal is to ease suffering, not to induce death. You (or the person to whom you've assigned your healthcare power of attorney) can ask the doctor to order medication at the end of your life to ease pain or difficulty breathing.

Another decision to consider is whether you want an autopsy that can help researchers understand more about how PD affects the brain. If terminal sedation or autopsy is part of your decision, you need to state this in your living will and make sure that a copy is on file with each doctor or hospital likely to treat you.

Last will and testament

A *will* states your choices regarding the distribution of your property and mementos after you die. This is a legal document, and although you may believe writing down your wishes (or telling them to your care partner) is enough, you can save everyone headaches (and probably a good measure of trauma) after you're gone if you take the time to create a legally witnessed and signed document that makes your wishes binding for your survivors. To help you in that, the Funeral Consumers Alliance offers a funeral planner entitled *Before I Go*, which is available under the Store link on their website at https://funerals.org.

Tough stuff, but even the healthiest of people need to address these seemingly gloomy issues. Getting on top of them early on is just one more way that you can take control and move forward with your life — on *your* terms.

IN THIS CHAPTER

» Staying in your home sweet (safe) home

» Expanding your sources of care: Community programs and services

» Taking that first (hardest) step: Deciding to move

» Choosing the right care community

» Rolling with the changes (and with your care partner)

Chapter **21**

It's Just Bricks and Mortar: Housing Options You Can Live With

In times of personal crisis, *home* often becomes a synonym for refuge or safe harbor. It's the one place most people can go and be themselves without feeling the need to keep up appearances or a brave front. It's also the place where people surround themselves with items that bring back memories of good times, successes, and even trials endured through the years.

The day will come when you and your care partner need to reassess your current living situation in terms of its safety and practicality. While time and your Parkinson's disease (PD) progress, you may develop balance problems that result in falls and fractures. In many cases, you can make adjustments to your present home that allow you to remain there in comfort. However, you may eventually need to choose between a building that represents your past and a place where you have the assistance you need for a productive and satisfying future.

And in the spirit of our mantra — prepare, don't project — you can get to work on these housing issues well before the need is imminent. This chapter helps you do just that. We first guide you through the safety issues of your present home and cover the community services that enable you to remain there. Then, we take you through the tough steps of deciding to move. Finally, the chapter breaks down the variety of residences you can choose from when you decide the time is right.

Making Your Home PD User-Friendly

Your first step in thinking through this whole nest quest is to take a good look at your current residence. You may be surprised to discover how even small changes can give you additional months, if not years, to enjoy your current home.

Safety first: Assessing your home

Accidents in the home are one of the most common causes of injury and death in America. With your PD and the meds that can make you more prone to falling (see Chapter 18 for more on this possibility), a check of your home is imperative. You may want to schedule a home safety check as often as you check the batteries in your smoke detectors — which is at least once a year, right?

TIP

Your local fire or police department may offer a home safety assessment at no cost. If so, take advantage of this great community service. There are also home safety assessments offered by trained nurses and home care providers, and this service is usually covered by Medicare and some insurance companies. If neither of those professional surveys is available for you, you can also perform your own home safety assessment.

Follow these steps to assess your home's safety specifically for the PWP:

1. **Check for adequate and safe lighting, both inside and outside the home.**

Keep in mind these lighting solutions:

- Consider installing motion-activated lights in dark places — outside, and in stairways and hallways.

- If you can't install motion-activated lighting, make sure that stairways and hallways have lighting controls at each end.

- Place nightlights in the bathrooms and along the path from bedroom to bathroom.

2. **Check the integrity and safe placement of cords for lamps and other electrical devices.**

   Apply these fixes for problems you identify:

   - If the cords and wiring show wear and need for repairs, get them fixed. Your local hardware store can help with any parts or repairs needed.

   - Avoid using extension cords, if at all possible; when they're absolutely necessary, anchor them to the wall (not the floor) to prevent tripping.

   - Bundle and tie up excess footage on computer and other electronics cords; then anchor them safely under the desk or along the baseboard.

3. **Evaluate your home for underfoot threats that can increase the potential for falls.**

   Identify the threats and plan for their removal:

   - Get rid of all scatter rugs (even those that have rubber backing) and carefully check for worn carpeting or edges that are coming free of their tacking; get the necessary repairs done.

   - Make sure floors (tiled, wood, or uncarpeted flooring) aren't slippery.

TIP

   Test floors in a pair of socks. If you can do the slide, the floors need to be stripped of the wax or compound that's making them slippery.

   - Remove any raised threshold strips that separate one room from another; make the transitions smooth.

   - Install nonskid runners on uncarpeted stairways.

REMEMBER

   Each stairway also needs a sturdy handrail on at least one side. And you can use bright neon tape to mark stairs in especially dark places.

   - This suggestion is not really for your home, but for your feet: Wear shoes that have nonskid soles and no laces, the kind that boaters prefer. (Chapter 17 has more hints for PD-appropriate apparel.)

4. **Examine your kitchen to ensure compliance with standard safety rules and make it PD-safe, too.**

   Kitchens can harbor accidents waiting to happen, so

   - Keep curtains or flammable materials away from the stove.

   - Test that all appliances are in good working order.

   - Assess whether items in the kitchen are convenient for you. For example, would glasses be easier to access if moved to a lower shelf? Can you move the skillet from the drawer under the oven to a hook or a higher cabinet?

5. **Comb through the bathroom for potential safety hazards.**

Bathrooms can also be dangerous places; to make them safer

- Place nonskid strips in the bathtub and shower.

- Install grab bars wherever they make life easier — bathtub, shower, and toilet.

- Set the hot water heater at 110 degrees or lower to prevent accidentally burning yourself with too-hot water.

Making repairs or additions that promote safety and security

If possible, make any modifications or additions for safety into a family project. List everything that needs attention — whether it's from your home assessment (see the preceding section) or just a necessary regular repair — and then subdivide that list into large and small jobs. Tackle any fairly extensive changes for improving movement (such as removing threshold strips) first. Structural barriers such as threshold strips — which usually exist in multiple places in your home — may put you in the greatest danger for falling.

Here are important items to include on your modifications-and-additions list:

» **Emergency contacts info:** Place emergency and other medical contact numbers next to every phone, or if you don't have landlines, on the refrigerator. Definitely include contact information for those emergency or other regular caregivers who help out you and your care partner.

» **Fire safety equipment:** Install smoke detectors (or check present ones) in every stairway and in the kitchen; place fire extinguishers in an accessible place on every floor level, including the basement; determine an escape route in the event of fire.

» **Hardscape elements:** Check for needed repairs to sidewalks and driveways, such as broken asphalt or concrete, uneven brickwork in paths and sidewalks, and so on. Consider installing ramps for the time when managing even a few stairs becomes difficult.

» **Home security features:** Are all locks on windows and doors working properly? Make sure that screens, storm windows, and doors are properly and securely installed. Get to know your neighbors and let one or two trusted neighbors know who to contact if they have concerns about your safety or the security of the property.

Decluttering and rearranging to go with the (traffic) flow

Take a good, long look at the contents of your residence. Address the clutter that may be hazardous and clean out unnecessary *stuff*. For example, does your son still play that drum set, or could it be moved into the attic or, better yet, sent to his house for the grandkids to use?

After you declutter your living space, you can consider repositioning the furnishings that are left. You want to create the best traffic flow, meet your needs for comfort, and still have some design appeal. (Wedging your television in the far corner may offer more space, but not a whole lot more!)

Some people seem to have an eye for positioning furnishings for maximum convenience and visual appeal. The rest of the world needs help — perhaps from a decorator, a particular family member, a friend, or a friend of a friend who has a real knack.

But you can do a little preliminary evaluating on your own. What suggestions can you incorporate from your assessment (see the section, "Safety first: Assessing your home," earlier in this chapter) and from the safety check by the police or fire department? For example, would a simple change in the placement of the sofa make it easier to access the doorway in the event of a fire or other emergency? Could you convert an underused room to a first-floor bedroom or consider installing a stair elevator?

TIP

Forget those room labels and think outside the box. How can you put the rooms of your home to better use — not just because you have PD, but because they may serve everyone better? If you're going to be spending more time on the computer — checking out information and staying in touch with family and friends — maybe that little-used guest room off the living room could become your headquarters. Even if you didn't have PD, chances are the rooms of your home could be far more user-friendly for the actual life you lead. Besides, change and playing around with new ideas can be fun and help keep your mind active.

Taking Advantage of Community Care Programs

If you choose to remain in your own home for as long as possible, you have some options for extending that timetable, even after your PD begins to put you at risk for falls or daily struggles (such as tackling the stairs). But staying at home and bringing in care services has financial considerations. Most services — even if your insurance or Medicare covers part of them — are for a limited period of time and focus on a higher level of care, such as the services of a nurse or physical therapist. The following sections help you weigh your options.

In-home services

In-home help may be your first line of defense against moving because it can provide two significant services:

>> **Household help:** Such as meal preparation, shopping, and home maintenance

>> **Personal and medical assistance:** Such as help with personal hygiene, dressing, or medications

Most large communities have agencies that offer in-home care-assessment services at no cost. They can suggest support options for you and your care partner. Smaller communities or rural areas likely have a well-known network of independent contractors — people experienced in offering the basic services you may need at some stage of your PD.

To find independent contractors and community services, consider the following strategies:

>> **People you know:** Talk to neighbors, friends, and the nurse or office manager in your physician's office for references.

>> **Local resources:** Check with your local librarian or search online for local agencies offering services. (See Appendix B for a list of state organizations focused on PD.)

>> **Social services:** Call the local hospital's social services department or your regional government's office that focuses on aging (search online for your state or your county and "office on aging").

>> **Websites:** Check out several websites that may be helpful; for example, the federal Administration for Community Living's Eldercare Locator (https://eldercare.acl.gov). Search the Internet by using keywords such as "home care" and your community's name.

Expand your search to the county level and surrounding communities if you live in a smaller town.

TIP

Even if taking these steps fails to offer the answers you need, don't stop there. Continue to seek contacts. If you're not computer savvy, your local librarian (or your child or grandchild) may be able to help.

Consider exploring the types of services in Table 21-1 for your area and file away that information for when you may need it down the road.

TABLE 21-1

Services for In-Home Assistance

Service	Contact Name and Number	Cost	Notes
Errand services			
Home repairs			
Transportation			
Meal programs			
Medical equipment and supplies			
Delivery: Meds			
Delivery: Groceries			
Housekeeping			

Some programs may involve little or no cost. For example, youth groups may offer snow-shoveling or routine home maintenance. Grocery stores and pharmacies may offer free delivery. Government-funded community meal programs for seniors can provide not only a hot, nutritious meal, but also the opportunity to get out and interact socially with other people.

On the other hand, some services may come with sticker shock that has you reeling and saying, "Are you kidding? I'll do it myself," or "If I can't, my care partner will!" But take care not to burn those bridges too quickly. What happens when you can't manage some tasks on your own? What happens when your care partner is ill, needs to go away, or has to work overtime and can't be there when you need the help? What about your escalating need for care? Are you really prepared to ask your care partner to assume all the household and personal care tasks that the two of you may have shared up to now?

REMEMBER

Don't be stubborn about accepting care from other people — even when you have to pay for it. If the service provides help for you *and* extra time for your enjoyable activities (not to mention independence!), it may be downright priceless.

Home healthcare services

Home healthcare is a higher level of medical assistance that isn't part of the normal services offered through either your doctor's office or the hospital. At the same time, it includes services that your doctor or the hospital's social worker and discharge planner might prescribe for you (such as having a visiting nurse come to your home and check up on you after you've had a fall). And keep these "news" items in mind:

>> **The good news:** If your physician orders or prescribes professional in-home care, your insurance or Medicare pays most, if not all, of the bill. After the professional (a nurse or physical therapist, for example) is approved, you may also become eligible for personal-hygiene care and housekeeping services that you need.

>> **The not-so-great news:** Such home health-services are finite — they continue for as long as medically necessary. If the necessity for professional service ends (hopefully because you have improved to the point of no longer needing that care), the personal in-home care also ends. Likewise, when you can reasonably travel to the site of the professional services (such as physical therapy), the home delivery ends.

REMEMBER

The most common situation in which you need home healthcare is following a hospitalization, often because of a fall that causes a hip fracture or other broken bones. Such services — whether they follow a hospitalization or another scenario — are finite and short-term, but they are available and might speed recovery.

Adult day care

Adult day care is relatively new in the United States and therefore not as geographically widespread as the need is. Day care programs for adults can offer an array of services in a variety of settings — from community rooms in religious or senior centers to free-standing facilities.

In most cases, day care programs focus on socialization, rather than healthcare services. Still, they offer more health support than traditional senior centers because day care programs have staff trained to provide nursing assistance and routine medical support, such as overseeing medication dosages, assisting with transferring a client from one position to another, and in some instances, providing personal care services (such as bathing, and barber or beautician services).

Day care can bridge an important gap in the continuum of care services. When your PD symptoms keep you from safely getting out and about on your own or when your care partner needs to work, day care offers an opportunity for you to be with other people and remain active safely.

WARNING

Keep the following facts in mind:

>> **Not all states license or certify day care centers for adults.** This means safety, cleanliness, and regular reviews of staffing and program standards aren't regulated.

>> **Programs can vary greatly.** Be sure you understand what services are included in the fee and what services you pay for on an as-needed basis.

>> **Some centers may offer a free trial day.** If they don't, then visit the center (if possible, more than once) before making your decision to participate in day care.

Adult day care isn't for everyone and may not be right for you if you're still an active participant in other social and community circles. But it's an option to consider while your PD progresses. Adult day care can lengthen the time you're able to remain in your own home, and it can provide occasional respite for your care partner.

Respite care

The concept of respite isn't just for your care partner. (Review Chapter 19 for this discussion.) When you have a chronic, progressive condition such as PD, you too need time off. Trying to keep up that brave and optimistic demeanor can be enormously exhausting. Managing symptoms and fighting for every bit of function and independence can sap the energy of even the strongest PWP.

You deserve a break — a regular timeout from thinking about PD at least once a week. (Although we cover this more completely in Chapter 19, the routine's important enough to reinforce here.) You also need (and deserve) the occasional longer R&R to:

>> Take a deep breath and be cared for without feeling like you're imposing on your family or living under their watchful eye

>> Come to terms with the progression of your PD

Believe it or not, respite-conducive places exist. In the early stages of your PD, when your symptoms are well managed by your treatment plan, consider traveling to

>> **A retreat center:** These facilities offer rejuvenation, often at a reasonable cost.

>> **A cabin or lodge in a state park:** Where you can spend a few days or a week for a reasonable cost in settings that inspire introspection.

>> **A major city:** If you really can't deal with all that quiet time, treat yourself to a stay in a hotel, tickets to a play or sporting event, shopping, dining (as opposed to simply *eating*), and letting strangers pamper you.

While your PD progresses, options for respite are available in an environment of safety and care appropriate to your needs. For example

>> **Adult day care programs** (see the preceding section) can give you and your care partner a few hours of respite.

>> **Programs at care facilities** such as hospitals, step-care communities (see the section "Taking a closer look at long-term care options," later in this chapter), rehabilitation centers, and dedicated Parkinson's centers on medical-center campuses, may offer overnight, weekend, or vacation respite care.

TIP

Even if you're not ready to make use of such programs right now, gather information about the ones in your area. You may find that such a service is handy when an emergency arises (such as when your care partner's mother needs help in another state), and your care partner worries about leaving you.

Deciding When It's Time to Move

One day in the future, your current residence may simply not work for you. (Frankly, that day comes for a lot of folks who aren't dealing with PD.) Certainly you've had other life passages when change wasn't necessarily welcomed, but it was required. You managed then — and perhaps you even thrived in the new setting. You can certainly do it again — especially if a move simplifies your care and frees you to enjoy other activities.

Bidding your abode adieu

The truth is that you're going to know in your heart of hearts when your home is no longer practical. You can't climb the stairs. Your bathroom — in spite of its maze of grab bars and safety features — is too small or difficult to use. Your wheelchair doesn't fit through the doorways or roll easily across the carpeted floors. You and your care partner are becoming isolated from friends, family, and the community activities that you love.

REMEMBER

The only problem may be your refusal to admit that the time is right. If you've prepared for this day (as we preach throughout this book), the struggle can be far less distressing. The decision won't be easy, but you can skip the panic and anxiety of not knowing where to turn because you already know your options. You're ready to pick one and get on with your life.

Weighing the pros and cons of moving

REMEMBER

Certainly, you don't want to move before you're ready, but you do need to let go of any fantasies about the future and face reality. Is it practical and safe to continue living in your home? More to the point, can your life, routine, and ease of functioning improve if you move?

One person with Parkinson's (PWP) didn't leave his home without a fight. Before he was willing to admit it was time, he tried everything — an alert necklace so he could call for help if he fell (which he did frequently), a hospital bed for his living room so he didn't have to go to the upstairs bedrooms, a portable commode next to the bed so he didn't have to walk to the bathroom during the night, and a private-duty aide at night so his wife could get her rest.

One day, he looked around the house and realized that it wasn't the refuge he had loved for so many years. The memories it held had been pushed aside to make room for the trappings of his illness — his home had become one giant sickroom. And he didn't want that for himself or his wife.

Moving is 90 percent attitude

However you come to the decision — willingly or kicking and screaming — moving day is tough. It's tough on you and on the people who love you and share the memories that made your house a home.

Further, this move is a major step in the progression of your PD — the admission that you need to (rather than *choose to*) move. This is the time to talk about your feelings with a counselor or trusted friend — one who has no stake in the emotional real estate of the home itself. In short, you need to take the time to grieve this passage, the same way you mourn any major passage in your life. Talking about your sadness and regrets eventually leads to acceptance and even (perhaps) anticipation of the next step.

Redefining Your Castle

Leaving the old homestead is the end of the world only if you say it is. Chapter 7 includes a discussion of your coping style — the old fight or flight scenario. Well, in this case, flight is turning your back on the positive possibilities of housing opportunities. Fight, on the other hand, is taking charge of this new challenge by considering the options you've researched and choosing the best one with your care partner.

You may be surprised at the possibilities after you begin to consider solutions for moving to a place that will permit you to continue to have as much independence and control over your routine as possible. The following sections describe some of the more common choices.

Moving in with a family member

Okay, stop shuddering. Moving in with a family member can work as long as both parties work through the details of the living arrangements and routines *before* making the decision to share living space. In every household, there are routine chores and schedules. What's yours and what's the schedule for the rest of the household? If you're moving in with an adult child, are there also grandchildren in the house? Then their schedules (and rights to privacy and socializing with friends) must also be taken into consideration.

Ideally, you have a specific space of your own in the house — your room (hopefully furnished with your things) and possibly (hopefully) your own bathroom. And the rules for you? Keep in mind that this is your relative's home — not yours. By all means, state your needs at the outset, but then settle in and do your part to become a welcomed member of the household.

Considering a more practical apartment, condo, or house

Some options aren't as drastic as moving to a care facility. If you're having mobility problems in your current residence, what can make that easier? Perhaps your home is multi-level, or the doorways are too narrow, or the rooms are too small to accommodate a wheelchair or the safe use of your walker. In such cases, consider a house, condominium, or apartment that's on one level and constructed for an aging population. Much new construction today offers wider doorways, smooth thresholds, and safety features in bathrooms as standard fare. Several other options are also available:

TIP

>> **Accessory dwelling units (ADUs):** ADUs are living spaces within an existing home or on the same property. (You may be familiar with the concept of a mother-in-law suite.) Can you remodel your present (and beloved) home to include a small apartment where you can live comfortably and safely while your adult child moves into the main house? Can you use the ADU as a residence for a live-in caregiver who, in exchange for room and board, provides care services for you?

An alternative is to move into an ADU within the home or on the property of your son or daughter who has been encouraging you to move in. An ADU gives you (and your child) privacy and autonomy while relieving the stress and care challenges of living some distance apart.

Check local zoning ordinances and assess the practicality of constructing an ADU. If you're determined to stay in your home for as long as possible, the ADU can help lengthen that stay.

>> **Subsidized senior housing:** In many communities, apartment or housing complexes use state and federal funding to accommodate middle- or low-income senior citizens. In such facilities, rents reflect a percentage of income.

>> **Board-and-care homes:** If you have no live-in care partner, a board-and-care home may be an option. Also referred to as *group homes,* these facilities are usually large homes that have been converted to serve people who can no longer manage on their own but who don't need a higher level of care such as assisted living or a skilled-care facility.

These homes are in residential neighborhoods, and residents have their own bedrooms and share common areas of the house. Sometimes, the makeup of the residents revolves around a common factor such as age, gender, or disability. A paid staff prepares meals, assists with some care, and may engage residents in group activities. *Note:* Such facilities aren't eligible for public funding such as Medicare or Medicaid.

Taking a Look at Long-Term Care Options

In response to the aging of America (and the rest of the world), in the last several decades, the options for long-term care have grown. Today, the most common types of services are grouped according to client ability: independent, needs some assistance, needs major assistance, and end-of-life. To locate services in your area (or in another community closer to adult children or a preferred climate), consider the following:

>> **Local government help:** Call your local government office that focuses on aging or check out its website.

>> **The federal Administration for Community Living (ACL):** Use the ACL's Eldercare Locator by calling 800-677-1116 or going online to https://eldercare.acl.gov. On this page, enter your zip code and click Search to get a list of your options.

REMEMBER

Whatever option you may choose, Medicare covers costs on the same basis as medically necessary services in a resident's private home (for example, if the doctor orders physical therapy for you, Medicare might cover such skilled home care with some possibility of personal care, as long as such services aren't already provided by the facility).

Long-term care facilities may have different names in different states, and the services and costs vary widely. The following sections discusses five basic types of long-term care facilities, along with their specific features, pros, and cons.

Continuing care retirement centers

Continuing care retirement centers (CCRCs), which are also called *step-care communities*, offer levels of care, from independent living through nursing care. The primary advantage is that you don't have to research new facilities, make a major move, or leave behind friends and staff when your needs change. You and your significant other can live together; if one partner needs a higher level of care, the other can remain nearby.

TIP

Services, levels of care, and admission procedures and requirements can vary widely in such facilities. Before you choose, get all the rules up front. Also, remember that if the time comes when you need a higher level of care, you want to be sure that the nursing part of any step community is a certified *skilled-care* facility (meaning they're qualified to accept Medicare payment for skilled rehabilitative services). The facility should also be certified for Medicaid (see Chapter 20 for more on this federal program). To be thorough, you may want to check their state inspection record. For more information about accredited care, check out the CARF International website at http://www.carf.org/aging/.

Some communities may not include a nursing care facility. If this is the case, ask whether they have an association with a nursing facility in the community and whether residents of the CCRC get preferential consideration if the nursing facility has a wait list. The same words of caution apply: Be sure this facility is certified so that you can ensure you receive the best possible care.

Independent apartment with services

Many step-community residents begin by residing in an apartment or cottage with their personal belongings. Such units may tie into the overall community through safety features (such as call bells in bathrooms), activities (such as field trips or book discussion groups), and meals in a common dining room.

Note: This level is similar to traditional freestanding apartment or condominium complexes. Residents come and go as they please, manage their own healthcare, and maintain roles of choice in the larger community.

Assisted living

These facilities can vary greatly in terms of standard services and those services offered at an extra cost. Be sure you ask for the specifics regarding both of them. In general, such facilities include assistance with activities of daily living (ADLs), such as bathing, dressing, and transferring from chair to bed and back.

Standard services may also include the management and administration of medicines, transportation to and from doctor appointments, and most meals. Residents usually live in their own efficiency or one-bedroom apartment within a building or complex of buildings that also houses common areas such as a dining room, activity room, and library. Most assisted living facilities have a standard monthly fee, and then additional services that you can purchase on an as-needed or as-wanted basis.

On the downside, if the facility isn't part of a step community that has an on-campus skilled nursing facility, if you fall and need extended rehabilitation, that will mean another move (plus having to pay for two places if you intend to return to the assisted living facility).

Skilled nursing facility (SNF) or rehabilitation center

Skilled nursing facilities or rehab centers are facilities that provide *skilled* care (services provided by professional medical staff such as nurses and certified nursing assistants) and must be specifically licensed to provide these professional rehabilitative services. Nursing facilities that aren't licensed for skilled care (as well as those that are) offer what's called *non-skilled, custodial,* or *maintenance care.* These non-skilled wings of the facility serve people in the advanced stages of illness by offering a wide range of support, personal care, routine health services, and social opportunities.

SNFs can serve a variety of populations — people of all ages who may reside there for varying lengths of time:

>> **People recovering from surgery** may spend several weeks in a nursing home or rehabilitation center before returning to more independent living.

>> **People who suffer from dementia,** such as Alzheimer's disease, often live in nursing home care centers when the community or their family can no longer manage the person's care. Often, the care centers have special memory care units that maintain the safety and dignity of people suffering from dementia.

>> **People whose care needs exceed the family's or community's ability** to meet those needs may live in this type of facility. Many facilities have special units where people who are frail but alert and relatively active can be safe and secure while taking part in the facility's activities and social opportunities.

>> **People in need of short-term care** occasionally stay here to give their caregiver a much-needed break.

TIP

The best nursing homes have full occupancy, so plan a tour well before you need such a facility and, if this is the place you want to be for any future rehab or residency services, get your name on the wait list now. *Note:* When your name comes to the top of the list, the administrator calls you. If you're not ready to move to the nursing home, you can request that your name stay on the list.

Hospice

Hospice care is becoming an increasingly preferred option for patients who are clearly coming to the end of life. Hospice programs provide personal care for the patient and also offer counseling for their families and friends. The program may be in a special facility, a hospital, or a nursing home, but in many cases, hospice services are also available in your own home. After the program accepts you, a team of doctors, nurses, home health aides, social workers, counselors, and even trained volunteers help you and your family cope with the final days, weeks, or months of your illness.

To find a program in your area, ask your hospital social worker, and remember that although Medicare may cover some costs, it won't cover round-the-clock care at home.

Assessing the options for a perfect fit

Only you and your care partner can describe in detail the needs you have as individuals and as a care team. But when you make that list together and use it to evaluate various housing options, keep these key factors in mind:

>> **Be realistic about your possible future needs** and the ability of you, your care partner, and your care team to meet those needs every day over what could be several years.

>> **List residential care options** in your area and in the area of an adult child, friend, or close relative where you may consider moving. Then assess and compare similar facilities for quality and consistency of care, as well as cost.

>> **Visit those facilities** (at all levels) that meet your criteria and assess them using the checklist in the following section.

>> **Talk to people.** Speak with staff and clients at the facility, people in the community, neighbors, and friends. Ask what they've heard, what they know, and what their Aunt Millie's experience was.

REMEMBER

Always choose on the basis of which facility best meets *your* needs.

Making a list, checking it twice: Evaluating the facilities

When you visit a facility, focus on the people in the program and note their interactions with staff. Two words of caution:

>> Don't let the *window dressing* (beautiful furnishings, plantings, free lattes, treats for prospective clients, and other such details) sway you.

>> Don't be taken in by an unusually warm welcome or excesses of flattery and interest from your tour guide.

These folks are in business to sell a product and a service. And you, dear reader, are their target buyers.

The items in the first column of Table 21-2 can serve as a checklist for your tours of various facilities. Use the table, or in a notebook, record and number each item in the first column, and then record any notes you have about that service (use a separate page or table for each facility you visit). Not all items apply to every location, and services offered by one facility and not others may influence your final decision depending on your current idea of what you will need when you first move to such a facility and the reality of what you might need further down the road.

TABLE 21-2   **Facility Ratings**

Facility Characteristic	Rating (1 to 5)	Notes
Entrance is user-friendly and attractive.		
Staff was welcoming and prepared for your appointment or tour.		
Light, doorways, and hallways are adequate to accommodate people who use wheelchairs or walkers.		
Facility is free of any noxious or unpleasant odor; clean and attractively furnished.		
Grab bars are in bathrooms, and handrails are in hallways.		
Temperature is comfortable for clients.		
Smoking is either not permitted or allowed only in clearly marked, designated areas.		
Exits are clearly marked; smoke detectors and sprinklers are throughout the facility.		
Furnishings are sturdy and appropriate for people who have movement disorders. For example, chairs have arms and are at a good height for ease of getting into and out of them.		
If meals are served, clients have choices, and special diets are available.		
Staff interact with clients and treat every client as an adult and with respect.		
Staff members are certified (where appropriate) or receive ongoing training; hiring includes background checks.		
Your tour guide calls residents by name and is clearly known to them.		
If appropriate, a registered nurse is on staff, in addition to the facility administrator.		
The ratio of staff to client is reasonable.		

Facility Characteristic	Rating (1 to 5)	Notes
Staff takes a team approach with the client and family in developing a plan of care.		
The administrative team has been in place at least one year.		
Ownership of the facility hasn't changed more than once in five years.		
In a residential facility, residents may bring personal furnishings.		
Resident living spaces have adequate and personal closet and dresser space, even if the room is shared.		
If rooms are shared, residents have a voice in choosing a roommate.		
Your tour guide offers copies of resident-rights documents and any reports of state or facility inspections for review.		
Activities are age-appropriate and conducted with respect to the experience and history of the clients.		
The facility has an outdoor area for client use; staff are available to assist the residents in accessing that area.		
Facility has an emergency evacuation plan that includes plans for unusual events such as tornadoes, hurricanes, and so on, if appropriate.		
Services alluded to in promotional materials are indeed included in the base cost; extra services and their cost are clearly spelled out.		

TIP

Consider placing a numeric value next to each item to reflect your overall observation of the service, amenity, or attitude (for example, a 5 is excellent and a 1 is very poor). Rating your impressions can help when you compare facilities with each other.

TIP

Certification and licensing isn't a requirement in all states or for all types of care facilities, but facilities that must meet such regulations (either state, federal, or both) should undergo regular (and unannounced) inspections to ensure compliance.

Certainly, any facility that accepts Medicare, Medicaid, or both must be licensed and inspected. The results of such inspections are a matter of public record. If you're considering a setting that provides full residential care and is licensed for payment through Medicare or Medicaid, you can view the most recent inspection results online at www.medicare.gov/care-compare.

A Few Words for You and Your Care Partner

The day may come (or it may never come) when your PD progresses to the point where you need constant round-the-clock care that's beyond the limits of what can be provided to you at home or in a semi-independent setting (such as an assisted living facility). If that day comes and you decide to move to a full-care facility, you and your care partner need to be prepared for some changes.

For example, the PWP must be prepared to accept help from strangers for even their most basic needs, including dressing, bathing, getting to and from the bathroom, and such, and they may need to rely on someone else to speak for them and make their wishes known. And the care partner will need to downshift their role from caregiver back to care partner (Chapter 19 explains the difference), which will involve monitoring the way care is provided by others, instead of providing that care themselves. The care partner also will need to advocate for the PWP, making sure that the PWP's wishes (especially as related to end-of-life plans) are followed.

WARNING

If the facility isn't used to caring for PWP, the care partner may also need to be firm about the importance of timing in the delivery of medications — even if that means the care partner must lobby for the staff to deliver meds outside of their normal routine rounds. Care partners, be prepared to have these tough conversations and stand your ground.

For both of you, this doesn't have to be a time of sadness. Instead, it can be a time to let go of the stresses of the last many years and look back instead at the triumphs of having maintained a full life in spite of having PD.

6

The Part of Tens

IN THIS PART . . .

Find ways to deal with negative feelings and work through difficult times.

Consider your care partner's needs and wants.

Take action and make a difference in the fight against Parkinson's disease.

Chapter **22**

Ten Ways to Deal with Difficult Feelings

oping with feelings has no hard and fast rules. Just like the wild elation of falling in love may seem impossible to control, the bouts of intensely negative feelings that can accompany Parkinson's disease (PD) may also appear beyond your control. Because of the depression, anxiety, and other symptoms of your PD, you may find these feelings more of a challenge over time. To top it off, other people don't easily recognize when you're upset, which only requires more of your limited patience at these troublesome times. This chapter offers ten ideas that may help you begin coping with these feelings.

Banishing the Concept of "Bad"

Placing some sort of value system on feelings is a no-win situation, yet people do it all the time. "I feel bad" doesn't mean that someone's physically ill, but rather that the person is wrestling with one or more emotions that make them feel out of sorts. By taking the time to examine and name this feeling, a person's more likely to find relief — and minimize the guilt. So, whenever you recognize that you're in a funk, consider these two tips:

>> Do identify the feeling (do *not* judge it as good or bad) by completing this statement: "I am _____ (angry/jealous/sad/other) because _____."

>> Don't resort to unhealthy comforts and cover-ups for the pain (such as binge-eating, popping a pill, or drowning the feeling in a stiff drink).

Halting the Isolation

Any chronic, progressive illness carries a measure of isolation — for you and your care partner. You get so tired of having to admit that you can't go here or do that. While your illness progresses and you truly have more trouble getting out and about, that sense of isolation can become overwhelming. Heal the feeling by

>> Meeting regularly with other persons with Parkinson's (PWPs)

>> Encouraging (and accepting) the offers of people to come to you to share an hour, a meal, or an entire evening

>> Connecting through e-mail and phone calls

>> Exercising — take a walk or take part in a sport such as golf or a game of ping pong

>> Tapping into whatever spiritual therapies work for you

Corralling the Anger

Anger at your PD is one issue, but anger at those who love you and are attempting to meet your needs is quite another. On its own, anger is a completely normal response to living with a condition like PD that hampers your control and freedom. And getting really ticked off once in a while can even be healthy. But generalized and unidentified anger that festers can do some real damage. So, get a handle on your anger from the outset by

>> Recognizing that your mask-like facial expression may compromise your efforts to convey your frustrations and anger

>> Naming the cause and then seizing the moment — rant and rage for a couple of minutes, punch a pillow, or count to ten

>> Putting your anger in perspective — talk it over with someone you trust to look for the actual underlying causes for the outburst

Taming the Guilt

Guilt is sneaky. It creeps up on you after a jealous, frustrated, or angry reaction. It chafes while you perceive people putting their lives on hold for you. Like anger, guilt can build on other difficult feelings. But just as you do with anger, you need to name the guilt and nip it in the bud by

>> Asking yourself whether you're being fair to people around you by accepting and appreciating their efforts

>> Taking stock and reassuring yourself that you're doing all you can to maintain your function in the face of your PD

Subduing Your Fears

Face it. We live in a pretty scary world, mostly because of the uncertainties that surround us — global warming, pandemics, threats of famine, and then some. As a PWP, your fears may be far more specific than these world events. You're concerned that you may have passed this disease on to your children; you worry that your PD will incapacitate you before you can achieve certain milestones, such as seeing your daughter married or taking that trip to Italy; quick trips to the hardware or grocery store become terrifying treks. Face your fears by

>> Reviewing the information on anxiety and depression in Chapter 13.

>> Accepting that life is uncertain for everyone. The best anyone can do is live each day to its fullest and *not* wait to celebrate and appreciate.

Venting Your Frustration

Frustration can arise from many situations. You may get frustrated with your inability to hold a comb or toothbrush. Or you may grit your teeth when you feel like your care partner's taking over tasks that you can do for yourself. Or maybe you gag with the lack of straight answers to your questions about PD and its progression. And on and on. Here's an excellent solution: Call or e-mail a trusted friend or one of the people in your support group and vent! Then get back to life.

Cooling the Jealousy

Jealousy is such a normal human reaction. You've dealt with it your entire life — when a friend got a bigger house or a better car; when a coworker got the promotion you wanted; when your sister lost 30 pounds without trying (or so she said!). As a PWP, odds are good that your green monster rears its jealous head when your family and friends are free to go and do as they please without even thinking about it. You, on the other hand, have to plan and time activities. Life is *not* fair. You know this one. Face it by

>> Reminding yourself of your successes. Could that coworker handle the challenge of PD with the kind of grace and humor that you do (most of the time)?

>> Expressing (in a kind and gentle way) your feelings of jealousy to the person. Chances are good that you'll discover the person is equally jealous of you.

Stopping the Spirals of Sadness

There's a little sad, and then there's a lot sad. *A little sad* is when you feel sorry for yourself, but the feeling passes quickly — usually within a few hours. *A lot sad* is when sadness spirals into full-blown mourning or grieving, the way you'd feel if you suffered some life-changing event, such as the death of a loved one or the break-up of a relationship. As Michael J. Fox once noted that while life continued to bombard him with lemons, he got awfully tired of making lemonade.

For PWP, intense sadness may be connected to the life you had planned before you learned you had PD. Left to its own devices, sadness of this magnitude can spiral into full-blown depression. You need to nip it in the bud by first acknowledging your right to mourn the life that will no longer be, and then by embracing the possibilities that are before you now.

TIP

If working your way through the sadness becomes overwhelming, seek professional support by talking to your clergyperson or the counselor you put on your care team to help you through tough times (see Chapter 6).

Caring About Apathy

"I just don't care anymore." "Nothing's going to change." Even if they feel true, neither of these statements is correct. You care; otherwise, you wouldn't have made it this far. So start by discussing these feelings with your doctor. If you're not already engaged in some form of talk therapy with a counselor, this is a good time to consider that option.

Dumping Depression

Short spurts of sadness can be healthy reactions while you adapt to life with a chronic and progressive condition. But when such feelings last weeks with no let-up, you may be facing depression. You need to treat it the way you'd treat any physical symptoms that don't go away after a short time. If feelings of helplessness, hopelessness, escalating apathy, or spiraling sadness persist beyond a few days, *get help*. Start by reading Chapter 13; then talk to your PD doctor about treatments for handling depression in PD.

Chapter **23**

Ten Ways to Care for Your Care Partner

L ife turned an unexpected corner for at least two people — you, of course, and most likely, your primary care partner — the day you were diagnosed with Parkinson's disease (PD).

Your care partner is your champion — speaking up when you can't, making sure that the medical community focuses on you as an individual (and not just as another case), and performing the thousand-and-one tasks that keep life running for both of you. Your care partner — if you are lucky enough to have one — deserves not only your empathy and understanding, but also your support and attention.

This chapter gives you ten ways to acknowledge their sacrifice and encourage a healthy form of selfishness for your care partner.

Honor the Partnership

A partnership is a two-way street. It's not all about you and your needs. You and your partner honor your partnership by recognizing it as a mutual exchange of ideas while you find your way together through this change in lifestyle. Initially, the focus is on you, and that's only right. But eventually, you need to get a grip on your own reaction to PD, and take a long, hard look at its effect on the people around you, especially the person next to you, your partner in care. These are some ideas for doing just that:

>> **Address the effect on your partner.** In any discussion about adapting daily life to your needs, address (via words and actions) how those needs will impact your partner's routine.

>> **Embrace help from others.** Be open to the idea of getting support and assistance from someone other than your care partner. For that matter, suggest calling in reinforcements yourself. Perhaps your sister (who's offered to help in the past) can drive you to the library so that your care partner can spend an afternoon alone.

>> **Listen to what your partner is really saying.** For example, suppose that you're discussing how your care partner is doing tasks that you can still manage (although it may take you longer). Perhaps your partner admits that doing the tasks themselves is just easier than waiting because of all you both have to do. That answer may give you a good clue that they're feeling overwhelmed, and the two of you need to discuss ways to get more help.

Acknowledge Life beyond PD

When every waking moment seems to focus on doctor's appointments, medications, maintaining function, and fighting depression, you need to stop and take a moment to really consider how much of your (healthy) care partner's life has been given over to your PD. Ask these questions:

>> How many of your conversations begin and end with PD?

>> How much of your and your care partner's days focus on managing symptoms and maintaining your independence?

>> What facets of your relationship before PD are beginning to slip through the cracks?

Address that imbalance right now before it's too late. Talk through just how you can work together to make sure PD doesn't become both of your lives.

TIP

Remind each other that there's more to life than your PD by declaring certain times of day *no-PD zones*. For example, agree to talk about topics other than your PD during and after dinner. You'll both sleep better if you spend the evening discussing lighter topics and catching up, in general.

Accentuate the Positive

Care partners may actually resist talking about pleasurable experiences in their lives. For example, because you can't ride any longer, your partner may avoid discussing the amazing bike ride they just completed. Or they may feel uncomfortable talking about some office-drama infighting at work for fear that the details seem so petty and silly to you. Or they may worry that if they talk about a friend's impending vacation, they may just remind you that you'll probably never make that trip to Paris that you dreamed of. You have a responsibility to encourage such sharing by making it clear that your partner is in some ways your extended eyes and ears, bringing you news and funny stories that have always entertained you.

Strike a Balance in Caregiving

Surely one of the most exhausting tasks for any care partner is trying to guess how much care is enough, and how much is too much. How is your care partner supposed to know whether you're too exhausted to do something for yourself or you're determined to complete a task, even if you take all day? Care partners have many talents, and they develop new ones over time, but mind-reading will never be on that list. If your care partner seems to be *doing* rather than *helping*, let that imbalance go for the moment, but find a time later to talk through the problems it may be causing. For example, your care partner may have feelings of resentment, or perhaps your sense of autonomy and independence are somehow threatened.

Ask, Don't Demand

Listen to yourself. When you need help, do you begin the request with a verb? "Get me the remote." "Come here." "Button this."

Your care partner isn't a private in your war against PD. Your care partner is right there in the trenches with you. Show some respect. This advice is not a request — it's a demand!

Use the Magic Words Often

Surely you learned them when you were a kid: *please* and *thank you*. Never have they had more power. In the grown-up version, you need to move beyond simple statements — you need to show, as well as tell. The smile, the touch of the hand, the small surprise that focuses just on your care partner all have magic in their own way. And the true magic is that you feel a little more like your old self if you can take care of your partner now and then.

Get Over Yourself

Yes, you've been dealt a really bad hand, but you're still here. For now, you have a life that includes this person who has put their life on hold to take this journey with you. You also have a choice: Live each day thinking about all the problems you may face while your PD progresses or *live each day!*

TIP

Check out Chapter 13 for helpful insights on dealing with anxiety, depression, and apathy.

Accept Services as a Gift for Your Care Partner

You may find asking other people to take care of needs that you once managed on your own depressing, especially if you're asking a stranger who's paid to deliver a service. (And especially if that service is so personal and private that you find it difficult to accept, such as bathing you or helping you to the bathroom.) Try to accept this help as one way of caring for your partner. Does paying for this service free your partner to attend to some other task or simply enjoy a break? Does the help that this outside person provides save time that both of you can put to better use?

Find Joy in Life

Caring for someone whose outlook is positive and hopeful — in spite of setbacks — is far less stressful than trying to bolster the spirit of someone constantly seeing the dark side. Your care partner has gone through all of the emotions you have: anger, fear, depression, the gamut. True, PD isn't attacking your care partner's ability to function, but PD is attacking both of your lives. Remember, you set the tone for how people respond to your PD. If you've shivered in the shadows for a while, try crossing over to that sunnier side of the street, and take your care partner with you.

Encourage Laughter and Dreams

Your care partner deserves a life beyond your PD, a life as full of pleasure and promise as possible under the circumstances, a life that keeps dreams alive. You can encourage and nurture that life for your partner. Start by flipping to Chapter 19. Post the Bill of Rights for the PD Care Partner list from that chapter somewhere that you and your care partner see it every day. And should your care partner resist self-nurturing and care, try reading the list aloud. Then talk about issues that can and must change so that you can help care for your partner — physically, mentally, and spiritually.

Chapter **24**

Ten Ways You Can Make a Real Difference

The Parkinson's community is unique in that most PD organizations at the national level are super-organized, well-connected, and have earned the respect of the powerbrokers who can affect change. Think of the benefits people with PD (PWP) have gained from the efforts of local chapters of the Parkinson's Foundation (www.parkinson.org), for example, and then multiply that by one million — the number of PWP in the United States alone. Those numbers have power. Here are ten ideas to get you started.

Read More About It

Start by making yourself a local expert on PD. Check out the resources in Appendix B — especially those that offer information to share with other people. A comprehensive and reliable source of information is the PMD Alliance (www.pmdalliance.org), which offers educational programs, support group search engines, and a number of other resources at the national and regional level. Get your friends, family members, acquaintances, and coworkers on board for a specific issue. Locally, that issue might be accessibility in local public buildings (where people vote or pay taxes, for example). Nationally, getting others involved might mean contacting elected officials when a key piece of legislation that could affect funding for research is up for a vote. And if you have the energy and the resources to travel, plan to attend the World Parkinson Congress, which every three years brings together PWPs, caregivers and medical experts around the world for a unique meeting of the minds. Check for the next date at worldparkinsoncongress.org.

Vote Early and Often

Americans are becoming increasingly apathetic about voting. How often have you heard someone say, "It doesn't matter — politicians are all the same"? Well, if you (as a PWP) don't care, who's going to care? The future of treating and curing PD rests on your elected officials' support for dollars for research and adequate care options.

REMEMBER

Absentee voting is always an option if getting to the polls is too difficult.

Get to Know Your Local Officials

Local elected officials work for you and often live in your community. Don't hesitate to talk directly to them about key issues that could impact you or others who have a chronic progressive condition such as PD. For example, if a zoning law prevents a rehabilitation clinic from opening in your community, let your elected officials know why this clinic is important. At a state or national level, consider making contact (by phone, e-mail, or letter) with an elected official's senior staff person. Use that link to get your message to the officials.

TIP

Never underestimate the power of a single note or phone call. And don't forget to follow up! If you write or call an elected official, and they say that someone will get back to you, but no one has, call again.

Don't Just Be Informed — Pass It On

Okay, you don't want to overdo this, but *carpe diem* — seize the day! Say you're at dinner with friends and the conversation has settled on politics. You know a key bill's coming up for a vote that can really impact PD research. Talk about it. Relate its importance to facts that will stick in people's minds and perhaps lead them to contact their congressperson to cast a key vote. A less in-your-face way to inform people while you go about your daily routine is to talk about projects and interests that you're involved in, even if they're not PD related. Why? Because you get an opportunity to show that PWP can be contributing members to society in spite of PD.

Support Your Local PD Support Group

Attend meetings and consider getting more involved in the group's effort to influence community leaders (or even national politicians). You can find power in numbers. Signing a petition, participating in a charity event, or raising money for research can all help you build a better future for PWP.

Rally Local Support

Consider ways you can build awareness through your local library, employer, and community organizations. For example, encourage your librarian to invest in informative books, DVDs, and CDs for people who have chronic, progressive conditions and their care partners. Ask your employer and community organization leaders to offer literature and seminars that help people who have these conditions and their families to manage their time and caregiving. Employers benefit from less absenteeism and a more focused and productive work force, and community groups become more engaged in the needs of the community. (Get things started by checking out the resources available at www.parkinson.org/get-involved.)

Pitch Your Story to Local Media Outlets

People who put together the local news (print, radio, and television) want to hear from you. Your story could help others who are struggling with chronic illness. Can you imagine how they would delight in a story about a 60-something doctor who has PD performing his first piano recital with a group of kids? What about the young onset Parkinson's disease (YOPD) person's care partner who also works full time, cares for their school-aged children, and volunteers? Before you call your local news desk, check with the person whose story you plan to offer (even if that's your care partner). In telling the story, include

>> **A local angle:** Offer a story about a person in your community.

>> **The key that makes it unique:** What makes it not just another health story (such as the piano-playing doctor).

>> **The visuals (for print and television):** For example, does the recital offer a photo op so that a photographer can attend along with the journalist?

Join the Fight to Find a Cure

In 2016, the Michael J. Fox Foundation for Parkinson's Research (MJFF) and the Parkinson's Action Network (PAN) announced that PAN would join MJFF. Today the two organizations operate as one to advance public policy priorities and better treatments for people living with Parkinson's disease (PD). Advocacy at any level requires conviction and passion for a cause. Finding a cure is *your* cause, so get off the sidelines and find ways you can contribute to the fight. Sign up for the MJFF newsletter and updates. Become an informed voter, meaning that you know where the candidates on the ballot stand when it comes to supporting research and affordable care options. Make a donation — even small amounts can make a difference.

Raise Money for Research

Research donations do not necessarily need to come from your pocket. You can raise awareness about PD, as well as dollars for research, in several ways. Work with your local or regional support network (see AIRPO listing in Appendix B) to organize a local event (walkathon or pancake breakfast, for example). Sign up to volunteer and get your friends and family on board, as well.

You also can be effective on your own. Haven't you read about someone biking or walking across America and collecting donations along the way to raise awareness of some cause? You don't need to plan a trek across America, but what else can you do? Try holding a yard sale with all the money going to PD research or ask family and friends to contribute in your name to a PD organization in lieu of gifts on holidays, birthdays, and other gift occasions. (After all, do you really need another book, t-shirt, or coffee mug?)

Celebrate National PD Month in April

PD gets its own month for national awareness — April (think springtime, renewal, and hope). How appropriate! How can you and your care partner mark this special month? Here are some easy ideas:

>> Donate a copy of this book (or another book about PD) to your local library.

>> Plan to schedule one of the events suggested throughout this chapter during the month of April.

>> Buy a couple dozen red tulips (a floral symbol of the fight against PD) and pass them out to your friends, family, and everyone on your healthcare team to thank them for making the journey with you.

Appendix A

Glossary

action tremor: An *involuntary*, rhythmic movement of the hand, arm, foot, or leg when a person performs a *voluntary* action such as lifting a fork, writing, or stepping onto a ladder. See *resting tremor*.

activities of daily living (ADLs): Routine activities that are part of a person's normal day (such as dressing, bathing, eating, toileting, transferring from bed to chair, walking from one room to another, participating in social and leisure activities).

advocacy: The process of influencing people via education, group actions, and publicity for a cause.

agonist: A muscle that contracts so the body can perform a specific movement; also a chemical or drug that stimulates a specific receptor to signal a desired action. See *dopamine agonist*.

akinesia: Also called *freezing*; temporary inability to initiate a desired movement.

antioxidants: Body chemicals that neutralize *free radicals*.

antiparkinsonian drugs: Drugs or medicines for the management and control of Parkinson's disease and its symptoms.

apraxia: The inability to execute a voluntary movement despite normal function and mental understanding of the desired action.

ataxia: Loss of balance and coordination.

athetosis: *Involuntary*, repetitive movements, especially with the hands, fingers, and (sometimes) feet.

basal ganglia: Groups of cells deep in the base of the brain that help the cortex in controlling *voluntary* movement and coordination.

bilateral: Occurring on or affecting both sides of the body or organ.

bradykinesia: The gradual slowing or loss of spontaneous movement that results in impaired abilities to perform a task or change positions.

bradyphrenia: The gradual slowing or loss of ability to process information.

CAM therapies: Techniques, medications, and therapies that take a holistic (mind, body, and spirit) approach to treatment of disease.

carbidopa: A drug that, when combined with *levodopa*, reduces the side effects of levodopa yet improves overall effectiveness of levodopa by allowing more of it to enter the brain.

care partner/caregiver: Usually a family member (spouse, adult child, parent, sibling, or close friend) who provides the emotional (and eventually physical) support and care for a person diagnosed with a chronic, progressive condition.

central nervous system (CNS): The network responsible for cueing the human body's mental and physical actions; consists of the brain and the spinal cord.

chronic: A medical condition that develops over time and can be managed or cured with treatment.

clinical trial: The research and testing required by the Food and Drug Administration (FDA) to determine whether new medicines, medical devices, and treatments are safe and effective before approving them for patients.

cognition: Those mental skills necessary to process information (such as perception, memory, reasoning, judgment, intellect, and creativity).

cogwheeling: The slow, jerky, or ratcheting sensation the doctor perceives when moving a patient's rigid limb at the joint.

computerized axial tomography (CAT or CT scan): A diagnostic computer procedure that uses a series of X-rays to produce a two-dimensional image of the body or specific body part.

catechol O-methyltransferase: (COMT:) inhibitors: Drugs that block an enzyme that breaks down *levodopa* before the levodopa can convert into *dopamine*, thereby increasing the therapeutic supply of levodopa to the brain.

deep brain stimulation (DBS): A surgical procedure that helps control symptoms of advanced PD; electrodes are implanted in the brain and controlled through a battery-operated device known as an implanted pulse generator (IPG) or pacemaker.

delusion: A fixed belief that is false, not proven by objective evidence.

dementia: The neurological condition or sign of progressive decline in intellectual ability (such as impaired judgment, memory loss, confusion, personality changes, and disorientation) caused by one or a combination of underlying conditions, such as Lewy Body disease, Alzheimer's disease, and stroke.

depression: Sustained, prolonged feelings of hopelessness, helplessness, and sadness.

diagnosis: A doctor's conclusions based on a patient's medical history and symptoms as well as the doctor's observations and tests.

DO: A doctor of osteopathic medicine focused on holistic treatment that considers environmental and lifestyle factors.

dopamine: The natural chemical substance present in areas of the brain that regulate movement, motivation, and feelings of pleasure. See *neurotransmitter.*

dopamine agonist (DA): *Antiparkinsonian drugs* that imitate and supplement the brain's naturally produced *dopamine.*

dysarthria: Difficulties with speech caused by impaired movement of muscles; results in slurred or muffled words or the inability to project one's voice or speak at a normal volume.

dyskinesia: Abnormal *involuntary movements* (examples are sudden muscle contractions; rapid, jerky, or lurching movements; fidgeting or restless movements of upper body, arms, legs, or head); may be a response to long-term use of *antiparkinsonian meds* and may worsen with stress.

dysphagia: The impaired ability to swallow.

dystonia: A movement disorder that causes significant and unexpected muscle contractions or spasms that result in abnormal and *involuntary* movement and posture. Can be a symptom of Parkinson's disease.

essential tremor (ET): More common than *primary PD*, this movement disorder causes an uncontrolled *tremor* of the hands, neck, head, or voice; most apparent when performing a *voluntary* action, such as lifting a cup. See *action tremor.*

executive function: The intellectual ability to set goals, make decisions, and perform multi-stepped processes such as balancing a checkbook.

festination: A series of progressively quicker, shuffling, almost-running small steps after walking is initiated; sensation of the upper body wanting to move forward but the legs are unable to follow appropriately.

Food and Drug Administration (FDA): The federal body charged with monitoring clinical trials and assuring the safety and effectiveness of a medicine or therapy before it's available to the public.

free radicals: Potentially toxic substances produced by the normal metabolism in all human cells; left uncontrolled, they can damage or destroy vital brain cells.

freezing: The sudden and temporary inability of a *PWP* to initiate a movement such as going through a doorway or exiting a car. See *akinesia.*

gait: Medical term for walking; includes the individual style of walking.

gene: The building block of inheritance contained in every human cell; a change in the gene can predispose the individual to a disease.

genetic: Anything related to genes or inherited characteristics, including diseases.

globus pallidus: One of the areas of the *basal ganglia* most affected by the lack of *dopamine* in Parkinson's disease.

hallucination: Unreal perceptions that a person may experience while awake; hearing or seeing objects or people that are not present. Sensory hallucinations may be a side effect of *antiparkinsonian meds* or a sign of disease progression.

hypokinesia: Decreased or reduced movement.

hypomimia: The lack of facial expression and absence of eye-blinking caused by Parkinson's disease. Also called *mask* or "facial mask."

hypophonic: Reduced vocal volume and clarity.

idiopathic: A diagnostic term meaning "of unknown origin or without apparent cause."

involuntary movement: Movement that happens without the person's intention or control.

levodopa (L-dopa): The most commonly used drug for treatment of PD; restores levels of *dopamine* in the brain.

Lewy bodies: Abnormal, round clumps of protein in damaged and dying *dopamine*-producing brain cells.

Lewy body dementia (LBD): The umbrella term for two forms of dementia associated with PD, namely Parkinson's disease with dementia (PDD) that usually occurs years after the initial onset of PD; and dementia with Lewy bodies (DLB) where symptoms appear within the first year or even before motor loss is detected.

magnetic resonance imaging (MRI): A noninvasive, diagnostic imaging tool that uses an electromagnetic field to create cross-sectional illustrations of particular organs and systems in the human body.

mask: See *hypomimia.*

micrographia: The small, cramped handwriting due to impaired fine motor skills in some *PWP.*

motor fluctuations: Daily variations of the benefits from *antiparkinsonian drugs.* Usually occur as PD progresses. Also called *on-off phenomenon* during which individuals can experience *wearing off* (or emergence of motor symptoms such as slowness and tremor), or *dyskinesia* (which can occur in the off or on state; the on state exists when motor features of slowness and tremor are well controlled).

movement disorders: A category of neurological conditions that impair normal control of movements; includes *Parkinson's disease* and similar disorders (*parkinsonism* disorders), *essential tremor*, *dystonia*, tics, chorea, and other less common diseases.

movement disorders specialist: Neurologists who have completed additional training to understand and treat conditions that affect certain brain regions.

multiple system atrophy: A neurological disorder characterized by *parkinsonism* that is poorly responsive to *levodopa*; typically associated early in its progression with signs of autonomic nervous system dysfunction including low blood pressure when standing, impotence, and urinary incontinence. It may also be associated with severe *gait* imbalance, slurred speech, and poor coordination.

National Institutes of Health (NIH): The primary federal agency charged with conducting and supporting medical research.

National Institute of Neurological Disorders and Stroke (NINDS): The branch of *NIH* that focuses on diseases and conditions that affect the brain and *central nervous system.*

neurodegenerative: A neurological disease (such as Alzheimer's and Parkinson's) marked by the progressive loss of *neurons*.

neurologist: A specialist in the diagnosis and treatment of neurological disorders of the brain, spinal cord, nerves, and muscles (such as PD, stroke, Alzheimer, and multiple sclerosis).

neuron: A type of cell (mainly in the nervous system) that processes and transmits information for specific functions.

neuroprotective therapy: Any treatment with the ability to prevent or slow the loss of vital *neurons* affected by a *neurodegenerative* disease.

neurostimulator: A surgically placed device about the size of a stopwatch that, for *PWP*, delivers mild electrical signals to the brain through one or more thin wires called leads.

neurosurgeon: A surgeon specializing in the treatment of neurological disorders.

neurotransmitter: The body's natural chemicals (such as *dopamine*) that send messages from one nerve cell to another or from nerve cells to muscles.

occupational therapy: Skilled rehabilitation techniques that help people with neurological conditions perform routine daily tasks at home; maximizes physical potential through lifestyle adaptations and possible use of assistive devices.

on-off phenomenon: Severe *motor fluctuations* that are particularly frequent, sudden, and unpredictable; also called "yo-yo" syndrome.

over-the-counter (OTC) meds: medication available without a prescription.

pallidotomy: A surgical procedure that lesions (burns) parts of the *globus pallidus* to lessen PD symptoms; now largely replaced by *deep brain stimulation* (DBS).

palsy: Also called "paralysis;" loss of the ability to move a body part. Parkinson's disease was originally called "shaking palsy."

parkinsonism: A group of movement disorders characterized by a variable combination of *tremor, rigidity, bradykinesia,* and *postural instability*.

Parkinson's disease (PD): A slowly progressing neurological disease resulting in the loss of *dopamine*-producing brain cells in the *substantia nigra*. The disease normally responds to the medication *levodopa, but at this time has no cure.*

person (or persons) with Parkinson's disease: See *PWP*.

physical therapy: The use of stretching and strengthening exercises and machines to help *PWP* maintain (or regain) strength, balance, coordination, flexibility, endurance, and function for as long as possible.

pill-rolling tremor: A characteristic finger *tremor* in which the thumb and index finger slowly rub against each other as if rolling something into a small ball. Typically (almost exclusively) seen in patients with *Parkinson's disease*.

placebo effect: A change or improvement (physical or emotional) in a patient who has been given a medication with no therapeutic benefits (as in clinical trials); there is no medical explanation for the change.

positron emission tomography (PET scan): A diagnostic imaging tool that uses an injected radioactive form of various compounds (such as glucose *levodopa*) to produce color maps of the sections of the brain and assist in the diagnosis of Parkinson's disease.

postural instability: A person's lack of balance or coordination when walking; usually results in awkward forward- or backward-leaning that may result in a fall as the person attempts to compensate for lack of balance.

postural tremor: *Tremor* or shaking that occurs when a person's arms are stretched outright to the front.

prognosis: A doctor's prediction of a condition's progression based on the patient's medical history and response to treatment as well as the doctor's knowledge of the disease.

propulsive gait: Also called *parkinsonian gait*; walking that is characterized by a stooped, rigid posture with head and neck bent forward; shorter and faster steps propel the person forward, placing the person at risk for falling. See *festination* and *retropulsive gait*.

PWP: Abbreviation for "person (people) with Parkinson's disease;" sometimes appears as "PLWP" for "person (people) living with Parkinson's."

range of motion (ROM): The measurement of a person's ability to fully straighten or bend a joint (knee, elbow, hip, ankle, shoulder, or spine).

receptor: The part of a nerve cell that receives a message from a *neurotransmitter* (*dopamine*, for example).

resting tremor: A *tremor* or shaking that occurs when a body part is relaxed and supported (hand resting on the arm of a chair) but not engaged in activity; typically tremor ceases or lessens if the limb is engaged in activity.

retropulsive gait: A movement characterized by persons propelling themselves backward in an attempt to maintain balance, thereby placing themselves at risk for falling. See *propulsive gait*.

rigidity: The abnormal stiffness of a joint or limb.

seborrhea: Increased volume of oily perspiration.

sialorrhea: Drooling.

side effects: Undesirable problems a patient experiences when taking a certain medication; prescription meds list major side effects in their printed information and over-the-counter products list them on the packaging.

sign: What the doctor observes and tests during an examination.

Sinemet: The brand name for *levodopa/carbidopa*, the most common medication for treating PD symptoms.

speech therapy: Rehabilitative techniques that help restore or strengthen speech and swallowing muscles affected by PD.

stem cell: Undeveloped or undifferentiated cells that can duplicate themselves or become cells of various body tissues; may originate from an adult tissue or an undeveloped embryo. Current studies consider these cells as potential cures for *neurodegenerative* diseases.

striatum: Part of the *basal ganglia* affected by the lack of *dopamine*. See *globus pallidus* and *subthalamic nucleus*.

substantia nigra: The small area of the brain that houses cells that produce the *neurotransmitter dopamine*; specifically affected by Parkinson's disease.

subthalamic nucleus: One of the small groups of cells in the *basal ganglia* primarily affected by PD; the most frequent surgical target for *DBS*. See *deep brain stimulation*.

support group: A gathering of people with a common connection (such as *PWP* or PD *care partners*) who meet regularly to share information, receive education, and sustain one another.

symptom: What a person feels or perceives as a reason to seek medical help.

thalamotomy: A surgical procedure intended to relieve *tremor*; now largely replaced by *DBS*. See *deep brain stimulation*.

transcranial magnetic stimulation (TMS): A procedure in which an electromagnetic coil briefly stimulates specific areas of the brain in order to modulate their activity; used experimentally to treat depression and PD.

tremor: A repetitive and involuntary movement such as trembling or shaking; usually in the hands but possible in feet, legs, arms, head, or voice.

trigger event: An event (a fall or head trauma), exposure (to toxins or other environmental materials), or unusual stress (loss of job or death of a loved one) that exposes a condition's previously unrecognized symptoms.

unilateral: Occurring on one side of the body.

voluntary movement: Movement performed with full intention and control.

wearing off: Reappearance of PD symptoms before the next dose of *levodopa* is due. See *motor fluctuations*.

young onset PD: PD diagnosed in people under the age of 50.

Appendix B
Additional Resources

E ven though this handy guide covers Parkinson's disease (PD) from A to Z and offers a world of suggestions in dealing with it, we realize you may not be satisfied with reading just one book. You may want to know everything you can, or you may want more information about a specific topic within this huge subject. So, to round out this all-purpose guide, our appendix highlights other valuable sources for credible information and practical tools. This is by no means an exhaustive list — but it does include some truly valuable *stuff* to broaden your understanding of PD.

Gathering Free Info Online

As soon as possible, bookmark the following Web sites on your computer. Visit them regularly for updates on the latest treatments, tips on managing symptoms, and suggestions for your care partner. You can even use the Web to locate a neurologist, a local support group, or a medical center that specializes in the treatment of PD.

TIP

Don't have a computer? Talk to your local librarian. Better yet, put a child or grandchild on the case. They're the experts at searching the Internet, and when you research a question or topic together, it can be great quality time.

Making national PD organizations your first stop

The PD community is well organized. Each of the following websites provides a full range of information from medical updates to tips for coping. On most sites, you can sign-up to receive a newsletter or updates to keep you in the know.

>> **PMD Alliance (Parkinson & Movement Disorder Alliance):** www. pmdalliance.org

Click the Getting Started link to find out where you fall in the PMD Alliance ecosystem, or investigate the Resources, Programs, and Blog links.

Other contact information: 7739 E Broadway Blvd #352, Tucson, AZ 85170; 800-256-0966.

>> **American Parkinson Disease Association:** www.apdaparkinson.org

Hover over the Education and Support link for a drop-down menu with selections for information in various formats (including videos and publications).

Find a list of local APDA groups by state or zip code under local resources.

Other contact information: P.O. Box 61420, Staten Island, NY 10306; Phone 800-223-2732.

>> **The Michael J. Fox Foundation for Parkinson's Research:** www.michaeljfox.org

Hover over the Understanding Parkinson's link and click on the Books and Resources link under the Education & Inspiration heading in the drop-down that appears. There, you find tools that can help you live with PD.

Click in the Email Sign Up box on the home page (near the top left) and enter your email address to receive the newsletter plus regular e-mail updates on research and other advances toward a cure.

Other contact information: Grand Central Station, P.O. Box 4777, New York, NY 10163; Phone 212-509-0995.

>> **Parkinson's Foundation:** www.parkinson.org

Hover over the Living with Parkinson's link to access a drop-down with a variety of materials plus links to care centers and local/regional chapters.

Other contact information: 1359 Broadway Ste 1509, New York, NY 10018; Phone 800-473-4636.

>> **Davis Phinney Foundation For Parkinson's:** https://davisphinney foundation.org.

Click on the Resources link for basic information and, especially, information for those dealing with Young Onset PD (YOPD).

Other contact information: 357 S. McCaslin Blvd, Ste 105, Louisville, CO 80027; Phone 866-358-0285.

>> **Lewy Body Dementia Association (LBDA):** www.lbda.org

Hover over the Resources link and then clink the Sign-up for the Lewy Digest link.

Other contact information: 912 Killian Hill Rd. S.W., Lilburn, GA 30047; Phone 800-539-9767.

>> **World Parkinson Coalition:** www.worldpdcoalition.org

Find news and events including the World Parkinson Congress; the sixth of these events is taking place in Barcelona in 2023.

Other contact information: 1359 Broadway Suite 1509, New York, NY 10018; 646-388-7688.

Finding local and regional resources

>> **The Parkinson's Foundation:** www.parkinson.org/search

Find information about local resources and services, such as support groups, exercise and wellness classes, education programs and more. Enter your zip code or state to search or call: 1-800-473-4636.

>> **AIRPO (The Alliance for Independent Regional Parkinson Organizations):** www.parkinson.org/get-involved/Local-resources/airpo.

>> **PMD Alliance (Parkinson & Movement Disorder Alliance):** www.pmdalliance.org/resources/support-groups.

Seeking assistance with your meds

Check out the Pharmaceutical Research and Manufacturers of America (PhRMA) at www.phrma.org. Click on the Patient Support link to find out more about financial assistance for meds. Click on the About link and then the Members link to locate the manufacturer of any medicine you're taking.

Finding tools that make your life easier

A number of devices are available to make life easier and to prolong independence for people with PD. The following resources offer places to check out as the need arises.

Exercise and speech tools

These resources offer exercise and speech programs you can use at home. They come in a variety of formats from printed booklet with illustrations to videos and audio tapes.

>> You can find a number of good videos on YouTube at www.youtube.com when you search for Exercises for Parkinson's Disease.

- » Check out LSVT Global at www.lsvtglobal.com for the LSVT LOUD (speech therapy) and LSVT BIG (physical therapy) programs.

- » Find the article *Exercise for People with Parkinson's Disease* online at the Cleveland Clinic website: https://my.clevelandclinic.org/health/articles/9200

- » Download an exercise book, such as *Fitness Counts*: www.parkinson.org/pd-library/books/fitness-counts

- » Learn about the key roles of exercise and nutrition (as they related to fighting PD) at the Johns Hopkins Medicine website: https://www.hopkinsmedicine.org

  On the Home page, scroll down and click the Health Information link. On the resulting page, click the Conditions and Diseases link, click the See Full List button, and then click Parkinson's Disease from the list. Scroll down the resulting page and click the Fighting Parkinson's Disease with Exercise and Diet link.

REMEMBER

Be sure you show any exercise or diet program or other therapy to your neurologist or rehab therapist before using that program on your own.

Clothing, medical alert systems, and other helpful aids

The following sites provide a range of aids from clothing with easy closures to canes that may help avoid *freezing* (legs locked, unable to step forward) to medic alert gear. New products come on the market every year.

- » **Wardrobe Wagon:** wardrobewagon.com

- » **Exerstrider:** www.exerstrider.com

- » **Healthline:** www.healthline.com/health/walking-canes

- » **Consumer Reports:** www.consumerreports.org/medical-alert-systems

Complementary and alternative therapies

If you and your neurologist decide that some form of alternative therapy may prove helpful, check out tai chi and yoga exercises available on YouTube at www.youtube.com, but also check out the website at the National Center for Complementary and Integrative Health at www.nccih.nih.gov.

Looking into financial and legal matters

Finances and legal matters are nothing to play around with. You need the help of (or at least a consultation with) an expert. These resources can help:

>> **American Association of Retired Persons:** www.aarp.org

>> **Medicare:** www.medicare.gov

>> **Medicare Rights Center:** www.medicarerights.org

Sharing sites with your care partner

Bookmark these sites for your care partner:

>> **Eldercare Locator:** https://eldercare.acl.gov

>> **National Alliance for Caregiving:** www.caregiving.org

>> **National Family Caregivers Association:** A resource you can find by searching for the acronym *NFCA* on the Caring Community website at https://caringcommunity.org

Other Books Worth the $$

New books on living with PD are published every year, and your local library may have these recent works. If it doesn't, suggest that the librarian add it to the library's wish list, or consider donating a copy yourself.

>> *No Time Like the Future: An Optimist Considers Mortality* by Michael J. Fox (Flatiron Books)

>> *Parkinson's Disease: Guide for the Newly Diagnosed* by Peter LeWitt, MD (Rockridge Press)

>> *Lucky Man: A Memoir* by Michael J. Fox (Ebury Press)

>> *Living with Parkinson's Disease: A Complete Guide for Patients and Caregivers,* by Michael Okun, MD, Irene A. Malaty, MD, and Wissam Deeb, MD (Robert Rose)

>> *Mediterranean Diet Cookbook for Beginners: Luscious Family-Friendly Recipes for Everyday Home Cooking* by Thea Garofalo

Index

festination, 306, 307, 402

fiber, in diet, 137

fight-or-flight mechanism, 217

financial advisors, recruiting, 91

financial and legal issues
about, 343
assessing financial health, 348–351
gathering information, 344–348
health insurance, 351–356
making wishes sacrosant, 356–358
resources for, 413
YOPD and financial planning, 123–124

fine motor movements, bradykinesia and, 38

fire safety equipment, 362

Fitness Counts, 412

flattening of affect, 220

flexibility, stretching and, 143–155

Flexion exercise, 158–159

focused ultrasound (FUS), 188

focused ultrasound (FUS) therapy, 190

Food and Drug Administration (FDA), 237, 402

Fox, Michael J., 82, 413

free radicals, 402

freezing, 38, 306–307, 402

friends
as caregivers, 324
relationships with, 262–264
sharing news with, 109–110
socializing with, 290
YOPD and relationship with, 122

frustration, controlling, 384

fundraising, 396

Funeral Consumers Alliance, 358

G

gait, 402

gait disturbances, 67

game plans, establishing, 92–96

Garofalo, Thea, 413

gastrointestinal (GI) problems, 35

GBA gene, 24

gender, as a risk factor, 28

gene, 402

gene mutation, 24

generalized anxiety disorder (GAD), 216

genetic, 402

genetic factors, as a cause of PD, 23–25

"The Genetic Link to Parkinson's Disease," 23

geriatrician, 86

Gilbert, Rebecca, 165, 221

glia cells, 26–27

globus pallidium, 190, 402

goal-setting, importance of, 79–82, 84

Gocovri, 177

government policies, 270–271

grandchildren, relationships with, 259–260

grooming, 284–285

ground rules, establishing, 102

guilt, controlling, 383

Guten, Gary, 142, 288

H

hallucinations, 314–315, 402

Hamstring Stretch, 149–150

handwriting, 39, 303–304

hardscape elements, 362

Head Tilt stretch, 144–145

head trauma, as a cause of PD, 22–23

Head Turn stretch, 144

health insurance, 351–356

Health Insurance Portability and Accountability Act (HIPAA), 354–355

Health Savings Accounts (HSAs), 355

healthcare team
about, 85
care partners and, 98–99
establishing game plans, 92–96
planning for hospital stays, 96–98
recruiting members for, 86–92

Healthline Media, 125, 412

help
accepting, 327–328, 337
from adult children, 257–259, 323
finding and accepting, 221–226

Hip Abduction exercise, 161

Hip Adduction exercise, 162

Hip Extension exercise, 162–163

Hoehn, Margaret, 64

Hoehn and Yahr rating scale, 64

home, managing medications at, 183–184

home healthcare services, 366

home security features, 362

Horizontal Pull exercise, 159–160

hospice, 374–375

hospitals
for deep brain stimulation (DBS), 195
managing medications at, 183
planning for stays in, 96–98

household help, 364–365

housing
about, 359–360
care partners and, 378
community care programs, 363–368
long-term care options, 372–377

P

pain, 41, 179

palilalia, 301

pallidotomy, 404

palsy, 404

panic attack, 217

Parcopa, 173–174

parents, 121–122, 260–262

Parkinson, James, 19

Parkinson & Movement Disorder Alliance (PMD Alliance), 409, 411

Parkinson Study Group, 242

parkinsonian gait, 405

parkinsonism, 67–68, 404

Parkinson's Disease (PD)
  about, 7–11
  causes of, 19–27
  compared with related conditions, 11–13
  comparing LBD to traditional onset, 126–129
  comparing YOPD to traditional onset, 114–116
  coping strategies for, 46
  defined, 404
  finding care for, 13–14
  impact of, 45–46
  managing, 15–17
  myths about, 12–13, 201–202
  risk factors of, 27–30
  signs of, 36–41
  stages of, 41–44
  symptoms of, 35
  terminology for, 34
  treating, 14–15
  unknowns of, 30–31

Parkinson's Disease: Guide for the Newly Diagnosed (LeWitt), 413

Parkinson's Disease Questionnaire (PDQ-39), 65

Parkinson's Foundation Center of Excellence, 21, 56, 57, 70, 77, 90, 225, 410, 411

Parkinson's Foundation's Young Onset Parkinson's page, 114

Parkinson's with dementia (PDD), 114

participants, qualifying and grouping for clinical trials, 239

pastoral counselors, 223

People with Parkinson's (PWP), 8, 405. *See also* Parkinson's Disease (PD)

personal assistance, 364–365

personal hygiene, 287–288

personal records, gathering and securing, 93–94

personal space, retaining, 254–255

pessimist, 212

Pharmaceutical Research and Manufacturers of America (PhRMA), 411

pharmacists, 89, 181–182

pharmacologic therapy, 171

PhRMA's Medicine Assistance Tool, 180

physical exam, 63

physical function, maintaining maximum, 80

physical therapist (PT), recruiting, 87–88

physical therapy, 405

pill-rolling tremor, 405

placebo, 239

placebo effect, 239, 405

PMD Alliance, 393

positive thinking, 212–213, 230–231

positron emission tomography (PET scan), 405

post-diagnosis
  about, 69–70, 83–84
  gathering information, 82–83

sorting through emotions, 70–76

taking action, 76–82

Posterior Shoulder Side Stretch, 148

Posterior Shoulder Stretch, 146–147

postural instability (P), 10, 38, 117, 207, 405

postural tremor, 37, 405

power of attorney (POA), 357

practitioners, finding for CAM, 210–211

prescription medications. *See also* medications
  about, 171
  changes caused by, 300–301
  cost of, 180, 237
  managing motor symptoms with, 172–178
  managing non-motor symptoms with, 179–180
  using, 180–185

presenting symptoms, 66

primary care physician (PCP), 57, 86, 98

primary caregiver, 319, 320–322

private health insurance, 354–355

proactiveness, importance of, 84

prodromal sign/symptom, 29

professional counselors, 222–224, 331

professions, possibly linked to PD, 22

prognosis, 405

progressive supranuclear palsy (PSP), 67

propulsive gait, 405

protein factor, 209–210

protocol, 238–239

pseudoparkinsonism, 12

psychiatric nurses, 223

psychiatrists, 222

psychological problems, as a symptom, 35

psychologists, 90, 223

public events, 291

Q

Quadriceps Stretch, 150–151

R

range of motion (ROM), 405

rasagiline, 175

rating scales, 64–65

realist, 212

receptor, 405

recreation, 165–166

rehabilitation center, 374

relationships
  about, 249–250
  changes in, 322–324
  with children, 255–259
  with friends, 262–264
  with grandchildren, 259–260
  with parents, 260–262
  with siblings, 260–262
  with significant others, 250–255
  YOPD and, 120–123
  with yourself, 264–265

relaxation, 205, 294

REM sleep, 139

REM sleep behavior disorder (RBD), 29, 140

Remember icon, 2

researching, 393–396

resources, 409–413

respite care, 367–368

rest and relaxation (R&R), 293–294, 331–332

resting tremor, 36–37, 308, 406

restless legs syndrome (RLS), 140

retropulsive gait, 406

reverse mortgages, 350–351

rights, 104, 341

rigidity (R), 10, 37, 67, 117, 306, 307–308, 406

risks, 27–30, 240–241

Rock Steady Boxing (RSB), 165

Rytary, 174

S

sadness, controlling, 384–385

safety, 180–185, 360–362

safinamide, 175

saliva increases, as a non-motor symptom, 179

Samuelson, Joan, 31

Schwab and England Activities of Daily Living, 65

seborrhea, 406

second opinions, 68

secondary caregivers, 319, 332–337

secondary dementia, 314

secondary parkinsonism, 11, 67–68

secondary signs/symptoms, 38–39

selegiline, 175

sensory neurons, 26

sequential movements, bradykinesia and, 38

sex, 253–254

sexual dysfunction, 41, 253–254

shakiness in hands, 35

shaking palsy, 36

sharing news
  about, 101
  care partners and, 104–105
  with close friends, 109–110
  with coworkers, 277–278
  with family, 106–109
  handling sticky conversations, 111–112
  with media outlets, 395–396

outside your inner circle, 111

preparing for, 102–104, 250–251

with your boss, 273–275

at your workplace, 271–273

Shoulder Roll stretch, 145

shoulder strengthening, 155–160

showering, 286–287

sialorrhea, 406

siblings, 260–262, 323–324

side effects, 309, 406

significant others, 120–121, 250–255, 322–323

signs, 36–41, 406. *See also* symptoms

Sinemet, 173, 406

single photon emission computed tomography (SPECT), 65–66

skilled nursing facility (SNF), 372–374

skin changes, as a secondary signs/symptoms, 39

sleep, 75–76, 139–141

sleep apnea, 140

sleep deprivation, lifestyle changes and, 228

sleep disorders, 139–140

sleep disturbances, 35, 40, 179, 310–312

sleep loss, 140–141

sleep stealers, 140–141

slowed speech, as a secondary signs/symptoms, 39

slowness of movement, as a sign, 37–38

slow-wave sleep, 139

slurred speech, as a secondary signs/symptoms, 39

smell, loss of, 29, 40

smoking, as a risk factor, 29–30

social phobias, 216

Social Security Disability Insurance (SSDI), 279

treatment group, 239

tremor, 67, 407

tremor at rest (T), 10, 36–37, 117

trigger event, 407

trips, as a respite, 294

turmeric, 209

23andMe, 24

U

uncontrollable movements, 300–301

uncontrolled shaking, 36–37

unexpected, managing the, 94–96

unilateral, 407

upper body stretches, 146–149

urinary issues, 40, 179, 312–313

U.S. Department of Health and Human Services, 77

U.S. Department of Housing and Urban Development (HUD), 351

U.S. Department of Veterans Affairs (website), 25

U.S. National Library of Medicine's Clinical Trials, 242

V

vascular parkinsonism, 11

vision, changes in, 305–306

visual hallucinations, 41

vitamin supplements, 210

voluntary movement, 407

volunteering, 241–243, 293

voting, 394

W

Wardrobe Wagon, 412

Warning icon, 3

water, in diet, 137

wearing-off effect, 173, 184, 407

wills, 358

workplace

about, 267

Americans with Disabilities Act, 276–277

disclosing diagnosis in, 271–273

homework about, 268–271

human resources (HR), 275–277

protecting income, 278–280

sharing news with coworkers, 277–278

telling your boss, 273–275

YOPD in the, 119–120

World Parkinson Coalition, 411

Wrist/Forearm Stretch, 148–149

Y

Yahr, Melvin, 64

yoga, 207–208

young-onset Parkinson's (YOPD)

about, 13, 24–25, 113–114

care partners and, 125

challenges of, 116–123

compared with traditional onset PD, 114–116

connecting with others with, 124–125

defined, 407

financial planning and, 123–124

yourself, relationship with, 264–265

YouTube, 412

About the Authors

Michele Tagliati, MD: As a clinician and clinical researcher investigating advanced therapeutics of Parkinson's disease, dystonia, and other movement disorders, Dr. Tagliati was among the pioneers developing the use of deep brain stimulation (DBS) in the United States. In addition, he has received research grants and support in excess of four million dollars from various agencies and foundations and has been a principal investigator in over 45 clinical trials exploring new medical and surgical therapies for Parkinson's disease and dystonia. Dr. Tagliati attended medical school and neurology residency in Rome, Italy, before moving to New York in 1993. He completed a second residency in neurology at the Mount Sinai School of Medicine, during which time he was chief resident. Later, he completed a fellowship in movement disorders at Beth Israel Medical Center and afterward joined the Department of Neurology at Albert Einstein College of Medicine. In 2004, Dr. Tagliati returned to Mount Sinai as Associate Professor of Neurology and Division Chief of Movement Disorders. In 2010, he accepted the position of Vice Chairman of Neurology and Director of Movement Disorders at Cedars-Sinai Medical Center in Los Angeles and, in 2015, was awarded the Caron and Steven D. Broidy Endowed Chair for Movement Disorders.

Jo Horne, MA: After receiving her master's degree in communications from the University of Cincinnati, Jo began her journey as the long-distance caregiver for her parents, becoming aware of the need for a comprehensive guide for caregivers and writing three such guides, all published by AARP. At the same time, she worked with her husband as he and others pioneered adult day care in Wisconsin. Jo was also a fellow of the Midwest Geriatric Education Center and was tapped to deliver the keynote address at the national meeting of the Association of University Professionals in Health Administration. Her later work was as communications manager in the dual corporate worlds of long-term care insurance and the pharmaceutical industry. Finally when her sister was diagnosed with PD, Jo found herself up close and personal with the impact PD can have on the PWP and those who love that person.

Dedication

Gary N. Guten, MD, MA, an original contributor to this work, died in 2018 and would be delighted to see our work updated. He felt qualified to contribute to this book for three reasons: Sports medicine orthopedic surgeon, author, and Parkinson's patient. As an orthopedic surgeon, he specialized in sports medicine, exercise, and nutrition. He was the founder of Sports Medicine and Orthopedic Center in Milwaukee, Wisconsin. As an author, he published six books on sports medicine and 27 medical journal publications. As a PWP, his insight and understanding of Parkinson's disease came from the fact that he developed PD in 1995 and his enthusiasm for research. He had to stop doing surgery — but continued to actively do office practice and consultations. Gary's battle for nearly quarter of a century was waged with humor, grace, and dignity, and always with the curiosity of one determined to push the limits of what was possible for anyone living with PD.

Author's Acknowledgments

Michele Tagliati, MD — I would like to thank Jo, whose enlightened spirit envisioned and inspired this book, and all my patients, who teach me a great deal about their disease every day. In addition, I would like to thank the Department of Neurology at Mount Sinai and Cedars-Sinai Medical Centers and the Bachmann-Strauss Dystonia & Parkinson Foundation for their continuous support.

Jo Horne, MA — Without the unique expertise and indefatigable dedication of Michele and Gary, this project would never have made it off the drawing board. I am indebted to both of them for their insights and humor as we made the original journey. I am also deeply indebted to Senior Editor Jennifer Yee, Editors Leah Michael, Laura K. Miller, and Dr. Katherine Amodeo, and everyone on the project team at Wiley Publishing. But as Willie Loman said in the Arthur Miller play *Death of a Salesman,* "Attention must (also) be paid" to the dozens of PWP, their care partners, and healthcare professionals who contributed to the work just by showing me what it means to live with PD. Finally I am profoundly indebted to those fearless and tireless warriors at the foundations and organizations who daily wage the battle to find a cure. My deepest wish is that they make this book obsolete in a very short time.

Publisher's Acknowledgments

Senior Editor: Jennifer Yee

Copy Editor: Laura K. Miller

Technical Editor: Katherine Amodeo,
    MD Movement Disorders Specialist

Production Editor: Tamilmani Varadharaj

Cover Image: © milan2099/Getty Images

Take dummies with you everywhere you go!

Whether you are excited about e-books, want more from the web, must have your mobile apps, or are swept up in social media, dummies makes everything easier.

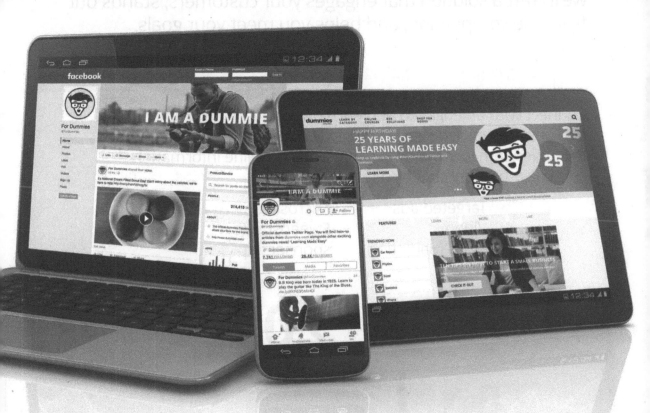

Find us online!

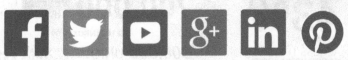

dummies.com

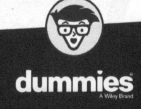

dummies
A Wiley Brand

Leverage the power

Dummies is the global leader in the reference category and one of the most trusted and highly regarded brands in the world. No longer just focused on books, customers now have access to the dummies content they need in the format they want. Together we'll craft a solution that engages your customers, stands out from the competition, and helps you meet your goals.

Advertising & Sponsorships

Connect with an engaged audience on a powerful multimedia site, and position your message alongside expert how-to content. Dummies.com is a one-stop shop for free, online information and know-how curated by a team of experts.

- Targeted ads
- Video
- Email Marketing
- Microsites
- Sweepstakes sponsorship

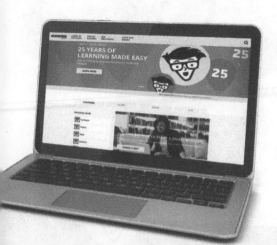

20 MILLION PAGE VIEWS EVERY SINGLE MONTH

15 MILLION UNIQUE VISITORS PER MONTH

43% OF ALL VISITORS ACCESS THE SITE VIA THEIR MOBILE DEVICES

700,000 NEWSLETTE SUBSCRIPTION TO THE INBOXES OF *300,000* UNIQUE INDIVIDUALS EVERY WEEK

# of dummies

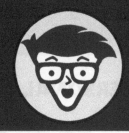

Custom Publishing

Reach a global audience in any language by creating a solution that will differentiate you from competitors, amplify your message, and encourage customers to make a buying decision.

- Apps
- Books
- eBooks
- Video
- Audio
- Webinars

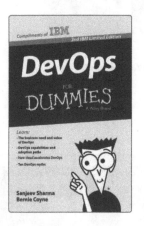

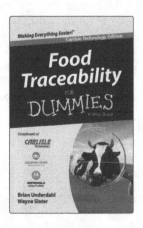

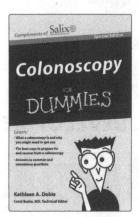

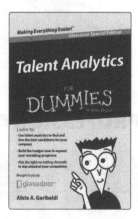

Brand Licensing & Content

Leverage the strength of the world's most popular reference brand to reach new audiences and channels of distribution.

For more information, visit **dummies.com/biz**

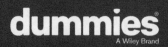

PERSONAL ENRICHMENT

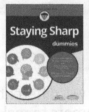

Staying Sharp
9781119187790
USA $26.00
CAN $31.99
UK £19.99

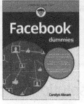

Facebook
9781119179030
USA $21.99
CAN $25.99
UK £16.99

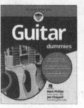

Guitar
9781119293354
USA $24.99
CAN $29.99
UK £17.99

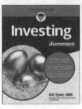

Investing
9781119293347
USA $22.99
CAN $27.99
UK £16.99

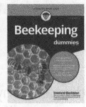

Beekeeping
9781119310068
USA $22.99
CAN $27.99
UK £16.99

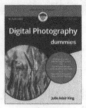

Digital Photography
9781119235606
USA $24.99
CAN $29.99
UK £17.99

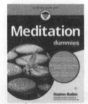

Meditation
9781119251163
USA $24.99
CAN $29.99
UK £17.99

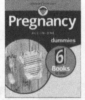

Pregnancy
9781119235491
USA $26.99
CAN $31.99
UK £19.99

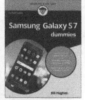

Samsung Galaxy S7
9781119279952
USA $24.99
CAN $29.99
UK £17.99

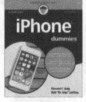

iPhone
9781119283133
USA $24.99
CAN $29.99
UK £17.99

Crocheting
9781119287117
USA $24.99
CAN $29.99
UK £16.99

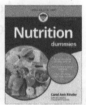

Nutrition
9781119130246
USA $22.99
CAN $27.99
UK £16.99

PROFESSIONAL DEVELOPMENT

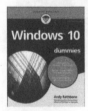

Windows 10
9781119311041
USA $24.99
CAN $29.99
UK £17.99

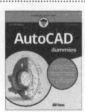

AutoCAD
9781119255796
USA $39.99
CAN $47.99
UK £27.99

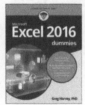

Excel 2016
9781119293439
USA $26.99
CAN $31.99
UK £19.99

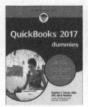

QuickBooks 2017
9781119281467
USA $26.99
CAN $31.99
UK £19.99

macOS Sierra
9781119280651
USA $29.99
CAN $35.99
UK £21.99

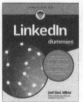

LinkedIn
9781119251132
USA $24.99
CAN $29.99
UK £17.99

Windows 10
9781119310563
USA $34.00
CAN $41.99
UK £24.99

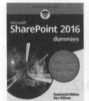

SharePoint 2016
9781119181705
USA $29.99
CAN $35.99
UK £21.99

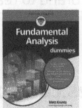

Fundamental Analysis
9781119263593
USA $26.99
CAN $31.99
UK £19.99

Networking
9781119257769
USA $29.99
CAN $35.99
UK £21.99

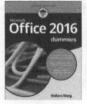

Office 2016
9781119293477
USA $26.99
CAN $31.99
UK £19.99

Office 365
9781119265313
USA $24.99
CAN $29.99
UK £17.99

Salesforce.com
9781119239314
USA $29.99
CAN $35.99
UK £21.99

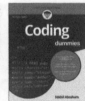

Coding
9781119293323
USA $29.99
CAN $35.99
UK £21.99